THE TOBACCO DEPENDENCE TREATMENT HANDBOOK

Treatment Manuals for Practitioners
DAVID H. BARLOW, *Editor*

Recent Volumes

THE TOBACCO DEPENDENCE TREATMENT HANDBOOK

A Guide to Best Practices

DAVID B. ABRAMS
RAYMOND NIAURA
RICHARD A. BROWN
KAREN M. EMMONS
MICHAEL G. GOLDSTEIN
PETER M. MONTI

Series Editor's Note by David H. Barlow

Foreword by Judith K. Ockene

THE GUILFORD PRESS
New York   London

Library of Congress Cataloging-in-Publication Data

The tobacco dependence treatment handbook : a guide to best practices /
David B. Abrams . . . [et al].
    p. cm. — (Treatment manuals for practitioners)
Includes bibliographical references and index.
  ISBN 1-57230-849-4 (pbk. : alk. paper)
 1. Tobacco habit—Treatment. 2. Smoking—Health aspects. 3.
Evidence-based medicine. I. Abrams, David B. II. Series.
RC567.T634 2003
616.86′506—dc21

                                   2002153857

About the Authors

David B. Abrams, PhD, is Professor of Psychiatry and Human Behavior and Professor of Community Health at Brown Medical School/The Miriam Hospital, and Director of the Centers for Behavioral and Preventive Medicine. He is a licensed clinical psychologist specializing in behavioral medicine and addictive behavior. For over 20 years Dr. Abrams has treated and conducted research on tobacco addiction, published over 200 articles, and directed numerous grants from the National Institute on Drug Abuse, the National Institute on Alcohol Abuse and Alcoholism, and the Robert Wood Johnson Foundation. He is Principal Investigator of a National Cancer Institute "Special Program of Research Excellence" in support of a Transdisciplinary Tobacco Use Research Center. President of the Society of Behavioral Medicine, Co-director of the Robert Wood Johnson Foundation's Tobacco Etiology Research Network, Chair of the Publications Committee of the Society for Research on Nicotine and Tobacco, and Fellow of the American Psychological Association and of the Society of Behavioral Medicine, Dr. Abrams received a Distinguished Scientist Award from the Society of Behavioral Medicine for his work in understanding, treating, and preventing tobacco use and dependence.

Raymond Niaura, PhD, is a clinical psychologist who has extensive experience in the study and treatment of addictive disorders, in particular alcohol and tobacco dependence. He has spent the past 18 years researching clinical strategies for treatment of tobacco dependence. Dr. Niaura is Professor of Psychiatry and Human Behavior at Brown Medical School/The Miriam Hospital, and Director of Research for the Centers for Behavioral and Preventive Medicine. He has served on the editorial boards of *Health Psychology* and the *Journal of Consulting and Clinical Psychology* and currently is associate editor for *Nicotine and Tobacco Research.*

Richard A. Brown, PhD, is Associate Professor of Psychiatry and Human Behavior at Brown Medical School and Director of Addictions Research at Butler Hospital. Dr. Brown has over 20 years of experience in the development of clinical approaches to treat tobacco dependence, most recently with a focus on co-occurring mood disorders. He is Principal Investigator of research grants from the National Cancer Institute, the National Institute on Alcohol Abuse and Alcoholism, the National Institute on Drug Abuse, and the American Cancer Society. He serves as a member of the Biobehavioral and Behavioral Processes Study Section of the National Institutes of Health, as Consulting Editor of *Psychology of Addictive Behaviors*, and as Chair of the Communications Committee of the Society for Research on Nicotine and Tobacco.

Karen M. Emmons, PhD, is Professor of Health and Social Behavior at the Harvard School of Public Health, the Director of Tobacco Control Research at the Dana–Farber Cancer Institute, and the Deputy Director of Dana–Farber's Center for Community-Based Research. Dr. Emmons is a clinical psychologist with a specialty in health promotion and cancer prevention. She has a long track record in the development and evaluation of motivational interventions for smoking cessation and in conducting smoking research with underserved and high-risk populations. Dr. Emmons has been Principal Investigator for numerous research grants from the National Cancer Institute and the National Heart, Lung, and Blood Institute and currently serves as Associate Editor of *Health Psychology*. Dr. Emmons is a member of the Academy of Behavioral Medicine Researchers, as well as a member of the Society of Behavioral Medicine, in which she has achieved Fellow status.

Michael G. Goldstein, MD, is Adjunct Professor of Psychiatry and Human Behavior at the Centers for Behavioral and Preventive Medicine, Brown Medical School, and Associate Director for Clinical Education and Research at the Bayer Institute for Health Care Communication. A board-certified internist and psychiatrist, Dr. Goldstein has served as Principal Investigator for several NIH-funded research studies to test the effectiveness of pharmacological and behavioral interventions for the treatment of nicotine dependence and to examine the barriers and facilitators of delivering brief treatments by primary care physicians. Dr. Goldstein served on the national panel that developed the definitive gold standard "Treating Tobacco Use and Dependence" Clinical Practice Guideline, and he was also a member of American Psychiatric Association's Task Force on Nicotine Dependence.

Peter M. Monti, PhD, is Professor of Medical Science and Director of the Center for Alcohol and Addiction Studies and the Clinical Psychology Internship Consortium at Brown University, Providence, Rhode Island. His research is supported by a Senior Research Scientist Award from the Department of Veterans Affairs, and he holds research grants from the National Institute on Alcohol Abuse and Alcoholism, the National Institute on Drug Abuse, and the Department of Veterans Affairs. Widely published, Dr. Monti is coauthor of *Treating Alcohol Dependence: A Coping Skills Training Guide, Second Edition*; and coeditor of *Adolescents, Alcohol, and Substance Abuse: Reaching Teens through Brief Interventions* and *Social Skills Training: A Practical Handbook for Assessment and Treatment*. He is a Fellow of the American Psychological Society and the American Psychological Association.

Contributing Authors

William G. Shadel, PhD, is currently Assistant Professor of Psychology at the University of Pittsburgh. He has spent his 10-year research career focusing on understanding basic psychological processes that underlie the development, maintenance, and cessation of smoking. He has devoted a significant proportion of his clinical time to delivering brief treatments to smokers in inpatient health care settings and intensive treatments to smokers in outpatient clinical settings.

Judith DePue, EdD, MPH, is Clinical Assistant Professor of Psychiatry and Human Behavior at Brown Medical School and the Centers for Behavioral and Preventive Medicine. Her research interests focus on public health approaches to delivering tobacco treatment and other preventive care interventions, especially using primary care channels. She has been an investigator on several primary-care-based research trials.

Laura A. Linnan, ScD, CHES, is a certified health educator; Assistant Professor in the Department of Health Education and Health Behavior at the University of North Carolina School of Public Health, Chapel Hill; and a member of the Lineberger Comprehensive Cancer Center. She has nearly 20 years of research and practice experience in public health settings at the national, state, and local level. Her research focuses on applied interventions that address individual, organizational, and community change in support of health, with a special emphasis on chronic disease prevention and control.

Series Editor's Note

The United States Government, through its Public Health Service, has decided that one of the most pressing and formidable risks to the nation's health is addiction to nicotine in its various forms. As such, they have unleashed considerable resources, augmented by settlements paid to the states by the tobacco companies, to treat and prevent nicotine addiction. Clinical practice guidelines outlining the most successful approaches have appeared. Now a distinguished clinical research group that has had much to do with the creation of these guidelines has put together a detailed, evidence-based practice guide. Led by David Abrams and his colleagues at Brown University and Harvard University, this guidebook will immediately become the authoritative source on treatment for all health professionals.

In nicotine addiction, we have perhaps the best example of the efficacy of combined psychological and pharmacological treatment. These approaches and their seamless integration are clearly outlined for the benefit of the provider. This insidious disorder also illustrates the power of psychological procedures to alter brain function. As the authors note, "nicotine is a subtle but powerful reinforcer that results in dependence among the majority of users through learned associations derived from the hijacking of the brain's central reward circuitry" (see Preface, p. xii). The fact that psychological procedures provide a proven method for altering this circuitry underscores the integration and interrelatedness of pathological processes and the power of psychological procedures to alter these processes. Every provider and health care setting should be aware of these approaches to treating nicotine addiction.

DAVID H. BARLOW

Foreword

Despite the enormous health consequences of tobacco use and the benefits of stopping, almost one quarter of Americans continue to use tobacco, and in many other countries tobacco use occurs in more than half of the population. As such, tobacco use is an important public health and treatment priority, both nationally and internationally. The treatment of tobacco use is one of the most effective disease prevention and health promotion maneuvers in clinical medicine and public health today. Health care providers, health care administrators, public health practitioners, policymakers, researchers, and teachers each play an important role in this effort.

As *The Tobacco Dependence Treatment Handbook* illustrates, there is a large body of evidence indicating that brief intervention delivered by health care providers is highly effective. Therefore, physicians, nurses, and other health care professionals must be able to deliver brief interventions within the course of routine health care contacts and be confident of their ability to do so. Such interventions could double the nation's quit rates. In addition, many tobacco users benefit from more intensive treatment, making it important that the complexity and intensity of tobacco treatment be matched to the needs of the tobacco user and that there are professionals specializing in tobacco treatment available to deliver care in such settings as community health centers, hospitals, social service agencies, and worksites. Lastly, the complicated tobacco user, who may be clinically depressed or alcohol dependent, may be best served by doctoral-level or licensed alcohol and drug addiction mental health providers, who can offer intensive treatment for drug dependence or mental health concerns in conjunction with treatment for tobacco dependence.

The comprehensive model proposed by David Abrams and colleagues in this book accounts for this need for different levels of treatment intensity delivered by a variety of clinicians. They recommend a stepped-care approach for the treatment of nicotine dependence and provide all of the strategies and materials necessary to implement and sustain each of the steps, utilizing evidence-based strategies consistent with the best practice recommendations identified by the latest Public Health Service (PHS) Clinical Practice Guideline for Treating Tobacco Use and Dependence (Fiore et al., 2000; *www.surgeongeneral.gov/tobacco/*). The strategies provided are tailored to a range of individuals with different problems and characteristics. This includes tobacco users who are at different stages of readiness to quit and those with comorbid psychiatric or medical conditions and substance abuse problems.

The challenge for treating tobacco addiction is for health care and public health professionals to know the best way to support, implement, and integrate treatment into existing systems on local, state, and national levels. Professionals who deliver care in diverse settings across the continuum of care—from community agencies for health, to inpatient services, to worksites and private practice offices—will find that mastery of this evidence-based clinical handbook's material will greatly enhance their capability and readiness to respond successfully to this challenge. As such, this book is of fundamental importance and will serve as an essential "state-of-the-art" reference and guidebook. It is unique in its comprehensiveness and the range of treatment material covered. It is an especially important resource today, given that most schools of medicine, public health, psychology, nursing, and other health professions responsible for training clinicians and public health specialists do not provide such training for their students and teachers but are becoming aware of the need to do so. This book will help them meet the important public health challenge of training providers to treat tobacco addiction.

In addition to providing information about treatment options and strategies, *The Tobacco Dependence Treatment Handbook* has valuable assessment instruments to assist in tailoring the interventions to particular patients and populations, handouts for patients, planning sheets for providers, information on factors and operations needed for effective treatment implementation in health care and public health delivery systems, and case studies to facilitate learning. All of the materials and handouts have been field tested and refined as part of research studies conducted by the authors at the Brown Medical School Centers for Behavioral and Preventive Medicine.

This book includes everything you need to know and all of the materials you need to have in order to set up and implement a comprehensive nicotine dependence treatment program, effectively translating research into practice. It is the first book of its kind to provide all of this information in one place, designed to appeal to clinicians with little time and experience as well as to those who are expert in the treatment of other addictions and have the time to deliver more intensive individual and group treatment in an outpatient or inpatient setting (e.g., psychiatrists, psychologists, psychiatric social workers, and nurse specialists).

Dr. Abrams and his colleagues are uniquely qualified to write this book. Each is a practicing clinician and researcher recognized nationally and internationally for his/her cutting-edge research, vision, and contributions to the field of nicotine dependence treatment. Much of the work that helps to provide the foundation for the Clinical Practice Guideline for Treating Tobacco Use and Dependence (Fiore et al., 2000) was conducted by the authors. They have worked together as a team for over 20 years, developing, testing, and refining the book's treatment and assessment materials in a variety of settings for different providers and patient populations in the real world.

This is an excellent "must have" textbook and a definitive treatment handbook, appropriate for providers of smoking cessation interventions as well as for students, teachers, researchers, and policymakers in health care and public health. The information and materials it presents are necessary for us to be able to meet the challenge of treating tobacco addiction on all levels.

JUDITH K. OCKENE, PhD, MEd
University of Massachusetts Medical School

Preface

The material covered in this clinical handbook is intended for an audience of professionals in health care, mental health and the addictions, and public health who are interested in delivering smoking cessation treatment. This book may be especially well suited to the rapidly expanding numbers of providers delivering treatments as part of recent state, federal, and third-party insurance initiatives to support local tobacco control efforts (e.g., using state tobacco taxes and/or funds allocated from the master settlement with the tobacco industry). The book is also strongly evidence based, consistent with the best practice recommendations identified by the latest Public Health Service (PHS) Clinical Practice Guideline for Treating Tobacco Use and Dependence (Fiore et al., 2000; *www.surgeongeneral.gov/tobacco/*). Because this book is consistent with the latest PHS guideline (Fiore et al., 2000), it can also be used as a textbook for students in training programs for medical, public health, and mental health professions, as well as by those providers already in practice who desire continuing education or to be trained and certified as smoking cessation counselors.

An effective approach to smoking cessation among diverse adult populations must be broad enough to make an impact on reducing population prevalence of smoking yet specific in guiding an individual through the treatment process. An effective approach must not only take into account the various backgrounds of treatment providers but also address the different treatment options, settings for delivery of care, resources, and costs involved. Thus the main focus of our book is somewhat broader than a typical clinical handbook in that it offers a range of treatment options, from brief to more intensive.

The conceptual approach to treatment planning (Chapter 1) provides the flexibility to implement treatment in settings that vary across the continuum of care—from community agencies for health, mental health, public health, and social services, to worksites and private practice offices, to inpatient and outpatient health and mental health clinics, substance abuse programs, and hospitals. Another helpful feature is the use of specific assessment instruments (Chapter 2) to tailor the interventions to the unique characteristics of the individual smoker, including his/her level of motivational readiness (Chapter 3) and pharmacological (Chapter 7) and cognitive-behavioral (Chapters 5 and 6) profiles. Assessment of each smoker's unique characteristics (e.g., severity of dependence, past quit attempts) also helps the provider determine the level of intensity of treatment (brief or intense) using a stepped-care framework.

Throughout this book, we assume that use of tobacco products reflects the underlying biopsychosocial theory that nicotine is a subtle but powerful reinforcer that results in dependence among the majority of users through learned associations derived from the hijacking of the brain's central reward circuitry (Koob & LeMoal, 2001; U.S. Department of Health and Human Services, 1988). The behavior is then erroneously associated with survival of the species and is placed on a par with food and water seeking and sexual reproduction (primary appetitive reinforcers). Over time, a cycle of hedonistic dysregulation emerges, producing several of the familiar self-destructive patterns of the drug addict, such as continued use despite personal harm (Koob & LeMoal, 2001). Once established in memory, this pleasurable but addictive pattern of smoking behavior is difficult to extinguish, as it becomes associated with hundreds of other secondary reinforcers (O. Pomerleau, Collins, Shiffman, & Pomerleau, 1993). The terms "nicotine addiction," "nicotine dependence," "tobacco addiction," "tobacco dependence," "smoking behavior," and "smoking" are used interchangeably in this book and are all intended to reflect the powerful biobehavioral mechanisms underlying nicotine addiction.

You (the provider) need to take into account biological, psychological, and sociocultural factors in order to break the cycle of nicotine addiction. Thus the material in this book aims to put what is known from research to date into a more comprehensive yet practical approach to treatment than is typically found in clinical guidebooks. A comprehensive approach that translates research into practice is especially timely. Since 1967, there has been a fivefold increase in the number of research articles on treating nicotine addiction (Hughes & Liguori, 1997). The PHS guideline panel reviewed more than 6,000 credible research papers, 3,000 of which were published between 1995 and 1999 alone (Fiore et al., 2000). Some recent research advances have not yet been fully incorporated into practice (see Niaura & Abrams, 2002). There is also an increasing array of commercial and alternative medicine programs and products available to help individuals stop smoking, for many of which little or no scientific evidence exists regarding their effectiveness. Finally, in order to make a population impact on reducing smoking prevalence, there is an urgent need to train students and all existing professionals, as we need many more providers to deliver quality cessation treatments. It is now recognized that smoking cessation treatment should be mainstreamed into public health and health care delivery at national, state, and local levels.

Children are exposed to nicotine early in life—over 80% of adult smokers become regular users before age 18 (Centers for Disease Control and Prevention, 2000b). There has been a 32% increase in youth adoption of smoking between 1991 and 1997 in the United States (Centers for Disease Control, 1998) and a 28% increase among college students (Rigotti, Lee, & Wechsler, 2000). The primary prevention of smoking initiation and progression to dependence among youth is not the focus of this book, although it is critically important in reducing the massive disease burden of tobacco. However, some of the techniques presented herein have been adapted (Abrams & Clayton, 2001; Monti, Colby, & O'Leary, 2001) for use in early cessation treatment efforts among youths and young adult (18- to 25-year-old) smokers, such as brief motivational interventions (Chapter 3) and brief cessation coping skills training (see Chapter 4). One published study reports promising preliminary results (Colby et al., 1998), and the issues and challenges facing researchers and providers of early treatment are explored in more detail in Chapter 9, on future directions. Every opportunity should be taken to slow, arrest, or reverse the tobacco industry's recruitment of these new tobacco users.

A comprehensive approach to successful treatment should incorporate "systems" considerations. Chapter 8 addresses some "delivery system" or contextual factors that can either strongly facilitate or create insurmountable obstacles to providers in delivering their best treatment efforts. Cost-effective treatment requires the support from administrators/gatekeepers, other stakeholders, and policymakers. Within the health care–mental health–public health delivery systems, treatment of adult nicotine addiction must be placed on an equal footing with the management of other chronic conditions that require persistent and long-term interventions, such as diabetes, bipolar disorders, and other substance abuse disorders (Abrams et al., 1996). A smoker, once identified, may have to be managed for many years, indeed for as long as it takes, to achieve continuous abstinence. This philosophy of persistence of treatment within a supportive framework is a special feature of this guidebook and stands in contrast to many of the "one shot at treatment" programs that are currently available.

Continuity of treatment of those at high risk for disease is in fact consistent with the latest trends in health care delivery (McLellan et al., 1998). Members of a health insurance plan who are at high risk or who have existing chronic diseases such as diabetes are assigned to a case manager or care management team. The care manager actively reaches out (i.e., is proactive) to maintain contact and improve adherence to prevention and treatment regimens. Maintaining an optimal lifestyle (good nutrition, physical activity, no smoking, adherence to medical regimens) can make an enormous difference in quality of life, not to mention the savings in health care utilization (McGinnis & Foege, 1993). The chronic refractory disorder of nicotine addiction has such devastating negative health consequences for so many people that it warrants the creation of long-term models of treatment planning such as care management and also deserves full coverage by federal and private health insurance (Curry, Grothaus, McAfee, & Pabiniak, 1998).

Only a few of the commercially available smoking cessation and alternative medicine programs have been evaluated for efficacy (see Fiore et al., 2000, pp. 49–50). The vast majority of treatments that have been rigorously evaluated in randomized controlled trials are based on behavior therapy (or modification) and on pharmacotherapy (e.g., nicotine gum or patch) or a combination of behavioral and pharmacological components (Abrams et al., 1996; Niaura & Abrams, 2002; Orleans & Slade, 1993). Behavioral and combined programs have consistently shown that they can outperform appropriate control groups (Shiffman, 1993).

The core treatment elements of behavior therapy programs (see Orleans & Slade, 1993) have been refined over 20 years in research studies undertaken across the world, including ours at Brown Medical School and The Miriam Hospital's Centers for Behavioral and Preventive Medicine (e.g., Abrams, Monti, Carey, Pinto, & Jacobus, 1988; Abrams & Wilson, 1979b; Brown et al., 2001; Goldstein, Niaura, Follick, & Abrams, 1989; Marcus et al., 1999; Niaura et al., 1999; Niaura, Brown, Goldstein, Murphy, & Abrams, 1996). Our Brown Medical School Centers have conducted research across a wide range of smokers and settings, including hospital clinics, worksites, primary care practices, and alcohol and substance abuse programs, and of underserved populations such as low-income Medicaid patients treated in public health clinics. The most recent randomized clinical trial that employs the intensive behavioral treatment programs presented in Chapters 5 and 6 achieved 12-month follow-up rates of 25–33% abstinence (Brown et al., 2001). These outcomes compare to the best outcomes reported in the PHS guideline (Fiore et al., 2000) and are likely to be improved if pharmacological interventions are added to the behavioral treatment (Goldstein et al., 1989).

We have used both our 20 years of clinical experience and our research studies to identify the treatment components used in this book. Each intervention component in this book has been evaluated as part of one or more of our clinical research trials but may have undergone revisions over the years to incorporate feedback from treatment providers and consumers. The suggestions for combining various components of our programs (e.g., from Chapters 3 through 7) have not been evaluated as a whole.

The interventions in this evidence-based clinical handbook are also firmly grounded in theory, specifically, Bandura's social cognitive learning theory (Bandura, 1997) and the neurobiological basis of nicotine addiction (Koob & LeMoal, 2001). The reader who is not familiar with the basic constructs of social cognitive learning theory (such as classical and operant conditioning, stimulus control, cognitive-behavioral coping skills, relapse prevention, and the central role of self-efficacy and outcome expectations in behavior change) may wish to consult a textbook on the subject (Bandura, 1997; Marlatt & Gordon, 1985; O'Leary & Wilson, 1987). The reader who wants a complete review of the entire field of nicotine dependence may wish to consult a comprehensive textbook such as Orleans and Slade (1993).

As previously mentioned, in 1996, a landmark review and meta-analysis of the available smoking cessation research studies was conducted and was updated by the PHS in 2000 (Fiore et al., 2000). A meta-analysis permits the identification of the most robust and consistent evidence about what treatments work and how well they work because the analysis is based on numerous studies rather than a single clinical trial. The PHS guideline now serves as the "gold standard" for evidence-based practice in the United States. One of us (M. G. G.) was a member of the PHS panel, and another two coauthors of this book (D. B. A. and R. N.) were external scientific advisors and/or reviewers. The American Psychiatric Association (APA) released its own "Practice Guideline for the Treatment of Patients with Nicotine Dependence" (Hughes et al., 1996). The APA guideline addresses specialized treatment for smokers who have failed first-line treatments and who have psychiatric or substance abuse comorbidity. Three of us (M. G. G., D. B. A., R. N.) were also involved in the development and scientific review of the APA guideline. Finally, the *Journal of the British Thoracic Society* published its comprehensive guideline for smoking cessation intervention (Raw, McNeill, & West, 1998). They used additional meta-analyses performed as part of the Cochrane Collaboration (Cochrane Collaboration Library, 1998). The British guideline has an extensive section on the health costs of smoking, the cost-effectiveness of treatment, and the benefits of successful reductions in prevalence. There is considerable agreement between the core recommendations from these three guidelines (Niaura & Abrams, 2002). We have made every effort to ensure that the treatment programs in this book are consistent with the consensus reports of the aforementioned three "best practice" clinical guidelines.

The first chapter in this book provides you with a brief rationale and a selective review of the research literature relevant to treating smokers. The chapter also presents some guiding principles for conceptualizing and developing a treatment plan. However, we stop short of presenting any specific algorithms for treatment planning (e.g., stepped care, stages of change) because there is not yet sufficient research support for a particular kind of treatment plan (Fiore et al., 2000). The conceptual principles should help enhance your own clinical judgment as you develop treatment plans that best fit into your own style and delivery setting. The eight chapters that follow cover assessment of the smokers' characteristics (Chapter

2); motivation to change (Chapter 3); brief behavioral treatments suitable for providers with only limited time available (Chapter 4); intensive behavioral treatments (Chapter 5) and the complications of comorbidities (Chapter 6); considerations for pharmacotherapy (Chapter 7); systems and contextual issues (Chapter 8); and future directions (Chapter 9). In order to develop the optimal treatment plan that can be tailored to the unique needs of the individual smoker, we recommend that you familiarize yourself with all the chapters and the "modules" available within each chapter. Selected handouts and forms used in the treatment sessions or homework assignments between sessions have been gathered in the appendix to facilitate ease of reproduction.

Continuity of care means that if your first attempt at treatment is unsuccessful, you have the option to reevaluate the treatment plan and develop the next intervention. In this manner, subsequent interventions for that smoker can be based on prior ones, and tailoring of treatment can be adjusted, based on the past responses. The subsequent intervention will generally be more intensive than the prior treatment. Thus, in some respects, the guiding principle for continuity of treatment most closely resembles a stepped-care model. Rather than viewing the previous treatment plan as a failure, you can reframe it to develop a better treatment for the next attempt (e.g., more work on motivation; more intensive treatment, such as increasing the frequency and duration of face-to-face or telephone contacts; adding new or different coping skills training components from Chapters 5 and 6; reevaluating pharmacological options).

The single most important message in this clinical handbook is that we must never give up on a current smoker until he/she has been helped to successfully maintain a tobacco-free life. It is literally a matter of life and death. An addiction is not simply a free choice made by adults, as the tobacco industry propaganda would have us believe, but rather is tantamount to enticing young people into a personal prison for the rest of their lives—a concentration camp that eventually kills over 430,000 of its U.S. inmates each and every year by toxic exposure to lethal poisonous gases.

NOTE

The research knowledge-base for this *Handbook* (see pp. xiii–xiv) is derived primarily from consensus of the independent Public Health Service (PHS) Clinical Practice Guideline for Treating Tobacco Use and Dependence (Fiore et al., 2000); from the American Psychiatric Association (Hughes et al., 1996), and from *Thorax: The Journal of the British Thoracic Society* (Raw, McNeill, & West, 1998). The cognitive-behavioral treatment materials are based on clinical trials sponsored by the National Institutes of Health and conducted at Brown Medical School/The Miriam Hospital's Centers for Behavioral and Preventive Medicine. Over the last 20 years, several authors of this book have collaborated with the pharmaceutical industry. We have made every effort to avoid recommendations that reflect competing interests of these sponsors. Some of us have served as consultants, served on advisory boards, or participated in sponsored clinical trials and other studies by Eli Lilly & Co., Bourroughs Wellcome, Glaxo Wellcome, SmithKline Beecham, GlaxoSmithKlein, DuPont Merck, Sano Corporation, Knoll Pharmaceuticals, Bristol-Myers Squibb, Pfizer, and Sanofi-Synthelabo.

Acknowledgments

We were fortunate to have had the talented assistance of Barbara Watkins, Senior Editor at The Guilford Press, whose advice and perseverance through several drafts and whose constant support during all phases of production are greatly appreciated.

David B. Abrams thanks his wonderful wife, Marion Wachtenheim, and children, Daniel, Aaron and Tanya, for their patience and loving support. He dedicates this book to his mentor and friend, Dr. Terence Wilson. Raymond Niaura acknowledges the unwavering support of his wife, Lynn, children, Amber and Alexandra, and parents, Jean and Al. Richard A. Brown dedicates this book to his wonderful children, Jessica and Jason, who have provided their unqualified love and support. Karen M. Emmons acknowledges the ongoing support of her husband, Donn, and her son, Max. Michael G. Goldstein acknowledges the loving support of his wife, Rebecca, and his children, Noah and Annie. Peter M. Monti dedicates this book to Sylvia Monti, with love and appreciation. William G. Shadel thanks his wife, Nicole, for her love and understanding and his children, Mila and Gus, for following him around the house and giving him an excuse to watch cartoons. Judith DePue thanks her husband, Tom Lamonte, for his ongoing support, which includes enduring long hours of her research projects over the years. Laura A. Linnan thanks her son, Stephen, who is great fun and a true blessing in her life.

We all wish to express our heartfelt appreciation to Dr. Amanda Graham for her careful review of the entire book as well as her suggestions and revisions, and to Dr. Brian Hitsman for his exhaustive work on the assessment measures and the figures, tables, and references. We also thank Dawn Risi for her help in preparing the tables and figures. There have been many faculty, psychology interns, and postdoctoral fellows at Brown Medical School and The Miriam Hospital who have taught us so much and helped to refine the treatment manuals and research protocols upon which this book is based.

A final word of thanks goes to Barbara Doll for her extensive work in preparing, editing, and proofreading the book for publication and obtaining all the copyright permissions. Barbara is a very special person; she has worked for us for many years and she still displays the same faith, thoughtfulness, and dedication to excellence as she did when she typed her very first manuscript for us. This book could not have been produced without her outstanding assistance.

Contents

1

Planning Evidence-Based Treatment of Tobacco Dependence

David B. Abrams
Raymond Niaura

This chapter gives you, the provider, a conceptual overview of the issues to consider in formulating a plan for treatment of tobacco dependence. We outline (1) a rationale for treatment based on the health-damaging consequences of smoking; (2) a selective review of the research evidence concerning mechanisms underlying reasons for smoking and effective treatments; and (3) the broad principles underlying the development of a treatment plan. Treatment planning includes two related but distinct considerations: (1) the "systems level" that determines continuity of care and the allocation of resources within a particular context and (2) the "individual level" that focuses on tailoring the treatment to the smoker's needs.

Systems-level factors can enhance the reach, enrollment, retention, effectiveness, and population impact of treatment. Systems factors include (1) the context or setting in which treatment is delivered; (2) the time and resources available to you to deliver a specific level of treatment in terms of amount and intensity, mode of delivery, and content; and (3) the smokers' resources and time available to access treatment (e.g., transportation, health insurance). Some systems-level factors may not be entirely under your control; this circumstance can constrain treatment options and continuity of care. These factors, together with the unique personal needs and characteristics of the smoker, are then weighed to formulate the treatment plan.

If the setting permits and the smoker is receptive, you can consider continuity of care to include a plan with several repeated treatments, perhaps delivered over years, rather than a "one-shot" treatment. Treatments may be arranged to fit the smoker's needs, as well as to take advantage of the principle of trying less intensive, less complex, and less expensive options first and adding more complex components only when the lesser options do not succeed (i.e., stepped care). When the smoker cycles back into treatment after a relapse, the new information from the previous cessation effort can be incorporated into a revised treatment plan that "steps up" the level of care and includes new components not previously delivered. You are encouraged to examine systems-level factors and look for opportunities to align the system to improve the delivery of your treatment(s) whenever possible (see Chapter 8 for more details).

Regardless of the systems-level factors, in the final analysis the treatment plan is driven by a focus on the individual smoker's needs and characteristics (individual differences) and, whenever possible, the smoker's own preferences. The planning process is facilitated by a knowledge of (1) the research evidence about the mechanisms involved in smoking (why people smoke and what motivates them to consider cessation); (2) the process of moving from smoking to cessation and relapse prevention; and (3) the treatments available and their efficacy. However, even this level of understanding, discussed in this chapter, is too general to effectively guide you in treatment delivery. The actual treatment plan for the individual smoker is based on an intake evaluation of that smoker using the assessment tools in Chapter 2. Based on that evaluation, you can connect the profile of the smoker's unique needs to the actual intervention components, contained in the subsequent chapters (3–7).

For many smokers, the treatments contained in Chapters 3–7 can be used with little modification. This is construed as a "one size fits all" or standard approach. However, one of the unique advantages of this book is that it provides you with a conceptual road map to create more tailored and flexible treatment plans. Thus you can mix and match some of the content within each chapter. For example, you may choose to include cognitive motivational enhancement strategies from Chapter 3 in either a brief (Chapter 4) or intensive (Chapter 5) clinical program. This intensive program (Chapter 5) can be enhanced with content from Chapter 6 (comorbid complications) that can either replace or supplement existing session content or that can be added on as extra treatment sessions. Most important, the pharmacological options delineated in Chapter 7 can and should be included in any treatment plan, from the briefest to the most comprehensive.

As you become familiar with the contents of this book, and as you gain more experience treating a range of smokers, you will feel more confident designing your own custom-tailored treatment plans. Ideally, systems and individual factors will come together in your treatment plan, with the smoker's personal profile taking priority in the plan and the "system" being positioned to fully support the plan. If every provider was able to reach and help every smoker to quit, the population impact on health and quality of life would be enormous. Why is it so important to reach every smoker and develop a plan to stay with them until they quit smoking?

SCOPE OF THE TOBACCO DEPENDENCE PROBLEM

This moment in time—the dawn of the 21st century—opens a window of extraordinary opportunity. If a substantial, sustained investment is made in efficient treatment, prevention, and policy, then the first half of the 21st century could be the host to a dramatic success story—reducing the enormous number of deaths and disproportionate disease burden that tobacco has caused among people of all backgrounds (U.S. Department of Health and Human Services, 1990). The reductions in population smoking prevalence from 1965 to 1990 are now for the first time translating into actual lives and dollars saved (e.g., male lung cancer rates that climbed from 1920 on, peaked in the 1990s, and have now reversed; reduced incidence of cardiovascular disease in California; Cole & Rodu, 1996; Fichtenberg & Glantz, 2000).

Unfortunately, women's rates of smoking prevalence have converged with those of men, and their later adoption of the habit in the 1960s has resulted in an epidemic rise in female lung cancer in the 1990s. More women are dying of lung cancer than breast cancer, and by 2003, twice as many women will die of lung cancer than breast cancer (American Cancer Society, 1999). The likelihood of surviving lung cancer five years after diagnosis is less than 15%. The best "treatment" available is smoking cessation to prevent onset of lung cancer.

Thus both promising and troubling trends emerged at the close of the 20th century. Tobacco use is still the leading preventable cause of death, disability, and disease burden in the United States (U.S. Department of Health and Human Services, 1990). If tobacco use were eliminated, over 430,000 lives could be saved every year in the United States alone and 2.1 million in the developed countries of the world (American Cancer Society, 1999). About one-third of all cancers (171,000 deaths per year) are directly caused by tobacco use, and, together with cardiovascular disease and pulmonary diseases such as emphysema, they account for the majority of the total preventable deaths attributed to tobacco use. Tobacco products are projected to be the *world's* leading cause of death and disability by the year 2020, far outstripping deaths from any single disease, most major wars, diarrheal syndromes, HIV–AIDS, substance abuse, suicides, homicides, and accidents (C. J. L. Murray & Lopez, 1996). If aggressive action is not taken worldwide, tobacco use will continue to be the human-created "bubonic plague" of the 20th and 21st centuries (Peto, Lopez, Boreham, Thun, & Heath, 1994).

The United States has witnessed an average annual reduction of 0.5% in prevalence of smoking, from 42% in 1965 to 27% in 1990. During the 1990s, the reduction leveled off. About 47–50 million American adults still smoke (24–26% of the U.S. population; American Cancer Society, 2000). Socioeconomic status is one overriding determinant of smoking patterns. Among white, non-Hispanic pregnant mothers with less than 12 years of education, over 50% smoke at the time of birth; in contrast, less than 10% of white mothers with more than 16 years education smoke (U.S. Department of Health and Human Services, 1998). Other populations of special concern include (but are not limited to) women, blue-collar and low-income workers, underserved ethnic and minority populations, and those without health insurance (Orleans et al., 1998; U.S. Department of Health and Human Services, 1998). Moreover, the sudden upturn in the 1990s of adoption of smoking among our youth (32% increase) and young adults (28% increase in college student smoking) will continue to add a diverse range of new smokers into the pipeline for decades to come (Emmons, Wechsler, Dowdall, & Abraham, 1998).

The past three decades of negative press about tobacco use have convinced millions of smokers to quit, many on their own or with self-help materials. With the exception of the new generations of young smokers, those adults who can quit have, for the most part, already done so. The older smokers of today are probably more highly dependent on nicotine and are more likely to have other comorbidities (Hughes, Goldstein, Hurt, & Shiffman, 1999). Nicotine dependence has the highest prevalence rate of all psychiatric and substance-abuse-related disorders in the United States. Almost 50% of psychiatric patients and over 85% of alcoholics are smokers (Zarin, Pincus, & Hughes, 1997). Nicotine dependence can complicate the treatment of psychiatric and medical conditions (American Psychiatric Association Work Group on Nicotine Dependence, 1996) because nicotine can change the bio-availability of other medications.

Contextual and environmental factors also are relevant to understanding smoking and cessation efforts. Exposure to secondhand smoke is associated with more than 3,000 cancer and 40,000 cardiovascular deaths annually among nonsmokers (Emmons, Hammond, & Abrams, 1995; U.S. Department of Health and Human Services, 1990). Maternal smoking is associated with low birth weight, and household smoking around children is associated with asthma, excessive pediatric ear, nose, and throat infections that often require unnecessary surgery, and a twofold risk of sudden infant death syndrome (SIDS; Ershoff, Quinn, Mullen, & Lairson, 1990; Marks, Koplan, Hogue, & Dalmat, 1990). Tobacco-related toxic exposure in utero is associated with conduct disorder and attention-deficit/hyperactivity disorder; the likelihood of becoming a smoker or an alcohol or substance abuser in adolescence; and criminal behavior and sociopathy (Griesler, Kandel, & Davies, 1998). Children who live in households in which parents or siblings smoke are much more likely to start smoking. Furthermore, having a household member who smokes makes it virtually impossible for another member of that household to quit.

Restricting or banning smoking in worksites, public buildings, homes, health care delivery settings, and transportation vehicles not only reduces the harm to nonsmokers but also may help smokers become motivated to quit (Emmons et al., 1995; Marcus et al., 1992). Thus the physical and social environment can be a powerful influence on individual behaviors, providing persistent, inescapable reminders and incentives to facilitate cessation and prevent relapse following cessation (see Chapter 8).

Cessation at any age has significant positive benefits—one is never too old or too young to stop (Rimer et al., 1994). After cessation, although the risk of disease does not return entirely to that of a person who has never smoked, much of the risk from cardiovascular diseases and some of the risk for cancers are reduced (U.S. Department of Health and Human Services, 1990). For chronic obstructive lung diseases such as emphysema, further damage can be slowed. Smoking complicates and speeds the progression of many medical problems, including (among others) heart disease, HIV–AIDS opportunistic infections, diabetes, vascular and peripheral vascular diseases, impotence, premature skin aging, and degeneration of vision (U.S. Department of Health and Human Services, 1990). For a summary of the major diseases and the benefits of cessation that are associated with each disease, see Table 1.1. Of all the possible preventive and palliative health measures available today, smoking cessation remains by far at the very top of the list as the most cost-effective per quality adjusted life years saved (Cromwell, Bartosch, Fiore, Hasselblad, & Baker, 1997; Parrott, Godfrey, Raw, West, & McNeill, 1998).

There is not a moment to lose. Because of its slow, silent process of destruction over decades, it is very hard for us as treatment providers, or for our society as a whole, to see the stark problem of tobacco addiction for what it really is—a catastrophic societal emergency requiring immediate aggressive intervention. Intervention must persist and be repeated over

TABLE 1.1. The Health Consequences of Smoking and the Benefits of Quitting at a Glance

Health consequences	Benefits of quitting
Overall mortality risk is two times higher in cigarette smokers than in nonsmokers.	Stopping smoking reduces the risk of premature death, with 50% of the risk eliminated within 5 years of quitting. After 15 years without smoking, former smokers' risk is nearly identical to that of lifelong nonsmokers.
Lung cancer risk in smokers is more than 20 times higher for men and 12 times higher for women than in nonsmokers.	After 10 years of abstinence, risk of lung cancer is reduced by 30% to 50%. With longer periods of cessation, the reduction in risk is greater.
Cancer of the oral cavity risk in men is more than 20 times higher in smokers. The risk in women smokers is between 5 and 10 times greater.	Compared with continued smoking, quitting halves the risks as soon as 5 years after cessation. Further risk reduction occurs over a longer period of abstinence.
Cancer of the esophagus risk among smokers is between 5 and 10 times higher.	Quitting significantly reduces risk: 5 years following cessation, risk is reduced by 50%.
Pancreatic cancer risk in smokers is two to three times higher.	Cessation reduces risk, although reduction may be measurable only after 10 years of abstinence.
Bladder cancer risk in smokers is between 2 and 4 times greater among both men and women.	Cessation reduces risk by about 50% after only a few years.
Cervical cancer risk among women who smoke is approximately 2 to 3 times higher.	Risk in women who quit smoking is substantially lower even in the first few years after cessation.
Coronary heart disease (CHD) risks due to smoking are higher in younger than older age groups. For both men and women under age 65 years, CHD risk in smokers is 3 times higher than in nonsmokers.	Risk reduced among men and women of all ages. Excess risk of CHD caused by smoking is reduced by about half after 1 year of abstinence. After 15 years of abstinence, risk of CHD is similar to that of persons who never smoked.
Individuals with *diagnosed CHD*	Risk of recurrent infarction or premature death is reduced by 50% or more.
Peripheral artery occlusive disease	Cessation substantially reduces risk.
Ischemic stroke and subarachnoid hemorrhage risks are between 2 and 5 times more common in smokers.	After cessation, risk is reduced to the level of those who have never smoked after approximately 10 years of abstinence.
Respiratory symptoms such as cough, sputum production, and wheezing.	Rates reduced after quitting smoking; often symptoms disappear within 6 months following cessation.
Persons without overt *chronic obstructive pulmonary disease* (COPD).	Pulmonary function can improve slightly (about 5%) within a few months after cessation.
Acceleration in *age-related decline in lung function*.	With sustained abstinence from smoking, rate of decline in pulmonary function of former smokers returns to that of those who never smoked.
COPD mortality rate among smokers is 10 times higher than among nonsmokers.	Sustained abstinence reduces COPD mortality rates in comparison with those who continue smoking.

(continued)

TABLE 1.1. *(continued)*

Health consequences	Benefits of quitting
Low-birth-weight babies	Women who stop before pregnancy have infants of same birth weight as those born to women who never smoked. Stopping smoking any time up to the 30th week of gestation results in infants with higher birth weight than continuing to smoke throughout pregnancy. Quitting before start of second trimester results in infants with birth weight similar to those born to never-smoking women.
Onset of menopause	Smoking causes women to have natural menopause 1 to 2 years early. Former smokers experience natural menopause at ages similar to those of women who never smoked.
Duodenal and gastric ulcers	The increased risk is reduced by smoking cessation. Smoking cessation is often medically necessary to promote healing.

Note. Adapted from Appendix 6-B by D. R. Shopland and D. M. Burns, from *Nicotine Addiction: Principles and Management*, edited by C. Tracy Orleans and John Slade, copyright 1993 by Oxford University Press, Inc. Adapted by permission of Oxford University Press, Inc.

time, because tobacco addiction is a chronic refractory problem (like diabetes, hypertension, or major bipolar disorder). One never knows at what point in time the toxins in tobacco will convert healthy human cells into an incurable cancer or trigger a heart attack or other medical malady. The sooner our treatments can reach, motivate, and assist smokers in quitting, the less their bodies will be exposed to the hundreds of highly toxic substances and carcinogens present in tobacco products (Jenkins, Guerin, & Tomkins, 2000). Reducing smoking prevalence among adults will also help future generations to avoid initiation, until we eventually have a smoke-free society.

REACHING AND TREATING EVERY SMOKER

The population perspective on the scope of the tobacco addiction problem illustrates the need to actively engage with your communities. Strive to capture the diversity of strategies needed to reach every smoker of every age and background, especially those who are hard to find, such as the unemployed, the uninsured, and other groups at disproportionate risk. Channels of access within the community, such as worksites or health care or social organizations, will have different systems factors that, in turn, will influence your decision making regarding what intervention(s) to use in what sequence, with which types of smokers, in what settings, and with what level of intensity (Abrams, Emmons, Niaura, Goldstein, & Sherman, 1991; Abrams et al., 1996).

The Public Health Service (PHS) Clinical Practice Guideline (Fiore et al., 2000) contains the best evidence-based information about treatment effectiveness. The PHS guideline provides an overview of the general flow, processes, and levels of intervention that are possible when one takes a "big picture," or population, perspective. The overall PHS model for treatment of tobacco addiction (adapted in Figure 1.1) is illustrated by a flow diagram that includes (1) reaching smokers within a larger population unit through various channels or delivery systems within the community and (2) screening and encouraging smokers at every opportunity to consider cessation. Once screened, smokers can then be (1) asked about their smoking habit; (2) assessed for motivation and readiness to set a quit date; (3) motivated to consider cessation if they are not ready to quit; (4) advised on how to quit if they are ready; (5) assisted with specific behavioral skills and pharmacological aids to achieve their cessation goals; and (6) given arranged follow-up care to prevent relapse. If they do relapse, they can be cycled back into treatment, and a new treatment plan can be developed. Thus treatment does not end until the smoker can maintain a tobacco-free life.

The sequence described herein and in Figure 1.1 employs what has become known as the "five A's"—Ask about smoking; Advise to quit; Assess willingness (motivation) to quit; Assist with quitting; and Arrange follow-up. The five A's are the basis for brief interventions (Chapter 4 in this book) primarily in the context of health care delivery settings, some of which are described in Chapter 8 of this book (e.g., medical office practices). Sample brief

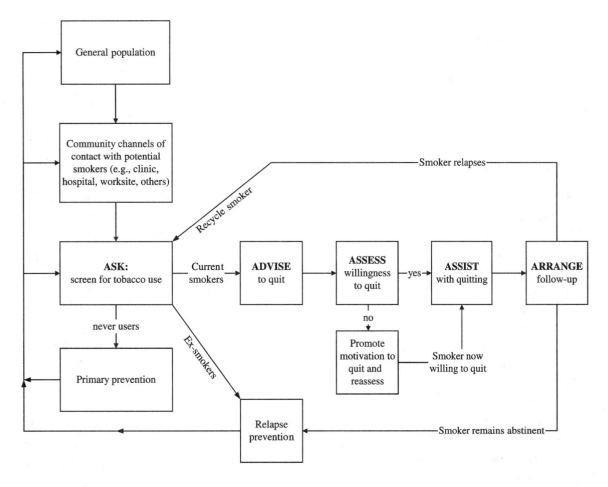

FIGURE 1.1. Population model for treatment of tobacco use and dependence. Adapted from *Treating Tobacco Use and Dependence. Clinical Practice Guideline,* by M. C. Fiore et al., 2000, Rockville, MD: U.S. Department of Health and Human Services.

treatment programs and other useful tools are readily available from the Public Health Service (PHS), the National Cancer Institute (NCI), various voluntary agencies (American Heart and Lung Associations and Cancer Society), and at the Surgeon General's website (*www.surgeongeneral.gov/tobacco/*).

This book is consistent with each step of the treatment process outlined in the PHS guideline. The skills needed for the assessment component (Ask) of the PHS guideline are described in Chapter 2, and the assessment results are then linked to the appropriate treatment. The different components of treatment are provided in Chapters 3–7. These chapters address the "Advise, Assist with motivation and Assist with quitting" steps in the PHS guideline, as well as with the "Arrange follow-up" components. Figure 1.2 will help you to link the PHS flow diagram of Figure 1.1 to the chapters in this book. At this point, we have provided you with one conceptual road map for treatment planning, albeit at the broadest level. In the next sections, we focus on developing the individual treatment plan by considering more specific smoker characteristics, treatment modalities, and outcome efficacy and related contextual factors.

WHAT WE KNOW ABOUT TOBACCO DEPENDENCE: WHY PEOPLE SMOKE

In this section, we review what is known about individual mechanisms in smoking relevant to the process of treatment planning. The principles are intended as guidelines rather than as a definitive set of rigid decision algorithms. The principles enhance but do not replace your own clinical judgement in tailoring treatment to the unique needs of each smoker.

The evidence base for the treatment principles in this book is derived from research on biobehavioral theories and mechanisms of addiction (see Abrams et al., 1991; Niaura & Abrams, 2002; Orleans & Slade, 1993) and the treatment recommendations of the PHS Clinical Practice Guideline (Fiore et al., 2000). A brief summary of the key conclusions in the PHS guideline is provided (see Table 1.2). You are encouraged to obtain a copy of the PHS guideline, become familiar with it, and use it as a reference source in conjunction with this book. The PHS guideline can be found online at *www.surgeongeneral.gov/tobacco/*. Printed copies of the PHS guideline are available from any of the following Public Health Service clearinghouses: the Agency for Healthcare Research and Quality (800-358-9295); the Centers for Disease Control and Prevention (800-CDC-1311); and the National Cancer Institute (800-4-CANCER); or write to Publications Clearinghouse, P.O. Box 8547, Silver Spring, MD 20907.

Individual Mechanisms

Biobehavioral Processes in Smoking and Cessation

A basic knowledge of the reasons for people becoming addicted to tobacco provides one set of guiding principles for treatment planning. Why do some people smoke and others do not? Why can some "chippers" (see Shiffman, 1989) smoke a few cigarettes per week and literally

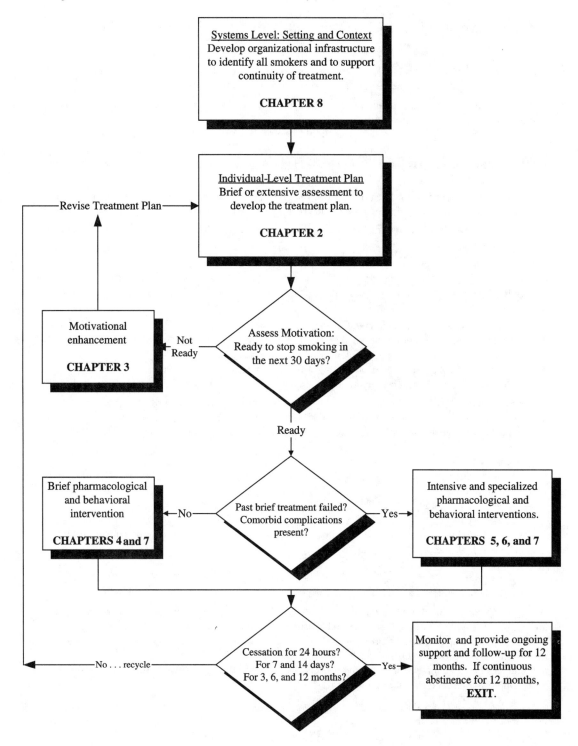

FIGURE 1.2. The process of treatment planning followed in this book.

TABLE 1.2. Major Findings and Recommendations of the PHS Smoking Cessation Clinical Practice Guideline

1. Tobacco dependence is a chronic condition that often requires repeated intervention. However, effective treatments exist that can produce long-term or even permanent abstinence.

2. Because effective tobacco dependence treatments are available, every patient who uses tobacco should be offered at least one of these treatments.
   - Patients *willing* to try to quit tobacco use should be provided treatments identified as effective in this guideline.
   - Patients *unwilling* to try to quit tobacco use should be provided a brief intervention designed to increase their motivation to quit.

3. It is essential that clinicians and health care delivery systems (including administrators, insurers, and purchasers) consistently identify, document, and treat every tobacco user seen in a health care setting.

4. Brief tobacco dependence treatment is effective, and every patient who uses tobacco should be offered at least brief treatment.

5. There is a strong dose–response relation between the intensity of tobacco dependence counseling and its effectiveness. Treatments involving person-to-person contact (via individual, group, or proactive telephone counseling) are consistently effective, and their effectiveness increases with treatment intensity (e.g., minutes of contact).

6. Three types of counseling and behavioral therapies were found to be especially effective and should be used with all patients attempting tobacco cessation:
   - Provision of practical counseling (problem-solving and skills training).
   - Provision of social support as part of treatment (intratreatment social support).
   - Help in securing social support outside of treatment (extratreatment social support).

7. Numerous effective pharmacotherapies for smoking cessation now exist. Except in the presence of contraindications, these should be used with all patients attempting to quit smoking.
   - Five *first-line* pharmacotherapies have been identified that reliably increase long-term smoking abstinence rates:
     —Bupropion SR
     —Nicotine gum
     —Nicotine inhaler
     —Nicotine nasal spray
     —Nicotine patch
   - Two *second-line* pharmacotherapies have been identified as efficacious and may be considered by clinicians if first-line pharmacotherapies are not effective:
     —Clonidine
     —Nortriptyline
   - Over-the-counter nicotine patches are effective relative to placebo, and their use should be encouraged.

8. Tobacco dependence treatments are both clinically effective and cost-effective relative to other medical and disease prevention interventions. As such, insurers and purchasers should ensure that:
   - All insurance plans include as a reimbursed benefit the counseling and pharmacotherapeutic treatments identified as effective in this guideline.
   - Clinicians are reimbursed for providing tobacco dependence treatment just as they are reimbursed for treating other chronic conditions.

Note. From *Treating Tobacco Use and Dependence. Clinical Practice Guideline*, by M. C. Fiore et al., 2000. Rockville, MD: U.S. Department of Health and Human Services.

"take one or leave one at will," whereas other smokers are so heavily addicted they cannot stop even after a laryngectomy due to throat cancer? Breakthroughs in research on the neurochemical and behavioral mechanisms in nicotine susceptibility and dependence (e.g., Koob & LeMoal, 2001; Niaura & Abrams, 2002; Shiffman, Mason, & Henningfield, 1998) are creating a deeper understanding of the mechanisms underlying this addiction and new opportunities for treatment and relapse prevention (Hughes, Goldstein, et al., 1999). At the basis of the diversity of smoking typologies is a complex gene-by-environment interaction that includes cellular and molecular differences in susceptibility to nicotine's reinforcing effects, differences in the way people metabolize nicotine—including gender differences—and a host of environmental factors, beginning with fetal exposure to nicotine *in utero* and onward throughout the life span. This gene–environment interaction makes smokers extremely diverse across the whole spectrum of patterns of tobacco use, degree of dependence severity, reasons for using, and reasons for wanting to stop using (for more details on genetics factors, see Cheng, Swan, & Carmelli, 2000; Lerman et al., 1999; O. Pomerleau & Kardia, 1999).

One useful view is that smoking is a form of "self-medication" to improve ability to cope with the stresses of everyday life, to avoid withdrawal symptoms, and to facilitate "self-regulation" of one's neurochemistry or physiology, psychological states, and other individual and social behaviors. Smoking is conceptualized as a learned behavior that is maintained primarily because of (1) the immediate positive reinforcing effects of nicotine, a central nervous system stimulant, and other tobacco-produced neurochemicals—they hijack the brain's most powerful neurochemical reward centers (mesolimbic area) and modify the availability of dopamine and other brain chemicals, including monoamine oxidase (MAO A and B; see Chapter 7 for more details); (2) the development of nicotine dependence and the negative reinforcement pattern smokers use to avoid unpleasant withdrawal symptoms; (3) nicotine's perceived "value" as a coping response to help regulate mood, stress, anger, anxiety, attention and concentration, memory, boredom, depression, and other psychological needs; and (4) nicotine's perceived interpersonal or social benefits, such as to identify a person as part of an "in crowd," to improve self-image, or to reduce social anxiety.

People also smoke for the immediate positive consequences that they come to expect or experience and to alleviate negative mood states or withdrawal. The expected positive benefits of smoking (outcome expectancies) and the learned habit (classical and operant conditioning) can create a psychological dependence on tobacco use as powerful as the neurochemical (biological) dependence derived from nicotine and other psychoactive constituents in tobacco.

The latest thinking is that the concept of dependence is best viewed as a continuum from low to high severity, that it is multidimensional, and that it is neither simply biological nor learned behavior but an interaction of the two (see Koob & LeMoal, 2001; Shadel, Shiffman, Niaura, Nichter, & Abrams, 2000). The biological aspects include cellular, molecular, and neurochemical components localized in the brain reward pathways (e.g., nicotinic acetylcholine receptors concentrated in the nucleus accumbens and amygdala). The cognitive-behavioral aspects of dependence include deeply entrained memory mechanisms of learned associations with pleasure, mood modulation, attention, and socialization. The interaction of biology and behavior then drives the typical behavioral expression of the dimensions of an addiction, such as compulsive use, stereotypic patterns, drug seeking despite negative consequences, craving, and avoidance of withdrawal.

There is evidence that lighter, perhaps less addicted smokers (< 25 cigarettes per day) are more than twice as likely to quit on their own or with low intensity self-change or brief treatment when compared with more heavily addicted smokers (Cohen et al., 1989). The current population of smokers may therefore be more severely nicotine dependent and/or may have other complications (e.g., comorbidity of mood disorders such as depression, alcohol or substance abuse, or adult attention-deficit disorder; see Hughes, Goldstein, et al., 1999). From a treatment planning perspective, smokers who have already tried unsuccessfully to quit on their own or with brief advice (Chapter 4) and over-the-counter nicotine replacement products (Chapter 7) will likely need more support and the more structured specialized treatments in Chapters 5 and 6 (see Figure 1.2).

The nature of nicotine dependence also means that withdrawal symptoms can begin as soon as 2 hours after the last cigarette, peak within days, and last up to several weeks (see Chapter 7). In some cases a protracted withdrawal has been noted that may last for months and include a subclinical level of malaise, low energy, poor concentration, and depressive features. The general implications for treatment planning are that (1) multiple modes of treatment (behavioral and pharmacological) are better than single modes; (2) more intensive treatments may be needed as dependence severity increases and as the multidimensional components of learned dependence become evident; and (3) repeated treatment and continuity of care are important not only in the immediate weeks following cessation, when vulnerability to relapse is greatest, but also for longer periods of time (3 months to 1 year).

Consistent with the "self-medication" model, smokers who come to rely on the psychoactive benefits of nicotine may also be less motivated to try to quit, knowing that they might have difficulty performing without their nicotine boost. A factory worker may be using nicotine to maintain performance while operating machinery that requires concentration and task repetition. Other smokers may smoke to help regulate body weight, especially women who are concerned about being overweight (Perkins et al., 2001). People smoke for many reasons, of which they may not even be fully aware at the onset of treatment.

There are also the learned behavioral and social components of dependence. People smoke simply because it is a learned habit, an automatic response. The habit is difficult to extinguish, in part due to the high frequency of use and the millions of repeated "doses" that a smoker administers as he/she goes through the lighting and puffing ritual. As a result of these repeated pairings, many previously neutral cues or stimuli can become conditioned to smoking (e.g., during phone conversations, at a celebration, when others are drinking). Situations that come to trigger a strong urge, craving, or desire to smoke are also likely to be considered as "high risk" in that they can provoke a relapse following an attempt to quit (Abrams et al., 1988; Shiffman et al., 1986). Situations that include smoking-specific cues (e.g., the sight and smell of a lit cigarette) are especially potent in triggering a craving to smoke (Abrams, 1986). However, treatment designed to directly extinguish reactivity to smoking-specific cues have yielded disappointing results, perhaps because the treatment itself may have provoked relapse due to its being delivered immediately after cessation (Niaura et al., 1999). Many of the psychological and situational factors that underlie the reasons for smoking are also the major variables that you need to consider when planning to prevent relapse immediately after cessation. If someone smokes to suppress anger and frustration at work, they will need to be taught alternative anger management skills to use in preparation for cessation and to prevent relapse after cessation.

Relapse and Recycling

Relapse is common: between 60% and 98% of attempts to quit end in relapse, with the greatest proportion (44%) occurring within 14 days (Garvey, Bliss, Hitchcock, Heinold, & Rosner, 1992). The relapse curves for nicotine are similar to those for heroin and alcohol addiction (Hunt & Bespalec, 1974). As many as 37% of smokers with a past history of depression will relapse the day they quit (Brown, Herman, Ramsey, & Stout, 1999). Relapse should be regarded as part of the learning experience along the pathway to cessation. Just like learning to ride a bicycle for the first time, persistent effort, practice, and openness to the correction of past mistakes will lead to eventual mastery and success (Bandura, 1997). If one falls off the bicycle, one has to get back up and try again to become proficient at negotiating the curves and the bumps in the road. Thus the idea of recycling smokers who have slipped back into smoking, who have not tried to quit for many years, or both is included in the treatment planning process (see Figures 1.1 and 1.2).

Key ingredients derived from self-efficacy within social cognitive theory (Bandura, 1997) predict successful maintenance of cessation and include: (1) the setting of small achievable goals (Borrelli & Mermelstein, 1994); (2) practicing successful use of coping skills to achieve these small goals; (3) gaining self-confidence that one can indeed achieve the goals (increasing self-efficacy expectancies); and (4) having a belief that the desired outcomes will result from executing the skills (increasing outcome expectancies). For example, a smoker feels confident (self-efficacy expectancies) that he/she can overcome social anxiety and resist the temptation to smoke at a birthday party where several close friends are smoking and everyone is drinking and having a good time. This person anticipates still having a good time (outcome expectancies) at the party by using social skills and relaxation training instead of smoking. Improved self-efficacy, in turn, helps the smoker to persist in trying to remain abstinent, even in the face of difficulties such as strong temptations (urges or cravings to smoke) or actual "slips" back into smoking. Thus a smoker's self-efficacy, his/her outcome expectations, and his/her motivation to break the addiction cycle (i.e., set proximal goals and adhere to them) are interrelated and must be monitored throughout treatment.

The process of quitting is only modestly influenced by the smoker's past history of attempts to quit. Longer previous periods of abstinence and very recent attempts (within the past year) may be prognostic of greater likelihood of success. One important general principle for treatment planning is that any past "relapse" and even a "failed" attempt to quit during current treatment should be reframed in the mind of the smoker. Rather than a "failure," it should be considered a learning experience and an opportunity to identify deficits in coping skills and to acquire new skills. A relapse is really a temporary "slip"; indeed, it is a *prolapse* along the pathway to eventual mastery of the coping skills needed for ultimate success (Brownell, Marlatt, Lichtenstein, & Wilson, 1986). Although many ex-smokers have quit on their own, most make several attempts before they finally succeed. They could have failed to quit during past attempts and become disillusioned, or they may never have seriously tried to quit before. Smokers who are low in motivational readiness to quit may benefit from a different treatment strategy and a supportive (client-centered) counseling style, one that collaboratively explores the smoker's decision making and risk perceptions rather than a counseling style that is more directive, in which the treatment focuses on action steps for cessation (motivational interviewing; see Chapter 3).

Smokers can also vary in their need for and reaction to social support (Mermelstein, Cohen, Lichtenstein, Baer, & Kamarck, 1986). Some prefer to be left alone; some react negatively to efforts that may be construed as "checking up" on them; others may welcome any support and encouragement (Fisher, 1997; Lichtenstein, Glasgow, & Abrams, 1986). Be aware that constructive social support for one smoker may be counterproductive for another (see Chapter 2). Having household members or close friends who are smokers can make it very difficult to quit. You may have to persuade other household members or friends to consider cessation at the same time as the smoker does. The sudden illness of a friend or relative who is a smoker or ex-smoker, especially if the illness is smoking related, can become a "teachable moment" that can increase a smoker's motivation to quit. Some smokers who are not at all motivated to quit may benefit from motivational counseling (see Chapter 3), whereas others may abruptly decide that it is time to quit and set a quit date.

In summary, the process of cessation can be variable and diverse; it can progress gradually and cumulatively; or it can be marked by fits and starts, sudden changes in motivation and behavior. There is no "typical smoker" or "tobacco addiction personality." The patterns of smoking, the reasons for smoking, and the reasons that motivate cessation can vary within a smoker over time and between smokers. Biological, psychological, behavioral, and sociocultural factors are involved in becoming motivated to quit, in making a quit attempt, and in the short- and long-term processes of resisting relapse after cessation. A smoker is most likely to relapse during the first 1–3 months following cessation, but he/she remains quite vulnerable for the 12 months following cessation. Your treatment plan should provide the flexibility to take these nuances into consideration. As the provider, your roles are (1) instilling and maintaining motivation to keep trying; (2) helping to set realistic short-term goals and boosting the smokers' self-confidence so that they can learn how to quit permanently; (3) providing the needed coping and problem-solving skills (cognitive, behavioral, and pharmacological); (4) giving continuous support and encouragement to persist in the face of setbacks for as long as it takes to quit; and (5) being willing to revise the treatment plan to add new components (including referral to specialists) as additional information about the smoker's characteristics is revealed by the process of trying to stop smoking (see also Figures 1.1 and 1.2).

TREATMENT PLANNING: IMPLICATIONS OF INDIVIDUAL SMOKER CHARACTERISTICS

You will need to evaluate each individual smoker's characteristics and history in order to decide on the treatment plan. The research literature reviewed herein suggests that at least six major areas should be evaluated: (1) intrinsic motivation and self-confidence in ability to quit; (2) level of nicotine dependence and severity of withdrawal on cessation; (3) degree of comorbidity; (4) past history of quit attempts and why they failed; (5) reasons for smoking, pattern of smoking (where, when, with whom), and reasons for wanting to stop; and (6) social and environmental supports and impediments (e.g., other smokers in the household). These domains are covered in detail in Chapter 2. The PHS guideline (Fiore et al., 2000) also reports the following variables associated with lower cessation rates: low motivation; low self-efficacy (confidence in one's ability to stop smoking by having and using coping skills); high nicotine dependence; psychiatric comorbidity (depression, schizophrenia, alcoholism, other substance abuse, anxiety, phobia); high environmental risks (e.g., other smokers in the household); and high stress levels or major life changes (e.g., divorce, job change, working in a stressful or boring job).

The process of developing a treatment plan for a smoker involves identifying the pattern of antecedent situational cues or stimuli that trigger smoking, as well as the consequences that maintain smoking through reinforcement—both positive (e.g., the pleasure of smoking) and negative (e.g., the alleviation of stress, depressed mood, or withdrawal). The analysis of Antecedent triggers that set the stage for the Behavior (smoking) that is then maintained by the reinforcing Consequences is easily remembered as the functional analysis of the ABC's of smoking. Behavioral techniques (Chapters 4–6), such as stimulus control and contingency management, are employed to assist in quitting and in preventing relapse (see O'Leary & Wilson, 1987, for details and the basic principles of behavior therapy). Treatment requires breaking of the learned automatic habit and helping the smoker learn alternative ways of coping with the antecedent triggers and with the reinforcing effects of tobacco, both biological and psychosocial. Because smoking is a learned behavior, it can be unlearned, and new, more adaptive, cognitive and behavioral coping skills can be substituted in its place.

Some smokers will need a treatment plan with provisions made for prolonged intervention and the use of several different treatment components and/or specialist providers (e.g., addiction specialists including disciplines in mental health—psychiatrist, psychologist, psychiatric nurse, social worker). A treatment plan may also have to incorporate the idea of stepping up the level of care in a number of possible areas to make successful cessation more likely on the next quit attempt (e.g., more frequent or longer sessions; support or group treatment; different pharmacological treatment options [see Chapter 7]; a specialist consultation or a referral for treatment of emergent psychiatric comorbidity or alcohol or substance abuse). In developing a treatment plan, you should also make a special effort to ensure that smokers with lower incomes, education, and no or inferior health insurance coverage do indeed have equal access to all the best levels of care available, including nicotine replacement and specialists.

Motivation

As mentioned previously, population surveys show that a small minority of smokers (14–28%) are highly motivated to quit in the following 30 days (Abrams & Biener, 1992; Velicer et al., 1995), although over 70% of current smokers will say they want to quit. Another 30–40% of smokers say they intend to quit in the following 6 months. Members of managed care groups such as health maintenance organizations (HMOs) show higher levels of motivational readiness than the general population, with as many as 70% planning to quit within 6 months

(Hollis, Lichtenstein, Vogt, Stevens, & Biglan, 1993). About 30% of all smokers say they do try to quit each year, but less than 1 to 5% maintain cessation (Centers for Disease Control, 1994b).

Some smokers come into treatment because of pressure from others. Motivation is best when it is intrinsic (comes from the smoker him/herself) and is tied to a realistic evaluation of the benefits of stopping versus the benefits of continuing to smoke (Curry, Grothaus, & McBride, 1997). When a smoker is not really ready to quit and lacks self-confidence to try, then it is not surprising that he/she will fail to quit when asked to try nor that you, the provider, will become discouraged from advising him/her to quit again in the future (see Chapter 3). Both smokers and their providers often have unrealistic expectations (Abrams, 1993; Abrams et al., 1996). The mismatch between smoker readiness (he/she is not ready) and provider enthusiasm (advising him/her to quit today) is most evident in settings that require a provider to proactively reach out to smokers who are not seeking treatment for their smoking. Such settings include nonvolunteer populations such as *all* the smoking members of a managed care organization, a worksite, a hospital, or a substance abuse rehabilitation program (Abrams & Biener, 1992; Abrams et al., 1996).

Thus a focus on *motivation* may be the only goal of the treatment plan for some time. The provider must be sensitive to the smoker's actual readiness and perceived barriers to cessation (see Chapter 3). Setting a quit date and providing instrumental coping skills or nicotine replacement therapy when a smoker is not yet fully committed to cessation is probably counterproductive.

Comorbid Complicating Characteristics

Many biobehavioral factors are related to a smoker's initial motivation to quit and to a smoker's likelihood of relapse. But for treatment planning purposes, few factors seem as compelling as severity of nicotine dependence and presence of comorbidity. The presence of nicotine dependence and comorbidity warrants consideration of more intensive treatment.

Nicotine Dependence

Nicotine withdrawal and dependence are considered to be distinct yet related disorders, each with specific diagnostic criteria (American Psychiatric Association, 1994). The 47–50 million smokers in the United States show a continuum of dependence from mild to severe (Shiffman, 1989). Dependence is defined by the American Psychiatric Association's 1994) *Diagnostic and Statistical Manual of Mental Disorders* (DSM-IV-R). These criteria and examples of nicotine dependence may be found in Chapter 7 (Tables 7.1 and 7.2). Depending on the number of symptoms used to define dependence and the response bias in the population of smokers surveyed, the percentage of dependent smokers can be as high as 87% (Hale et al., 1993). Greater nicotine dependence is related to lower motivation to quit, difficulty trying to quit smoking, failure to quit, and better treatment outcome with nicotine replacement (Hughes, 1996; Shiffman et al., 1998). Withdrawal symptoms are also related to severity of dependence, and these symptoms may increase temptations to smoke to alleviate the withdrawal, especially in the first 30 days after cessation.

Most studies to date have examined various nicotine replacement delivery systems either alone or in combination with behavior therapy. Nicotine replacement increases all smokers' chances of quitting. The PHS guideline (Fiore et al., 2000) therefore recommends that all smokers be advised to use nicotine replacement (gum or patch) when trying to quit except when contraindicated (see Table 1.2 and Chapter 7).

Psychiatric and Substance Abuse Comorbidity

Depression, alcohol and other substance abuse disorders, adult attention-deficit/hyperactivity problems, psychotic disorders, and anxiety disorders are associated with increased prevalence of smoking (Hughes, 1993). Smokers with a history of depression are more likely to be diagnosed as nicotine dependent and to progress to more severe levels of dependence than persons without a history, and they are less likely to quit smoking (Glassman, 1997; Patten, Martin, Myers, Calfas, & Williams, 1998). Smoking rates of over 85% are observed in alcoholics, opiate addicts, and polydrug users (Fertig & Allen, 1995). More alcoholics die of tobacco-related causes than from their alcoholism (Hurt et al., 1994). Smokers with a history of alcoholism are more likely to be nicotine dependent.

The presence of comorbidities must be considered in treatment planning (Patten et al., 1998). Among smokers with susceptibility to depression, both nicotine replacement therapies and antidepressant therapies may be needed (Hughes, Stead, & Lancaster, 2002). Specialized behavioral coping skills training programs have been developed to address areas such as mood management (see Chapter 6). Smokers with a past history of comorbidity, as well as those with current or emerging signs of comorbidity during a quit attempt, may benefit from the highest levels of intensity of behavioral and pharmacological treatments and the involvement of specialists in addictions, psychiatry and psychology, or other mental health professions (American Psychiatric Association Work Group on Nicotine Dependence, 1996).

Medical Comorbidity

Opportunities for treating nicotine dependence arise in the course of treatment for a medical condition (Gritz, Kristeller, & Burns, 1993). An acute illness can provide the context for a "teachable moment" and can result in very high quit rates. Many chronic diseases (e.g., cardiovascular disease) are complicated or worsened by smoking. By contrast, smokers with smoking-related illnesses who continue to smoke are very difficult to treat by any method. Programs that are tailored to medical groups have proven more effective than "generic" cessation interventions. Interventions tailored for pregnant smokers, smokers with cardiac disease, and cancer patients have been developed by Gritz (Gritz et al., 1993), Ockene, and others (Ockene et al., 1992; Orleans, Rotberg, Quade, & Lees, 1990; Taylor, Houston-Miller, Killen, & DeBusk, 1990). Special interventions can also be used to boost motivation among hospitalized smokers (Fisher, Haire-Joshu, Morgan, Rehberg, & Rost, 1990; Hurt et al., 1992; Orleans et al., 1990). In some cases (pregnancy, after a heart attack), the decision about the safety of nicotine replacement must rest on a careful assessment of the risk–benefit equation (N. L. Benowitz, 1993; Fiore, Jorenby, Baker, & Kenford, 1992).

Gender Differences and Weight Gain

Possible gender differences in ability to quit smoking, with and without treatment, have come under increasing scrutiny (Wetter, Fiore et al., 1999). Several studies suggest that women have more difficulty quitting smoking than men do, despite evidencing less nicotine dependence (Wetter, Kenford et al., 1999). Moreover, women in particular may be less responsive to nicotine replacement therapy. Some evidence exists to suggest that women smokers may be influenced more by non-nicotine-related stimuli related to smoking, which may explain in part decreased responsivity to nicotine replacement therapy (for review, see Perkins, Donny, & Caggiula, 1999; Perkins et al., 2001). However, very little is known regarding the array of factors, ranging from drug sensitivity to sociocultural influences, that may ultimately explain potential gender differences in smoking initiation, prevalence, risk for relapse, and response to treatment. Understanding gender differences in smoking cessation, including depression (e.g., Borrelli et al., 1999), smoking for weight control, response to nicotine, and treatment response, may lead to improved interventions for smoking cessation for both women and men (U.S. Department of Health and Human Services, 2001).

Concern about post-cessation weight gain is prevalent among some men but primarily among women smokers. The weight control benefits of smoking appear to be an important motivator for continued smoking (Gritz, Klesges, & Meyers, 1989) and for smoking relapse (U.S. Department of Health and Human Services, 2001). The smokers' beliefs about the importance of smoking in preventing weight gain (i.e., their cognitions of self-efficacy and outcome expectancies) may be more potent than the actual weight gain, which is modest in most smokers (Borrelli & Mermelstein, 1998; Perkins et al., 2001). In addition, accumulating evidence suggests that women smokers may evaluate their bodies more negatively than nonsmoking women (King, Matacin, Bock, & Marcus, 1997). Women smokers also reported feeling less attractive and perceived themselves as heavier than comparison samples (King, Matacin, Marcus, Bock, & Tripolone, 2000). It is possible that body image evaluations play an important role in smoking behavior (e.g., women who negatively evaluate the size or shape of their bodies may be more likely to smoke to lose weight or to prevent weight gain).

Dietary intake may play a role in postcessation weight gain (U.S. Department of Health and Human Services, 2001). Caloric consumption increases after smoking cessation but tends to return to precessation levels with longer abstinence. Dietary interventions to prevent weight gain during smoking cessation have not been effective in increasing quit rates or reducing postcessation weight gain (Hall, Tunstall, Vila, & Duffy, 1992; Pirie et al., 1992). This lack of success may be due to the complex demands of working on two extinction behaviors simultaneously (Klesges, Benowitz, & Meyers, 1991).

Pharmacotherapy can be tailored to address weight concerns (see Chapter 7). In addition, there is accumulating evidence that increasing physical activity may reduce postcessation weight gain (Kawachi, Troisi, Rotnitzky, Coakely, & Colditz, 1996; Marcus et al., 1999). The Commit to Quit trial, conducted at our Centers for Behavioral Medicine at Brown University Medical School and The Miriam Hospital, found that vigorous exercise training improves cessation rates and may be a useful strategy for short-term maintenance of smoking cessation (Marcus et al., 1999). Smokers participated in a regular program of supervised, group-based vigorous activity in a hospital outpatient setting. Space does not permit us to reproduce the Commit to Quit program here, but essentially this program employs the cognitive-behavioral treatments outlined in Chapters 5 and 6 in concert with a formal super-vised exercise program. After approval by their physicians, smokers can be encouraged to participate in a supervised, group-based vigorous physical activity program, especially if they have concerns about weight gain. If this is not possible, smokers should be encouraged to en-gage in a home-based physical activity program. For an excellent self-help guide to increas-ing physical activity, see Blair, Dunn, Marcus, Carpenter, and Jaret (2001). Physical activity is a healthful alternative to smoking that has been shown to yield many physical and psycho-logical effects that could be beneficial to smokers.

ADDITIONAL TREATMENT, PROVIDER, AND SETTING CONSIDERATIONS

Treatment programs vary in intensity, duration, content, and modality of delivery, as well as in cost, degree of professional specialty training required for delivery, and effectiveness. Set-tings vary according to the infrastructure of the delivery system. The delivery system can ei-ther constrain or facilitate smoking cessation treatment depending on the degree of support received from administrative management and supervisors and on the policies, values, costs, cost offsets, and incentives—the "culture and context" of the setting. The smoker's living sit-uation (home environment, social support, smokers among household members, coworkers, close friends, disposable income, access to health insurance) also must be considered in plan-ning treatment.

Treatment Characteristics

Available treatment elements range along the continuum of treatment intensity, complexity, cost, and duration. Self-change guides, Internet (World Wide Web) resources, and tailored print materials require no face-to-face contact. Brief telephone or computer-assisted counsel-ing strategies or brief face-to-face treatments (such as in medical offices) can be used. Volun-tary agency programs (e.g., American Lung Association, American Cancer Society, American Heart Association) offer individual or group meetings with trained volunteer staff or paid pro-fessional counselors (usually ex-smokers). There are also more formal specialty outpatient clinics or alcohol and substance abuse programs (Bobo, McIlvain, Lando, Walker, & Leed-Kelly, 1998; Martin et al., 1997). For example, the formal and more intensive programs developed by our research group at Brown University Medical School (Chapters 5 and 6) consist of eight or more outpatient group treatment sessions and yield 1-year cessation rates at follow-up of 24.7–32.5% (Brown et al., 2001). At the most intense and expensive end of the treatment continuum are inpatient programs. Hurt and colleagues (1994) have described an inpatient treatment for smokers who have failed in formal outpatient programs or have prom-inent nicotine dependence, psychiatric, substance abuse, or medical comorbidity (Hurt et al., 1994).

Commercial and "alternative medicine" programs are also available. All programs for which credible research evidence supports efficacy are included in the PHS guideline (Fiore et al., 2000). Most commercial and alternative medicine programs are not supported by sufficient evidence (Fiore et al., 2000). The PHS guideline (Fiore et al., 2000) points out that both stepped-care models and tailoring using the "stages of change" or transtheoretical model (Prochaska, Redding, & Evers, 1997) hold promise for enhancing treatment efficacy, but neither has sufficient empirical support. Although more research on stepped care is needed to improve cessation outcomes, considering the level of intensity of treatment within a stepped-care framework provides a useful general principle for treatment planning.

The main components of treatment, derived from behavior therapy, form a common core for most treatment programs regardless of intensity (Abrams & Wilson, 1986; Orleans & Slade, 1993). The core components are used in self-change guidebooks such as the American Lung Association's *Freedom from Smoking* (Strecher & Rimer, 1999) and the *Clear Horizons* manual for smokers over 50 years of age (Orleans et al., 1997). Decades of research support the cognitive-behavioral approach that we use in this book (Orleans & Slade, 1993).

On a broad level, treatment programs can be categorized into minimal, moderate, and maximal, depending on intensity and duration and modality of treatment (e.g., behavioral, pharmacological, multiple providers). This simplifies the continuum of treatment options into three "steps" and corresponds to self-change, brief provider interventions, and more formal multisession smoking cessation programs (for details, see Abrams et al., 1996). The PHS guideline (Fiore et al., 2000) also provides strong evidence for a dose–response relationship between intensity (duration, frequency, and modality) and effectiveness. Programs with greater intensity and time allocation that combine different providers and modalities of treatment (e.g., problem solving, behavioral skills, social support and pharmacotherapy) have better outcomes. Table 1.3 summarizes the key recommendations from the PHS guideline

TABLE 1.3. Findings Relevant to Intensive Interventions

- There is a strong dose–response relation between counseling intensity and cessation success. In general, the more intense the treatment intervention, the greater the rate of smoking cessation. Treatments may be made more intense by increasing (1) the length of individual treatment sessions and (2) the number of treatment sessions.

- Many different types of providers (physicians, nurses, dentists, psychologists, pharmacists, etc.) are effective in increasing rates of tobacco cessation, and involving multiple types of providers may enhance abstinence rates.

- Proactive telephone calls and individual and group counseling are effective tobacco cessation formats.

- Particular types of counseling and behavioral therapies are especially effective. Practical counseling (problem-solving and skills-training approaches) and providing intratreatment and extratreatment social support are associated with significant increases in abstinence rates, as are aversive smoking techniques (e.g., rapid smoking).

- Pharmacotherapies such as bupropion SR or nicotine replacement therapies consistently increase abstinence rates. Therefore, their use should be encouraged for all quitters, but special consideration is required with some populations (e.g., pregnant smokers, those who have had a heart attack, adolescents).

- Tobacco dependence treatments are effective across diverse populations (e.g., populations varying in gender, age, and ethnicity).

Note. From *Treating Tobacco Use and Dependence. Clinical Practice Guideline*, by M. C. Fiore et al., 2000. Rockville, MD: U.S. Department of Health and Human Services.

(Fiore et al., 2000) regarding the positive dose–response relationship between treatment intensity and outcome efficacy. As a general rule, treatment outcomes at 6- to 12-month follow-up range from under 10% for minimal self-change programs to 14–20% for brief interventions to over 25–35% for more intensive formal treatments with pharmacotherapy, repeated contacts, social support, and cognitive behavioral coping skills training.

In summary, according to Fiore et al. (2000), the relationship between treatment and successful outcome is as follows:

1. When added to either a brief or a more intensive behavioral program, nicotine replacement and other proven pharmacotherapies can almost double success rates.
2. Greater frequency and duration of treatments (number of sessions and length of sessions) significantly improve outcomes.
3. Behavioral coping skills training, problem solving, and social support all improve outcomes.
4. Intervention by multiple treatment providers improves outcomes.

Intervention sessions can be scheduled more or less frequently for varying durations and using a variety of modalities (telephone, face-to-face, computer-assisted, group or individual sessions, Web-based).

Reach, Impact, and Cost of Treatment

The treatment plan may be enhanced by considering that different levels of program intensity attract different populations and that these populations also vary dramatically in their motivation to quit. Minimal self-change and brief-contact programs usually take place or are disseminated *proactively* to a "defined" population in which the vast majority of individuals are *not motivated to quit* and are not seeking any help for their tobacco addiction. For example, treatment might be delivered proactively to a whole region or a community via mass media, to all smoking employees at a worksite (Abrams, Boutwell et al., 1994), or to all smokers who are members of a primary care office practice or of a health maintenance or managed care organization (Curry et al., 1998). In contrast, intensive clinical programs (e.g., 6- to 20-week outpatient smoking cessation classes) usually wait for *highly motivated* smokers to call them and schedule individual or group treatment sessions (Cooper & Clayton, 1993). Clinics therefore enroll their participants in a *reactive mode*, resulting in self-selection of individuals who are already motivated to quit and are also typically higher in socioeconomic status and education. The latter are usually seen as part of a more "clinical" treatment approach and the former as part of a broader "public health" intervention. A treatment plan for individuals who are proactively recruited (using a public health model) may require a different emphasis (less intense treatment, more focus on motivation, at least initially) compared with smokers coming into a clinic.

Compared with public health treatments, clinical interventions typically are more effective but also more intensive and costly, and they need to be delivered by trained specialists. Clinic programs reach a very small selective proportion of the population. In considering clinical versus public health treatments (that can range from minimal to moderate in intensity and can reach very large numbers of smokers), a standard measure is needed to evaluate their respective contributions to smoking cessation outcomes at a population or societal level. A common metric is needed to help place different intervention options in proper perspective. One useful way of comparing interventions is to refer to their *impact* (see Table 1.4). Impact is the efficacy of an intervention (E) multiplied by its reach (R), where reach is defined as the percent penetration of the intervention into a defined target population (e.g., a worksite or a community). In Table 1.4, the result $(E \times R)$ is multiplied by 100 to produce a range of impact from zero (no impact) to 100 (ideal or perfect). Two extreme situations could hypothetically result in zero impact: (1) a very effective, expensive program (100% efficacy) that fails to attract any clients (0% reach); or (2) a self-help brochure delivered to every smoker at no charge (100% reach) that does not work at all (0% efficacy). In actual practice, a "clinical" intervention might have a high efficacy (40%) but reach only 5% of the population (impact $= 40/100 \times 5/100 \times 100 = 2$). A "public health" intervention that has a modest efficacy of 5% but reaches 80% of the population will double the impact of the clinical approach (impact $= 4.0$). A "middle of the road" intervention with efficacy of 30% and a reach of 70% would have an impact of 21—5 times that of either the clinical or the public health approach.

Cost considerations can also be considered in your treatment plan. In general, cost is directly proportional to intervention intensity. The impact variable provides a standard metric to compare the efficiency (or the cost-effectiveness) of interventions designed for different samples of the population (proactive versus reactive). Shiffman and colleagues (1998) point out that in absolute numbers an intervention with modest efficacy but broad reach (e.g., brief treatment combined with over-the-counter [OTC] nicotine replacement) can be highly efficient and can produce a very large number of quitters per year compared with the more intensive and expensive options (see Table 1.5). A recent analysis of cost-effectiveness also indicates that more intensive and expensive programs may actually be *more cost-effective* than less intensive and less expensive programs (Cromwell et al., 1997). You may have to take impact, cost-effectiveness, cost offset, and return on investment factors into consideration when designing a treatment plan (for more information, see Parrott et al., 1998).

TABLE 1.4. Hypothetical Impact of Different Levels and Types of Interventions Along the Clinical–Public Health Continuum

Intervention type/tobacco control	Efficacy (% quit)	Reach (% pop)	Impact[a] $100(E \times R)$
Reactive: clinical treatment, behavioral + pharmacological	30–40	3–5	0.9–2.0
Reactive: clinical treatment, behavioral group	20–30	5–10	1–3
Reactive: self-help programs	5–10	10–20	0.5–2
Proactive: brief primary care, behavioral + pharmacological	10–20	10–30	1–6
Proactive: interactive computer interventions	10–20	40–60	4–12
Proactive: stepped-care (hypothetical) intervention	25	80	20
Ideal, perfect intervention	100	100	100

[a]Impact = Treatment efficacy (E) × population reach (penetration; R) × 100; range: 00–100.

TABLE 1.5. Estimated Efficacy and Utilization of Approaches to Smoking Cessation

Intervention	Efficacy (% quit at 6 months)	Reach/Utilization (No. using method annually)	Impact (total no. quitters)
None (unaided)	3	22,800,000	684,000
Rx nicotine replacement therapy (1995)	14	2,500,000	280,000
OTC nicotine replacement therapy (1996)	14	6,300,000	560,000
Behavioral counseling	24	395,000	94,800
Inpatient treatment	32	500	160

Note. From "Tobacco Dependence Treatments: Review and Prospectus," by S. Shiffman, K. M. Mason, and J. E. Henningfield, 1998, *Annual Review of Public Health, 19,* p. 337. Reprinted with permission from the *Annual Review of Public Health,* Volume 19, ©1998 by Annual Reviews *www.AnnualReviews.org.*

Provider Counseling Style and Continuity of Care

An important treatment planning principle is the emphasis on a collaborative approach to treatment that empowers the smoker to be a full partner in the development of the treatment plan (patient- or client-centered counseling). This approach encourages joint responsibility, improves adherence, and provides the kind of relationship that is central to long-term continuity of care. This philosophy mirrors the treatment of other chronic conditions such as diabetes or schizophrenia. An open, trusting relationship between you and the smoker creates the best climate for success. This principle also permits care to be delivered over relatively long time periods (as long as is necessary until the smoker quits), and the plan can include continuous quality improvement via a self-correcting process by which setbacks (e.g., relapse) can be "reframed" as part of a learning experience on the pathway to permanent cessation rather than as a "failure" (Brownell et al., 1986). In other words, if an initial treatment is unsuccessful, then you can revise the prior treatment plan and try again.

The smoking status of providers and key staff members within the delivery system can influence the degree of support for a treatment plan. For example, the smoking status and beliefs of substance abuse counselors can strongly influence their ability to advocate for smoking cessation (Bobo, Anderson, & Bowman, 1997). In particular, substance abuse counselors who are current smokers and may have had a history of substance abuse themselves are likely to believe that smoking cessation can undermine successful substance abuse treatment. Indeed, contrary to these counselors' beliefs, there is evidence that continuing to smoke after ceasing to drink may actually *promote* relapse back into alcoholism (Abrams, 1995; Abrams, Marlatt, & Sobell, 1995).

Ideally, delivery systems such as managed care organizations or mental health clinics should be designed to support and track the quality of care delivered over time and even by multiple providers. For example, a managed health care organization may have a policy that requires all providers in all settings (e.g., emergency room, primary care, specialty care) to screen for smokers and to develop, document, and implement an individualized treatment plan for each smoking member of the health plan. In medical, psychiatric, and substance abuse treatment settings, the Health Plan Employer Data and Information Set (HEDIS 3.0) report cards are designed to track the mandate of the National Committee for Quality Assurance (National Committee for Quality Assurance, 1996). Surveys that inform these report cards evaluate whether all providers are asking about tobacco abuse as a *vital sign* (along with taking temperature and blood pressure) at each and every contact with the health care system (see also Fiore et al., 2000). Chapter 8 addresses some of these systems-level components in support of the individual treatment planning process. We highly recommend that you work with your organizations to create the infrastructure, policies, and reimbursement incentives to ensure that the context of care affords the best chance of reaching all smokers and following them for as long as it takes them to stop smoking.

Provider Goals and Expectations

Setting realistic goals and knowing what specific results might be expected from the treatment plan are important considerations. This concept is best illustrated with examples drawn from the hypothetical extremes of treatment outcomes. At the one extreme are goals that result in outcomes that reflect the earliest movement toward cessation. At the other extreme are the outcomes following years of abstinence. Generally, an acceptable initial outcome for a proactively recruited smoker who is not at all motivated to quit might be simply to retain that smoker in ongoing care. A second outcome at a later phase of intervention may be to look for ways to motivate that smoker so that he/she moves from not being ready to stop smoking in the foreseeable future to being willing to try to stop smoking within the following 6 to 12 months. Note that neither you the provider nor the smoker would discuss or entertain making an overt attempt to reduce or to quit smoking during this period of the treatment plan. You can still regard the smoker as making progress within your treatment plan because he/she has achieved two early outcomes: (1) he/she has remained willing to discuss smoking over time; and (2) he/she has moved from being not at all motivated to quit to being willing to at least consider cessation in the near future.

For a smoker who is a little closer to making a quit attempt, goals and outcomes of treatment planning can include intermediate behavior change (e.g., cutting down by 50% or an "experimental" 12- or 24-hour quit attempt) and short-term abstinence (e.g., continuous abstinence of 7 to 30 days). Moderate (i.e., brief treatment) to high intensity treatment programs (behavioral plus nicotine replacement therapy) should achieve 24-hour cessation rates of 40–70%, and 25–50% should be able to maintain cessation for 7 days. The gold standard for successful treatment outcome is abstinence over longer time frames (6 or ideally at least 12 months of continuous abstinence). Specific cessation rates for 6–12 months of abstinence using minimal, moderate, or maximal intensity treatment can range from 8 to 15 to 30%, respectively (see Fiore et al., 2000). Finally, even more distal direct or indirect outcomes can also be considered as part of successful treatment planning (e.g., 5 years' continuous abstinence, improvements in health status, quality of life, reduction in use of health services; see Parrott et al., 1998; Shepard, Stason, Perry, Carmen, & Nagurney, 1995). You should try to follow smokers you have treated for at least 1 year to provide support, to prevent relapse, to recycle them back into treatment if relapse occurs, and to track your success rate in terms of 12-month outcomes.

Harm Minimization

Smokers may not quit for a long time, and it is estimated that as many as 50% of smokers will never quit (Hughes, Cummings, & Hyland, 1999; Hughes, Goldstein, et al., 1999). Many smokers repeatedly fail after trying the very best interventions available. Because any amount of smoking is harmful, it is hoped that continued engagement in treatment will eventually lead to longer periods of abstinence rather than to a reduced amount of smoking. For a subgroup who will not quit even with the highest levels of care, the treatment emphasis may have to change from abstinence to *harm minimization* (Baer, Marlatt, & McMahon, 1993; Hughes, Cummings, & Hyland, 1999; Marlatt, 1998; Shiffman et al., 1998; Warner, Slade, & Sweanor, 1997).

A harm minimization approach is controversial because it can be misinterpreted as accepting continued smoking, albeit at a lower level of harm. One potential negative consequence should be considered. Although it may be argued that reduced rates of smoking constitute "harm minimization," there is evidence that smoking topography (e.g., depth of inhalation) may change to compensate for the reduced nicotine levels (L. Kozlowski & Ferrence, 1990; L. T. Kozlowski, Pope, & Lux, 1988). This behavior could *increase* harm to the smoker. Moreover, most smokers who try to reduce their level of smoking cannot sustain the reduction and will return to their previous higher rates sooner or later.

Eventually, you and the smoker may conclude that everything has been tried and may be tempted to give up. In the era of effective and safe alternative nicotine delivery systems (e.g., patches, gum, nasal spray, inhalers), harm minimization for recalcitrant smokers may become a realistic alternative to total abstinence from nicotine (N. L. Benowitz, 1996; Zevin, Jacob, & Benowitz, 1998). Nicotine replacement is preferable to reduced cigarette smoking as a means of achieving "harm minimization," as the risks of even long-term nicotine replacement therapy are smaller than the risks of reduced smoking frequency (Shiffman et al., 1998). The idea of using some form of nicotine replacement as an alternative to obtaining nicotine from a highly toxic delivery system (the cigarette) has been termed "exposure reduction" (see Chapter 9 for more details).

Harm minimization or exposure reduction involves a client-centered approach of accepting small steps toward reducing the harm caused by smoking as a method of last resort. Within a treatment plan, the time frame can be thought of as the entire lifespan of the smoker. This provides for a flexible rather than an "all or nothing" approach. Harm minimization can become a viable option when the treatment plan is negotiated with full involvement of the smoker and consideration of the alternatives, both beneficial and detrimental.

CONCLUSION

In summary, the treatment plan approach is used here to identify the areas of consensus in our current knowledge base. Sufficient theory, research, and clinical evidence support the basic assumptions of the planning principles, including the notion that more treatment (and combined pharmacological and behavioral skills and support) is better than less treatment. If the setting where you provide treatment is public health oriented as opposed to clinical, with access to a large population of smokers the majority of whom are not motivated to quit, then it may be helpful to consider the treatment options as fitting into a stepped-care approach. Stepped-care considers less complex, intensive, and expensive treatment options first and then "steps up" care to more intensive options if those fail. This approach is also appealing if expense and resource allocations are limited. One can reach larger numbers of smokers in a relatively effective manner with a middle-of-the-road level of treatment intensity. In one view of health care delivery, this provides efficient and value-based services.

Smoking cessation treatment, despite being the most cost-effective preventive intervention of the current preventive and palliative medical interventions (see Table 9.1 in Chapter 9), is still not integrated into the financial reimbursement base nor into the organizational infrastructure of health care and of public health delivery systems (Parrott et al., 1998). The benefit of coronary bypass surgery or even the needs for lifetime medication use to manage cholesterol, diabetes, hypertension, or schizophrenia are accepted, whereas cessation services are not. Medical care is based not only on costs and profits alone but also on the value of improved quality of life and quality of care. Of great concern is how to ensure a safety net of appropriate levels of quality and quantity of services for low-income and uninsured smokers. These fellow members of our society are in reality denied access to even moderate levels of cessation interventions (Orleans et al., 1998). Poverty itself is a major risk factor for tobacco use, and it clusters with other poor lifestyle habits, breeding drug abuse, violence, and unrest (Brennan, Grekin, & Mednick, 1999). Smoking is increasingly a problem of the poor, and these smokers are challenging: They are hard to reach, hard to motivate, hard to treat, and hard to follow over time.

This selective review of the field of tobacco addiction proposes a treatment planning approach that combines systems and individual treatment factors using concepts such as stepped care, the tailoring of interventions to individual smoker profiles, and a smoker-centered (i.e., client- or patient-centered) philosophy. We believe the treatment planning guidelines presented here summarize the best theory and scientific evidence known to date. The optimal treatment strategy will move us closer to being able to (1) reach all smokers and engage them in intervention; (2) deliver the most effective interventions for individual smokers; (3) provide continuity of care and ongoing treatments and support for as long as it takes to help a smoker stop; and (4) achieve the greatest social and financial benefits to individuals, families, communities, and society.

2

Assessment to Inform Smoking Cessation Treatment

Raymond Niaura
William G. Shadel

Depending on the setting, from 26% (primary care setting) to 90% (substance abuse treatment program) of your caseload could be composed of smokers. The PHS guideline (Fiore et al., 2000) and the Health Plan Employer Data and Information Set (HEDIS) report cards of the National Committee for Quality Assurance (National Committee for Quality Assurance, 1996) require that smoking status be considered a "vital sign" (see Chapter 8, Table 8.2) like temperature, blood pressure, height, and weight. Identification of the smokers in your setting, *regardless* of your specialty or discipline, is the important first step toward helping those individuals improve their health and well-being.

Once a smoker has been identified, the next step is to assess those factors important for helping them to quit and to formulate an initial treatment plan (see Chapter 1). The purpose of this chapter is to inform you how to assess smokers' characteristics and how to use the results of these assessments to inform treatment. First, we consider the context in which assessment can occur. Second, we discuss key elements of using assessment information to develop a treatment plan. Third, we review triage assessments, that is, those assessments that can be utilized to make a determination as to whether motivational counseling, a brief treatment, or a more intensive treatment is most appropriate for the smoker. Finally, we review assessments that can be administered to smokers in the context of treatment in order to better tailor that treatment. We also provide case examples culled from our own experience to illustrate key points.

THE CONTEXT OF ASSESSMENT

What Is Assessment?

Each individual smoker has a different smoking pattern; each may smoke at different rates, "use" smoking in different ways, and think about smoking and quitting differently. As a result, each smoker will have different concerns regarding motivation and a different experience with stopping smoking and sustaining abstinence over the long term. Because of these inherent individual differences between smokers, the same treatments will not work equally well with every smoker. Assessment is a process of (1) discovering the individual difference factors (e.g., biology, thoughts, emotions, behaviors) that can have the greatest impact on motivation, initial cessation, and relapse prevention; and (2) using knowledge of these individual differences to ensure that the smoker receives the most effective treatment that meets his/her particular needs.

Where Should a Smoking Cessation Assessment Take Place?

Assessment does not necessarily have to take place in the context of a smoking cessation clinic but can occur in the context of *any type* of treatment or even at *any contact* with a smoker. Think of contacts with smokers as teachable moments during which assessment (and treatment) is a priority. An adequate assessment of factors related to smoking can take place in diverse contexts, such as outpatient primary care clinics, both in- and outpatient psychiatric and substance abuse treatment centers, hospital units, emergency rooms, physician or dental offices, worksite health promotion programs, rehabilitation (e.g., cardiac, occupational, physical) programs, or psychological treatment and community centers, to name just a few such settings. In short, assessment can take place in any treatment context following the guidelines outlined in this chapter, even if the focus of that treatment is not on smoking cessation per se. Chapter 8 details the steps that can be taken in order to develop and integrate smoking cessation programs in such alternative contexts.

The degree of complexity of the smoker's profile and the amount of time available to administer an assessment should determine the degree and number of assessments that are administered. One of our main goals is to provide feasible assessment options that can be used whether you have only a few minutes or considerably more time with a smoker. In an ideal setting, the more time that you feel you can allocate, the more thorough the assessment, and the more accurately the smoking cessation intervention will be tailored to the specific and unique profile of the individual smoker. Additional assessments can be conducted during subsequent visits.

Assessment Is a Dynamic Process

Smoking cessation is a process that often requires several unsuccessful attempts before a lifetime of nonsmoking is achieved (Cohen et al., 1989). Moreover, smoking patterns and motivation to quit can change markedly during treatment or after a cessation attempt. Put another way, smoking is a chronic, relapsing condition. A provider with whom a smoker has multiple contacts therefore has a unique opportunity to monitor and assess motivation and smoking and cessation behavior throughout the course of treatment.

It is useful to think of assessment and treatment of smoking in the same way that one may think of assessment and treatment of chronic medical or psychiatric conditions, such as diabetes or bipolar disorder. Over time, between 50% and 80% of diabetics will become nonadherent to their medications, diet, or exercise regimens (for reviews, see Abrams et al., 1998; Shumaker, Schron, Ockene, & McBee, 1998). In cases of nonadherence with treatments for these chronic conditions, providers try to examine the patient/client barriers to adherence (e.g., medication side effects) and continue to work with the patient over his/her entire lifetime if necessary in order to achieve proper control of the condition. A provider would never give up on a diabetic patient who is nonadherent with his/her medication schedule and monitoring. This same level of monitoring and attention is necessary for the smoker during the course of treatment.

Constant monitoring of the smoker is important, but a word of caution is necessary. Despite the fact that the assessments reviewed in this chapter have demonstrated consistent scientific support, it is important to recognize that due to factors outside of your control, some level of measurement error can be expected. Factors not yet discovered or those that have not been studied nearly enough may influence the overall success of treatment. Therefore, you should recognize that repeated assessment of a smoker's history and quitting may sometimes yield conflicting results or new information.

What Format Should an Assessment Take?

The assessments are usually administered in a written format, though in certain settings (e.g., consultation-liaison inpatient service) oral administrations of some of the shorter assessments are more than adequate. A provider can, with appropriate training, use a more formal interview-type of format to administer some of the specialized assessments discussed later in this chapter. Most of the assessments can be completed and scored quickly, and decisions about treatment can be made within a very short period of time (i.e., within 15 minutes of the smoker's time and literally 2 minutes of the provider's time).

The Importance of Trust and Collaboration

Oftentimes, providers administer assessments to smokers, evaluate results, and determine treatment with only minimal input from the smoker. Although there certainly is merit to this approach, developing a successful treatment plan for the smoker requires a collaborative approach to assessment and to the treatment decision-making process. During the process of assessment, the provider should establish a trusting relationship with the smoker and set the stage for maintaining this relationship.

Establishing strong rapport requires the provider to "meet the smokers where they are" in terms of their smoking and desire to quit, and rapport is best established by being an empathic listener and communicating to the smokers that you understand their needs and concerns. This step in a care management approach to smoking cessation is especially important for smokers who are not yet ready to quit smoking, though even smokers who are ready to quit benefit from this sort of patient-centered approach. Chapter 3 provides more detail on the steps that should be taken to ensure that a trusting and empathic relationship is established with the smoker.

Once a collaborative relationship has been established, the results and rationale for the assessments should be made explicit to the smoker and the results explained in detail and discussed. Treatment options should be explored with the smoker, and his/her preferences for treatment (e.g., group vs. individual; brief vs. intensive; with or without pharmacotherapy) should be solicited. The treatment plan can then be decided on. The assessment information that we provide and the decision rules we suggest should be considered *guidelines only*. The key to utilizing assessment information to guide treatment planning is based on four factors: (1) the relationship that you have with the smoker; (2) the combination of assessment information that you are able to gather; (3) your own clinical judgment as to the most appropriate course of action; and (4) the smoker's treatment preferences and reactions to treatment.

TRIAGE: THE FIRST STEP

Triage is generally defined (from military medicine) as the process of "sorting" injured patients into different treatments according to a set of decision rules that are designed to maximize the number of survivors (i.e., the most critically injured receive top treatment priority; those with less serious injuries may wait for treatment). The purpose of triage is to identify which smokers are not ready to quit and to identify which smokers of those who are ready would be more likely to achieve abstinence with a briefer treatment or with a more intensive treatment. Those not ready receive motivational counseling (Chapter 3) until they become ready. As was reviewed in Chapter 1 (see Figures 1.1 and 1.2), brief treatments (see also Chapter 4) are defined by both the length of time spent with the smoker and the intensity of skills training that is to be provided. Intensive treatments (see Chapters 5 and 6), by contrast, are longer in duration, require the provider to take a more active role in teaching the smoker cessation skills, and suggest that some special treatment issues need to be considered (e.g., psychiatric comorbidity). In general, briefer treatments are appropriate for smokers who are "less complicated," and more intensive treatments are recommended for smokers who are "more complicated." This distinction will become more apparent as we move through our review of assessment tools. Conducting a brief treatment as a first line of intervention does not preclude the use of a more intensive treatment at a later point in time (i.e., stepping up to a higher level of care depending on the smoker's reactions to the earlier treatment plan).

Triage assessments can be thought of as brief screening tools that allow informed decisions to be made about the best course of treatment for smokers. As such, these assessments generally take very little time to complete and can be administered as part of a battery of questionnaires (e.g., family history of presenting problem, demographics, insurance) that smokers typically complete as part of an intake program in any sort of treatment. Five clinical areas are measured during smoker triage: (1) *motivation*; (2) *nicotine dependence*; (3) *past quit attempts and smoking history*; (4) *substance abuse comorbidity*; and (5) *psychiatric comorbidity*. The final area that should be assessed but that is not necessarily thought of as a clinical area per se is the *smoker's preference* for treatment type. We provide assessment options in each of these areas for both minimal amounts of time and for lengthier times.

Table 2.1 illustrates triage assessment decision rules and suggestions for disposition in terms of treatment intensity, possible indication for considering pharmacotherapy, and additional specialized assessments (described in more detail later in this chapter).

Motivation

In the general population of adult smokers, 70% say they want to quit, but the vast majority (80%) are not ready to quit within 30 days, and 30–45% are not intending to quit even within 6 months (Abrams & Biener, 1992; Centers for Disease Control, 1994a). Motivation appears to be an important predictor of whether or not someone will quit smoking (W. R. Miller & Rollnick, 2002).

Addressing issues of motivation and how to engage the smoker who is not yet ready to quit is so important that it merits its own chapter. A more intensive review of assessment of and methods for increasing motivation appears in Chapter 3. For purposes of triage, however, the *Readiness to Quit Ladder* (Figure 2.1) is a good measure, with 10 response options that assess motivation along a continuum, from not considering quitting smoking at all in the near future to having already quit smoking (Abrams et al., 1992). A higher score on the ladder is associated with greater motivation to quit smoking. The Readiness to Quit Ladder has been shown to be associated with objective measures of readiness to quit smoking (e.g., intention to quit, nicotine dependence, number of prior quit attempts; Abrams & Biener, 1992) and with actual quit attempts. Thus, the ladder has the advantage of being a short, efficient, and face-valid measure that is generalizable for use with many diverse populations (e.g., it can be easily understood by populations low in literacy). Smokers who score below a 7 on this scale (i.e., not ready to quit in the next 30 days) may wish to consider interventions that specifically address motivational issues (see Chapter 3), whereas smokers who score 7 and above may wish to consider more active behavioral and pharmacological treatments (Chapters 5–7).

Nicotine Dependence

A smoker who is more dependent on nicotine (that is, more addicted) may have more difficulty quitting smoking (Fagerstrom & Schneider, 1989) and may benefit from more intensive treatment with nicotine replacement therapy than smokers who are not as dependent (Niaura & Abrams, 2002). Table 2.2 presents two options for assessing nicotine dependence.

A brief and valid assessment of a smoker's current dependence level can be done with two questions from the Heaviness of Smoking Index (HSI; Heatherton, Kozlowski, Frecker, Rickert, & Robinson, 1989). One item assesses time to first morning cigarette, and the other assesses the individual's daily smoking rate. An individual who smokes within 30 minutes of waking and who smokes more than 25 cigarettes per day on average is probably more dependent on nicotine and in need of more intensive treatment—at the very least, some behavioral skills training (see Chapter 5) and nicotine replacement therapy (see Chapter 7).

These two items from the HSI are actually taken from a more lengthy, though still brief,

TABLE 2.1. Triage Assessments: Suggested Decision Rules and Disposition

Triage assessment instrument	Results	Disposition
Motivation		
Readiness ladder	Score < 7	• Motivation enhancement
	Score ≥ 7	• Active brief *or* intensive behavioral and pharmacological treatment
Nicotine dependence		
HSI	1st A.M. cig: > 30 min *or* # cig per day: < 25	• Brief behavioral treatment • Consider intensive behavioral treatment • Consider pharmacological treatment
	1st A.M. cig: ≤ 30 min *or* # cig per day: ≥ 25	• Intensive behavioral treatment • Pharmacological treatment • Administer specialized assessment module 1: Biochemical measures
FTQ	< 7	• Brief behavioral treatment • Consider intensive behavioral treatment • Consider pharmacological treatment
	≥ 7	• Intensive behavioral treatment • Pharmacological treatment • Administer specialized assessment module 1: Biochemical measures
Length of past quit attempts		
	> 14 days	• Brief behavioral treatment • Consider pharmacological treatment
	≤ 14 days	• Intensive behavioral treatment • Pharmacological treatment
Other substance use		
Past use and treatment questions (see Table 2.4)	No	• Brief behavioral treatment • Consider pharmacological treatment
	Yes	• Intensive behavioral treatment • Pharmacological treatment • Refer for behavioral and pharmacological treatment for current substance use • Administer specialized assessment module 3: Other substance use
Psychiatric disorders		
Past psychiatric treatment questions (see Table 2.5)	No	• Brief behavioral treatment • Consider pharmacological treatment
	Yes	• Intensive behavioral treatment • Pharmacological treatment • Refer for behavioral and pharmacological treatment for psychiatric disorders • Administer specialized assessment module 2: Psychopathology
Smoker preference		
		• Prior experience with pharmacotherapy and behavioral treatment may help guide current choice

Note. HSI = Heaviness of Smoking Index; FTQ = Fagerstrom Tolerance Questionnaire.

INSTRUCTIONS: Below are some thoughts that smokers have about quitting. On this ladder, circle the one number that shows what you think about quitting. Please read each sentence carefully before deciding.

10	I have quit smoking and I will never smoke again.
9	I have quit smoking, but I still worry about slipping back, so I need to keep working on living smoke free.
8	I still smoke, but I have begun to change, like cutting back on the number of cigarettes I smoke. I am ready to set a quit date.
7	I definitely plan to quit smoking within the next 30 days.
6	I definitely plan to quit smoking in the next 6 months.
5	I often think about quitting smoking, but I have no plans to quit.
4	I sometimes think about quitting smoking, but I have no plans to quit.
3	I rarely think about quitting smoking, and I have no plans to quit.
2	I never think about quitting smoking, and I have no plans to quit.
1	I enjoy smoking and have decided not to quit smoking for my lifetime. I have no interest in quitting.

FIGURE 2.1. Readiness to Quit Ladder.

measure of nicotine dependence, the *Fagerstrom Tolerance Questionnaire* (FTQ; Fagerstrom, 1978). The FTQ is a popular 8-item self-report scale that generally assesses nicotine dependence levels. Table 2.2 provides the actual items for the FTQ. Smokers' responses are coded and added together to produce a total score. Scores on this scale range from 0 to 11, with lower scores indicating low dependence and higher scores indicating high dependence. Scores greater than or equal to 7 are considered high dependence (Fagerstrom & Schneider, 1989). In any case, smokers who receive higher scores on the FTQ should be considered highly dependent and should receive intensive treatments, whereas smokers who receive lower scores on the FTQ should consider briefer treatments. Ideally, all smokers will benefit from using nicotine replacement therapy (e.g., gum, patch), but those with high dependence may benefit more from pharmacological adjunctive therapy (see Chapter 7).

Past Quit Attempts and Smoking History

An assessment of past attempts to quit smoking is important because certain characteristics of past quit attempts can have an impact on a smoker's success in quitting. The absolute number of past quit attempts does not seem to be critical to determining cessation success (Cohen et al., 1989). Rather, the *length of the longest past* quit attempt and the *length of the most recent*

TABLE 2.2. Triage Assessments: Two Options for Nicotine Dependence

	Criterion	Score
Option 1. FTQ: Fagerstrom Tolerance Questionnaire[a]		
1. On average, how many cigarettes do you smoke per day?[a]	< 15	0
	16–25	1
	> 25	2
2. Which brand of cigarettes do you consider your regular brand? Nicotine content:	< .5	0
	0.6–1.1	1
	> 1.1	2
3. Do you inhale?	Yes, all of the time	2
	Some of the time	1
	No	0
4. Do you smoke more in the morning than during the rest of the day?	Yes	1
	No	0
5. How soon after you wake up do you smoke your first cigarette?[a]	≤ 30 minutes	1
	> 30 minutes	0
6. Of all of the cigarettes you smoke each day, which cigarettes would you hate most to give up?	1st of day	1
	any other	0
7. Do you smoke if you are so ill that you are in bed most of the day?	Yes	1
	No	0
8. Do you find it difficult to refrain from smoking in places where it is forbidden, e.g., in church, at the library, in cinemas, etc.?	Yes	1
	No	0
	Total score (max = 11)	☐
Option 2. HSI: Heaviness of Smoking Index[b]		
1. On average, how many cigarettes do you smoke per day?	< 15	0
	16–25	1
	> 25	2
2. How soon after you wake up do you smoke your first cigarette?	≤ 30 minutes	1
	> 30 minutes	0
	Total score	☐

[a]From "Measuring Nicotine Dependence: A Review of the Fagerstrom Tolerance Questionnaire," by K. Fagerstrom and N. G. Schneider, 1989, *Journal of Behavioral Medicine, 12,* 159–182; and "The Fagerstrom Test for Nicotine Dependence: A Revision of the Fagerstrom Tolerance Questionnaire," by T. F. Heatherton, L. T. Kozlowski, R. C. Frecker, and K. O. Fagerstrom, 1991, *British Journal of Addiction, 86,* 1119–1127.
[b]Items from the Heaviness of Smoking Index (Heatherton, Kozlowski, Frecker, Rickert, & Robinson, 1989).

quit attempt are the strongest determinants of smokers' success with quitting (Farkas, Pierce, Gilpin, et al., 1996). The critical indicators for predicting smoking cessation success seem to be a lifetime past quit attempt of 1 year or more and a most recent attempt of more than 5 to 14 days (Farkas et al., 1996). These data make sense clinically. The more time that a person abstains from smoking, the more practice he/she has and the more he/she learns what it is like to be a nonsmoker. The longer the most recent quit attempt, the better the individual should be able to remember what it was like to be a nonsmoker and the skills that it took to remain a nonsmoker.

Assessments of past quit attempts can be made using four simple questions that take no more than 1 minute. Table 2.3 provides a list of these questions. In general, the less time that a smoker has been abstinent in the past, the more likely it is that he/she will benefit from more intensive treatment. However, if the smoker has never made a serious attempt to quit, it is difficult to predict his/her treatment needs, and brief treatment may be considered if there are few other complicating factors (e.g., high dependence, comorbid substance abuse).

Other Substance Use

Drug- and polydrug-abusing populations have high smoking prevalence. Smoking rates over 85% have been noted in alcoholics (Battjes, 1988; Hughes, 1994b), opiate addicts [Rounsaville, Kosten, Weissman, & Kleber, 1985] and polydrug users (Burling & Ziff, 1988). Alcohol use and abuse and possibly abuse of other drugs is also associated with difficulty giving up smoking. Drinking alcohol is a significant precipitant of smoking relapse (Shiffman, 1986). Moreover, alcoholics are considerably less likely to be successful than nonalcoholics in their attempts to quit smoking (DiFranza & Guerrera, 1990).

Assessment of other substance use (e.g., marijuana, opiates) can be very difficult during a brief screening. This difficulty is due to the inherent unreliability of self-reports of persons who use illegal drugs or substances to excess (Washton, Stone, & Hendrickson, 1988), despite assurances of confidentiality. Nonetheless, questions about past and present drug use should be asked (see Table 2.4). At the level of triage, it is appropriate to ask about past use and past treatment for problems with alcohol, illegal drugs, and/or overuse of prescription medications. Smokers who indicate any past or current difficulties with substances (i.e., a "Yes" to any of the triage questions) should consider more intensive treatment, whereas persons who deny such a history should consider briefer treatment options.

TABLE 2.3. Triage Assessments: Past Quit Attempts

1. How many times in the past have you made a serious attempt to quit smoking?
2. What was the longest period of time that you were able to quit smoking?
3. a. When was your most recent serious attempt to quit smoking?
   b. How long were you able to stay quit during your most recent quit attempt?

Note. From "Addiction Versus Stages of Change Models in Predicting Smoking Cessation in California," by A. J. Farkas, J. P. Pierce, S. H. Zhu, B. Rosbrook, E. A. Gilpin, C. Berry, and R. M. Kaplan, 1996, *Addiction, 91,* 1271–1280.

TABLE 2.4. Triage Assessments: Drug and Alcohol Use

1. Have you ever used more of an illegal substance or a prescribed medication more than you intended?

       No   Yes

2. Have you ever used alcohol more than you intended?

       No   Yes

3. Have you ever received treatment for drugs or alcohol use?

       No   Yes

Comorbid Psychiatric Disorders

About 40–70% of psychiatric patients smoke, as we discussed in Chapter 1. Studies have demonstrated significant relations between self-reported depression, the frequency of smoking, difficulty with cessation (Covey, Glassman, & Stetner, 1997), and subsequent relapse to smoking (Glassman et al., 1988). A number of studies have established that psychiatric patients, especially those with so-called psychoses (e.g., schizophrenia), are much more likely to smoke than the general population or than nonpsychiatric patients (Hughes, Hatsukami, Mitchell, & Dahlgren, 1986). Given the multiple complex issues that need to be addressed with psychiatric patients who smoke (due to the interactions between smoking and psychotropic drug levels; see Glassman, 1993) and the likelihood that patients with psychiatric disorders may have more difficulty quitting smoking (Niaura & Abrams, 2002), an assessment of comorbid psychiatric involvement is necessary.

A number of good instruments allow individuals to be diagnosed across a range of psychiatric syndromes, but these lengthy and often complicated assessments are not appropriately administered as part of a triage assessment. However, these assessments may prove useful during treatment of the smoker, and we review some of these psychiatric assessment tools in detail later in the chapter. Therefore, a brief triage option for assessing mood disorder involves asking about current or past history of treatment for mood disorders and psychiatric treatment (see Table 2.5).

TABLE 2.5. Triage Assessments: Psychiatric History Questions

1. Have you ever received treatment for a mental health problem?

       No   Yes

2. Has there ever been a time in your life when you were down or depressed most of the day, nearly every day for a period of 2 weeks?

       No   Yes

SMOKER PREFERENCES

One important, and perhaps often neglected, element of triage is assessing smoker preferences and opinions about different treatment options. That is, treatment recommendations are often made by the provider with the expectation that the smoker will follow through with those recommendations. More often than not, however, the smoker does not follow these prescribed treatment recommendations. The reasons for this lack of adherence are many, but at the heart of the matter is usually a lack of what the smoker feels is an appropriate match to his/her needs (Abrams et al., 1998) or lack of motivation (W. R. Miller & Rollnick, 2002). We will not review these reasons here. The important point is that the smoker's views about treatment should be solicited, and the treatment plan tailored as much as possible to these perceived needs (see also Chapter 3). In fact, smoker input into treatment choice may actually improve clinical outcomes (see Bayer, 1995; Marlatt, 1999). This process can begin with a dialogue with the smoker about the assessment results and what direction the clinician sees the treatment moving. Table 2.6 provides a sample dialogue. The key is not to be too directive with the smoker but rather to collaborate with him/her in the approach. The smoker is guided to a treatment by the provider, using the techniques of motivational interviewing (see Chapter 3).

Often, during the course of negotiating preferences for treatment, smokers will inquire about treatments for which there is little or no consistent research support. We generally do not discourage smokers from seeking these other treatment resources, but we provide them with information on the specific unsupported treatment about which they inquire so that they may make an informed decision about the best course of treatment (see Fiore et al., 2000, pp. 67–70). A balance needs to be struck between reinforcing smokers' desire to seek treatment in general, providing accurate information about those treatments, and suggesting more appropriate (i.e., scientifically supported) treatments. If a smoker insists on pursuing one of these options, we typically encourage him/her to use these other treatments as adjuncts to a more scientifically supported treatment (see Chapters 3–7). We review several of the more common alternative treatments in this section.

TABLE 2.6. Sample Dialogue of Negotiation of Treatment Directions with Smokers

"Our goal is to decide together what type of smoking treatment would be best suited to your needs. This is best accomplished by two means: (1) Sharing with you the results of some of the smoking assessments that you completed earlier, and (2) getting a sense from you as to what your preferences and thoughts about treatment are.

"You completed a few brief smoking assessments earlier, and I would like to give you some feedback on your results. In general, we looked at areas like your level of nicotine dependence, prior substance use and treatment, and psychological treatment history because we know that these areas are important to determining how successful someone will be with quitting smoking."

[Review of assessment result specifics]

"What do you make of these results? You have several types of treatment options available to you. I would like to explain in some detail what those options are and which ones might be best suited to helping you to quit smoking. Please stop me at any time to ask questions or to indicate whether you think that a particular treatment would be of interest to you."

Nicotine Anonymous (NICA) is an international organization, closely modeled after other, more familiar groups, such as Alcoholics Anonymous (AA). Similar to AA, NICA approaches smoking cessation in a spiritual fashion, appealing to a higher power to progress through 12 steps on the road to successful smoking cessation (or recovery, as it is referred to). In addition, smoking or nicotine addiction is thought of as an incurable, yet manageable disease that the smoker does not have the power to control alone. Smokers or ex-smokers attend meetings at which personal accounts and testimonials are given in a supportive group context to other smokers and ex-smokers. NICA does not endorse any formal treatment program or quit-smoking methods, but it does provide a number of publications with tips on quitting smoking that interested individuals can order at a minimal cost from the central offices (for a review of NICA, see Lichtenstein, 1999).

The past 5 years have seen a virtual explosion in development, proliferation, access, and use of the Internet. At the time of this writing, a search on the term "smoking cessation" reveals no fewer than 60 sites for information on smoking and nicotine addiction, help with quitting smoking, and referrals. Much of the smoking cessation material provided consists of tips for helping smokers quit, managing withdrawal symptoms, high risk situations, and support. Although few have been evaluated, it is our impression that QuitNet (*www.quitnet.com*) offers a number of treatment options derived from the evidence-based literature. Because of their ease of access, convenience, and constant availability, Web-based programs can be used to supplement more formal treatment plans such as the ones offered in this book. Other sites provide information, instructions, and decision trees to help the interested smoker choose the most appropriate form of pharmacotherapy. However, ultimately, questions about pharmacotherapies for smoking cessation should be directed to the appropriate medical professional (e.g., see Chapter 7).

Hypnosis in reference to smoking cessation can be defined in any number of ways—for example, intensive relaxation, group suggestion, and individualized induction. A few studies have been conducted to examine the effect of hypnosis on smoking cessation, but these studies collectively have indicated that hypnosis alone is not particularly effective in helping individuals quit smoking (Fiore et al., 2000, pp. 67–70).

A number of other alternative treatments are advertised as aids for smoking cessation or "cures" for nicotine dependence (e.g., acupuncture, herbal remedies). However, as with the other options that we reviewed in this section, the data are inconclusive on the effectiveness of these particular treatments (Fiore et al., 2000).

TRIAGE ASSESSMENT: CASE EXAMPLES

Results from the six domains that are assessed provide sufficient information for the provider to make an initial determination as to whether a motivational (Chapter 3), a brief (Chapter 4), or an intensive treatment (Chapters 5 and 6) is most appropriate for the smoker's cessation efforts. A difficulty arises when thinking about how to best weight each piece of this information and make the most appropriate treatment recommendation. In part, the difficulty comes from the fact that we have no clear algorithms or rules concerning how smokers who exhibit various characteristics at triage fare with particular cessation treatments; we have only broad knowledge of their likelihood of success. In the absence of rigorous, research-derived rules, experience teaches the most appropriate weights to assign to each of these factors in order to maximize the smoker's chances of successful cessation. We have provided some case examples derived from our own clinical experiences that can be used as starting points in this triage process.

CASE EXAMPLES

TRIAGE CASE EXAMPLE 1: MR. N.

Background Information

Mr. N. is a 60-year-old divorced Caucasian man whom you have been seeing on an ongoing basis in your outpatient alcohol treatment practice. Because you have been seeing Mr. N. for 2 years, you know that he has a 38-year history of abusive alcohol consumption (diagnosed with alcohol dependence) and that he quit drinking for the first time about 1 month prior to entering treatment with you (he voluntarily entered an inpatient treatment facility at this time). He has reported to you feelings of regret and guilt when he stopped drinking (e.g., "I lost so much because I was drunk so much"), but he has never been treated for depression or other psychiatric disorder. A referral to a psychiatrist revealed that Mr. N. had never experienced any diagnosable affective disturbance. He reports to you that he occasionally drinks an alcohol-containing beverage, but he claims that these drinking episodes have never led to intoxication. You know that Mr. N. smokes because you have seen him light up on leaving your office, but he has never mentioned to you that he would like to stop smoking. You have no other information about his smoking, but you feel that your relationship with him is developed enough that you can mention it to him. Given that you see him only once per month for about 30 minutes, you decide to ask him during your next visit if he has "ever thought about his smoking or about quitting smoking." He replies, "I'm willing to listen to what you have to say."

Triage and Disposition

With respect to the triage domains that you need to assess, you already know two important facts about Mr. N.: he has a positive alcohol history, and he has never had another psychiatric disorder or problem. You have no solid information about his motivation to quit smoking, his level of nicotine dependence, or his past attempts to quit. Because you have so little time with him per visit and because your main treatment charge (mandated by his health insurance) is for alcohol dependence, you decide to administer the Readiness to Quit Ladder (to test motivation; Figure 2.1), the HSI (to test nicotine dependence; Table 2.2), and questions about his most recent quit attempt (Table 2.3) during the first 3 minutes of his next visit.

You do not need to "score" any of the triage assessment results. You are able to scan his responses very quickly and you find the following:

Ladder: 5 ("I often think about quitting, but I have no plans to quit.")
HSI: Smokes within 2 minutes of waking; smokes 2–3 packs of cigarettes per day
Most recent quit attempts: Never made any attempts to quit smoking

Treatment Plan

Your examination of these responses, along with your prior knowledge of Mr. N.'s past history, suggest to you that he is a "more complicated" smoker: He has a past history of alcohol abuse, has never made any attempts to quit smoking, and, based on his HSI responses, appears highly dependent. Moreover, his score on the Ladder indicates that he is not really ready to actively consider smoking cessation. Even though he has no prior history of psychiatric disturbance, you feel that the weight of the evidence suggests that he probably would benefit from more intensive cessation treatment when he is ready to quit. You decide that the best course of treatment action at the present time is not to refer him for this more intensive treatment but rather to periodically work into your regular sessions some principles of motivational interviewing (see Chapter 3) in order to potentially enhance his desire to stop smoking. You also decide to readminister the Ladder to him at every clinic visit so that you may monitor his progress and be prepared to take more definite action when he becomes more motivated to stop smoking, that is, when a Ladder assessment reveals a score of at least 7 ("I definitely plan to quit in the next 30 days").

Comment

As a substance abuse treatment provider, you were in an advantageous position because you had knowledge of Mr. N.'s prior psychiatric and substance abuse histories. However, at the same time, despite this knowledge, you had no real idea of his thoughts about smoking or quitting. The assessment results suggested that Mr. N. would benefit from more intensive treatment, yet you refrained from suggesting more intensive treatment because he clearly was not ready to stop smoking (based on his Ladder score). Because of your seemingly good rapport, you could potentially have been more assertive in suggesting treatment options or at least discussing them with him; however, the more conservative approach was to use the relationship as a basis to motivate Mr. N. to quit smoking by using motivational interviewing techniques.

TRIAGE CASE EXAMPLE 2: MS. A.

Background Information

Ms. A. is a 36-year-old single woman who was referred to you, a psychologist, by her physician for an assessment and possible treatment of an anxiety disorder (she first reported "feeling nervous all the time" to her physician). In the packet of information that you have all of your patients complete prior to their first assessment visit with you (i.e., insurance forms, general health background), you include all written forms of the triage assessment (if the person does not smoke, they simply indicate this fact at the beginning of the triage form and answer no further smoking-related questions). Ms. A. has mailed the information packet back to you (as requested), and you note that she is in generally good health. You notice also that she is a smoker.

Triage and Disposition

You quickly turn to the results of her triage assessment and spend 2 minutes scoring it. Her scores reveal the following:

Ladder: 8 ("I still smoke, but I have begun to change, like cutting back on the number of cigarettes I smoke. I am ready to set a quit date.")
FTQ score: 7
Most recent quit attempts: Made two attempts to quit smoking: the first was 5 years ago (lasted about 3 days) and the most recent was last year (lasted for 6 months)
Substance use: None (answers "no" to all questions)
Psychiatric history: None reported

Treatment Plan

You are pleased to see that Ms. A. is motivated to quit smoking. In thinking about what sort of treatment would most benefit her, you note that even though she is probably highly nicotine dependent, she has a recent lengthy quit attempt, and, significantly, no complicating comorbidity (based on the screening questions). However, you recall that she has been referred to you for possible treatment of an anxiety disorder. In your mind, the possible presence of an anxiety disorder is a complicating factor in your thoughts about smoking cessation treatments. Your initial thoughts are therefore to conduct your intake for the referral question (i.e., a typical psychosocial and behavioral assessment for anxiety). If the results of that assessment suggest that she has an anxiety disorder, you will discuss with her the possibility of intensive treatment; if the results of that assessment are negative for an anxiety disorder, you will discuss with her brief treatments for smoking. You decide not to miss this opportunity to talk about smoking cessation with her (it is a teachable moment) despite the fact that she may have an anxiety disorder.

Comment

Ms. A. presents a mixed picture for triage. On the one hand, she presents as a highly nicotine dependent smoker, but one who is motivated to quit and who has considerable experience with not smoking (due to prior quit attempts). On the other hand, she presents with a possible anxiety disorder (or problem) that may be related in some way to her continued smoking (i.e., it is possible that anxiety is a trigger for her). Your assessment of her anxiety will thus be a critical factor in your assessment and disposition of her smoking treatment.

INCREASING ASSESSMENT INTENSITY

The results of the triage assessments provide the bare minimum of information that can be used to determine whether a motivational, a more intensive treatment, or a briefer treatment is warranted. Now, let's assume that the smoker is motivated and in treatment and that you are responsible for delivering a cessation intervention, whether brief or intensive. What is your next step? What direction should your intervention take?

It is difficult, if not impossible, to appropriately treat the smoker without knowing something more about him/her. The next step in assessment is to find out as much about the smoker as you can, even during your treatment, in as efficient and effective a manner as possible. Think of this next step as an information-gathering expedition; the results of this expedition will allow you to treat the smoker in the optimal fashion.

Myriad domains can potentially be assessed, and within those domains there are many assessment instruments. Based on research (Fiore et al., 2000) and our own clinical experience, we have organized the treatment component of assessment into modules (see Table 2.7). Each module is designed to summarize a different domain that is important for guiding a particular facet of smoking cessation treatment. The assessment instruments that we provide within each module can be used to measure different domains and to guide treatment. The numerous assessments that can be administered have been broadly categorized by content area into two broad types of modules: *basic assessment modules* and *specialized assessment modules*.

Basic assessment modules can generally be delivered by any provider with minimal training. We have hierarchically organized our review of assessments within each of the basic modules from those that take the least time to those that take the most time. You are encouraged to make your own determination as to which assessment device or strategy fits your time needs and constraints. There are four basic modules:

TABLE 2.7. Basic and Specialized Assessment Modules

Basic assessment modules	Purpose of assessment and treatment strategies

Module 1. Smoking Triggers and Coping Skills

Triggers
  Option 1: Questions (Table 2.8)
  Option 2: Self-monitoring (see Figure 5.1)

Purpose: To identify high-risk situations for smoking
• Functional analysis, self-management, nicotine fading, problem solving for relapse prevention

Coping skills
  Option 1: Open-ended questions and Coping with Temptations Inventory (Table 2.9)
  Option 2: Self-monitoring (see Figure 5.1)

Purpose: To identify thoughts and behaviors that help or hinder cessation
• Coping skills training, reworking skills that are ineffective or less effective, problem solving for relapse prevention

Module 2. Stress, Withdrawal, Cravings, and Urges

Stress
  Perceived Stress Scale (Table 2.10)

Purpose: To detect high levels of stress
• Stress management training (e.g., relaxation exercises)

Withdrawal symptoms
  Option 1: Past experience
  Option 2: Shiffman–Jarvik Scale (Table 2.11)
  Option 3: Minnesota Withdrawal Scale (Table 2.11)

Purpose: To identify smokers at high risk for distress while quitting
• Pharmacotherapy (e.g., NRT, clonidine)
• Nicotine fading

Cravings and urges
  Option 1: Craving single item (Table 2.12)
  Option 2: Questionnaire on Smoking Urges (Table 2.12)

Purpose: To assess potential high-risk situations and need for pharmacotherapy
• Pharmacotherapy (e.g., NRT, clonidine)
• Nicotine fading

Module 3. Cognition

Self-efficacy
  Option 1: Single-question assessment (Table 2.13)
  Option 2: Self-Efficacy/Temptations Scale (Table 2.13)

Purpose: To assess confidence regarding cessation and abstinence
• Develop cognitive-behavioral strategies to cope with high-risk situations (e.g. confidence-building exercises via role play)

Outcome expectancies and beliefs
  Option 1: Decisional Balance Scale (Table 2.14)
  Option 2: Smoking Consequences Questionnaire (Table 2.14)

Purpose: To assess beliefs regarding reasons for smoking, quitting
• Target irrational, maladaptive beliefs and distorted thinking with cognitive restructuring strategies

Self-concept
  Option 1: Adjective Identification Task (Table 2.15)
  Option 2: Smoker Self-concept and Abstainer Self-concept questionnaire (Table 2.15)

Purpose: To assess self-images (smoker versus abstainer)
• Cognitive restructuring techniques to increase self-awareness of smoking identity

Intrinsic and extrinsic motivation
  Reasons for Quitting Questionnaire (Table 2.16)

Purpose: To assess degree to which reasons for quitting are intrinsic vs. extrinsic
• Cognitive restructuring and motivational interviewing to increase intrinsic motivation to quit

Module 4. Social Environment

Social support
  Option 1: Counting number of supportive individuals (Table 2.17)
  Option 2: Partner Interaction Questionnaire (Table 2.17)

Purpose: To identify the degree of social support available for quitting
• Intratreatment supportive environment and encouragement
• Group support
• Exercises in engineering social support (buddy system)
• Assertiveness training

(continued)

TABLE 2.7. *(continued)*

Specialized assessment modules	Purpose of assessment and treatment strategies

Module 1. Biochemical Markers

Carbon monoxide
Cotinine

Purpose: To assess heaviness of smoking and nicotine intake for treatment planning.
- Indication for intensive pharmacotherapy, tailoring dose of NRT

Module 2. Psychopathology

- Center for Epidemiologic Studies—Depression Scale (CES-D)
- Structured Clinical Interview for Non-Patients (SCID-NP)
- Schizophrenia and Affective Disorders Schedule (SADS)
- PRIME-MD
- Psychiatric Diagnostic Screening Questionnaire (PDSQ)
- Daily Mood Rating Form (see Table 6.2)
- Inventory of Thoughts (see Table 6.8)
- Top 20 Pleasant Events (see Table 6.11)

Purpose: To identify psychopathology and negative moods/thoughts that may be hinder cessation or be exacerbated during cessation
- Cognitive restructuring techniques
- Referral for treatment
- Increased vigilance during cessation

Module 3. Other Substance Use

- CAGE questions
- Alcohol Dependence Scale (ADS)
- Cocaine Abuse Assessment Profile (CAAP)
- SCID-NP
- SADS

Purpose: To identify substance use that may hinder cessation
- Refer for treatment of other substance abuse/dependence
- Increased vigilance for difficulties during cessation attempt

---

Basic Module 1: Smoking Triggers and Coping Skills
Basic Module 2: Stress, Withdrawal, Cravings, and Urges
Basic Module 3: Cognition
Basic Module 4: Social Environment

Specialized assessment modules require additional, more intensive training and are most appropriately administered and interpreted by clinical specialists. The specialized assessments are, by definition, designed for smokers who have been assigned to more intensive treatments and are, in fact, more intensive versions of the screening assessments that are administered during triage; thus, they take more time to administer. There are three specialized modules:

Specialized Module 1: Biochemical Markers
Specialized Module 2: Psychopathology
Specialized Module 3: Other Substance Use

In general, all of the modules are designed either to stand alone or to be additive, and they can be combined in any way that the provider sees fit, depending on the presenting concerns of the smoker. Note, too, that the results of the triage assessments can provide guidance as to the modular assessments that need to be administered to a particular smoker. For example, if it seems as though a smoker has a current or past history of alcohol abuse, based on positive responses to history of substance abuse questions, a more intensive assessment of alcohol use or dependence is probably warranted.

BASIC MODULES

Basic Assessment Module 1: Smoking Triggers and Coping Skills

Triggers

Background and Rationale

Smoking is a behavior that has distinct triggers or cues. Triggers can lead to a number of physical, cognitive, and emotional reactions in the smoker (Abrams et al., 1988; Niaura et al., 1998) that eventually lead to smoking or to relapse (Abrams et al., 1987). It stands to reason, then, that assessing and understanding a particular smoker's triggers can lead to controlling those triggers and thus controlling the patient's smoking through the use of coping and self-management strategies (Chapter 5).

Trigger Assessment Option 1

You can ask the smoker a series of questions directly, or the smoker can respond to self-report questions about smoking triggers. We typically ask smokers to think of three times during the day that they are 100% certain that they smoke. In almost all cases, smokers are able to readily name those times that they smoke. Once the situations have been identified, we typically ask the smoker what he/she feels or what happens to trigger his/her urges or cravings to smoke.

Sometimes smokers will respond that "nothing triggers my smoking; I smoke all day." In these cases, we ask the smokers about the cigarette that they would most hate to give up. Once this cigarette is identified, we ask them why it would be so difficult to go without this cigarette. This process usually leads to identification of triggers or precursors to their smoking. At the very least, it helps to identify the reasons that they smoke. Table 2.8 presents a representative sample of these questions.

TABLE 2.8. Basic Assessment Module 1: Smoking Triggers

Option 1. Ask smoker directly:
  a. "Tell me three times during the day that you know that you smoke 9 out of 10 times."
  b. "What causes you to smoke in those situations?"
  c. "What cigarettes would you hate to give up most? Why?"

Option 2. Self-monitoring forms (see Figure 5.1 for sample Pack Wraps form)

Trigger Assessment Option 2

Self-monitoring, or keeping a record of factors related to smoking, serves to establish baseline data, to increase knowledge about the factors that trigger and maintain the smoking habit, and to track progress throughout the cessation attempt (Shiffman, 1988). Self-monitoring also may have an added treatment benefit of actually serving to reduce the total number of cigarettes smoked per day (Abrams & Wilson, 1979a). A preprinted card or sheet that can be attached to the cigarette pack (Pack Wraps; see Figure 5.1) facilitates self-monitoring. Smokers are instructed to record each cigarette prior to smoking it and to record the time of day, the situation in which the cigarette was smoked (e.g., with coffee), associated mood (e.g., tense, relaxed), and urges prior to smoking (Shiffman, 1988). The situational notations reveal the environmental and emotional influences that trigger smoking as they occur. These events or triggers that are associated with smoking need to be delineated, as they may become future high-risk situations for relapse that require effective coping responses (Marlatt & Gordon, 1985; see also Chapter 5). It is best to have smokers record situations throughout the duration of treatment.

Coping Skills

Background and Rationale

Relapse prevention theory (Marlatt & Gordon, 1985; see also Chapter 5) proposes that the ability to cope with high-risk situations determines an individual's probability of maintaining abstinence. Failure to cope initiates a chain of events that may lead to a slip and perhaps to a full-blown relapse. In these instances, participants are taught to avoid self-defeating attributions and resulting negative emotional reactions (i.e., the abstinence violation effect) that promote continued smoking (Marlatt & Gordon, 1985). In any case, increased use of both cognitive and behavioral forms of coping predicts increased chances of abstinence (Shiffman et al., 1996; Shiffman et al., 1997). An assessment of coping can be conducted using a number of formats to identify any coping skills deficits that may exist and to address those deficits with specific skills training strategies (Chapter 5).

Coping Assessment Option 1

As with an assessment of triggers, the clinician can ask the smoker what he/she does to manage cravings or urges to smoke when in situations in which he/she cannot smoke, for example, movies, church, or restaurants. Table 2.9 presents a list of these open-ended questions. A smoker who is unable to generate strategies independently or who responds with "I just don't smoke" is likely lacking in the coping skills necessary to successfully quit smoking. A more detailed picture of the smoker's coping repertoire may be obtained by using the Coping With Temptations Inventory (CWTI), a lengthy list of behavioral coping strategies (e.g., physical activity, distraction) and cognitive coping strategies (e.g., willpower, delay thoughts). The CWTI can indicate where coping deficits exist and whether sufficient skills are being executed in order to manage cravings and "high risk" situations. This list can also be used

TABLE 2.9. Basic Assessment Module 1: Two Options for Coping Skills Assessment

Option 1. Ask the smoker directly and supplement discussion with CWTI
    a. "What do you do when you are in situations where you cannot smoke?"
    b. "How do you manage your smoking when you are in places that do not permit you to smoke?"

Option 2. Self-monitoring forms (see Figure 5.1).

The Coping with Temptations Inventory (CWTI)

INSTRUCTIONS: For each of the items below, please indicate whether you have used this strategy to manage cravings or urges to smoke when you are trying not to smoke.

Behavioral coping responses	Yes	No
Used alternative consumption		
• Food and drink (e.g., allowed yourself to eat more to avoid smoking, chewed gum, drank water/juice)	☐	☐
• Nicotine (e.g., chewed nicotine gum or used snuff)	☐	☐
Used alternative activities		
• Exercise (e.g., lifted weights, took walks)	☐	☐
• Distraction (e.g., kept busy, doodled when talking on phone)	☐	☐
• Relaxation (e.g., practiced deep breathing exercises, took hot shower to relax)	☐	☐
Engaged in self-care activities		
• Stress reduction (e.g., isolated yourself for a relaxing weekend, kept out of stressful situations)	☐	☐
• Other self-care activities (e.g., ate better, took more time for yourself)	☐	☐
Practiced stimulus control		
• Cigarettes and smoking paraphernalia (e.g., bought cigarettes by the pack rather than the carton, got rid of ashtrays, refused to keep cigarettes in the house)	☐	☐
• Other substances (e.g., avoided alcohol and coffee, drank fruit juice)	☐	☐
• People (e.g., avoided friends who smoke, did not visit with smokers)	☐	☐
• Situations (e.g., sat in nonsmoking section of restaurants, avoided situations in which you typically smoke, change places of relaxation at home)	☐	☐
Asked for help from others		
• Social support (e.g., asked your children to throwaway your cigarettes, called a "buddy" for support, talked with an ex-smoker for support)	☐	☐
• Wagers, dares (e.g., made a bet or wager with a friend as a motivator for quitting)	☐	☐
• Treatment (e.g., attended a stop smoking clinic, enrolled in a clinic)	☐	☐
Practiced direct control of smoking		
• Cut down (e.g., bought low tar cigarettes, cut back, stopped smoking in the car)	☐	☐
• Satiation (e.g., smoked a cigar or chain smoked to make yourself sick)	☐	☐
Used other techniques		
• Self-reward (e.g., put $1 in jar for each day quit, rewarded yourself for 3-hour periods of abstinence)	☐	☐
• Cognitive cueing (e.g., reread your list of reasons for quitting, hung list on refrigerator)	☐	☐
• Other behavioral responses? (list here):	☐	☐

(continued)

TABLE 2.9. *(continued)*

Cognitive coping responses	Yes	No
Thought about the positive health consequences for yourself		
• Future (e.g., living longer, being alive for grandchildren, improved health with quitting)	☐	☐
• Immediate (e.g., being able to breathe deeply, no longer waking up coughing, feeling better physically if you quit)	☐	☐
Thought about the negative health consequences for yourself		
• Future (e.g., getting cancer, dying, leaving children or spouse alone)	☐	☐
• Immediate (e.g., getting frequent colds or chest pains from smoking, feeling sick often)	☐	☐
Thought about the health consequences of smoking on others		
• Realized that the health problems of children are due to your smoking, decided that it would be nice for them to have fresh air in the house and car	☐	☐
Thought about the social consequences		
• Positive (e.g., setting a good example for pregnant daughter, making family members happy/proud)	☐	☐
• Negative (e.g., getting nagged by friends, disappointing family members)	☐	☐
Thought about financial consequences		
• Thought about having additional money for other purposes, saving more money each month	☐	☐
Thought about other consequences		
• Realized that food would taste better, house would smell cleaner if you quit	☐	☐
• Decided you wanted to improve your complexion, feel less nervous/jittery by quitting	☐	☐
• Decided smoking smells bad and is offensive to others	☐	☐
• Thought about yellow teeth and discolored fingers from smoking	☐	☐
• Thought about having bad breath and not being "kissable"	☐	☐
Downplayed the value of smoking		
• General devaluation (e.g., told yourself "It's not worth it; smoking is gross; I'm sick of cigarettes")	☐	☐
• Disappointment in smoking habit (e.g., realized that cigarettes are not a solution to daily hassles, smoking doesn't make you feel better, smoking doesn't improve anything)	☐	☐
• Sensory devaluation (e.g., reminded yourself that smoking tastes bad)	☐	☐
Used self-talk		
• Self-motivation (e.g., kept telling yourself that you don't want cigarettes and don't need them, reviewed your reasons for quitting)	☐	☐
• Willpower (e.g., gave yourself orders not to smoke, told yourself "no" when you were tempted)	☐	☐
• Self-redefinition (e.g., told yourself "I'm a nonsmoker" and visualized yourself as a nonsmoker)	☐	☐
• Positive thoughts (e.g., told yourself "I can do it," gave yourself pats on the back for each period of abstinence, reminded yourself that quitting smoking would get easier each day)	☐	☐
• General positive attitudes (e.g., kept a positive attitude toward the process of quitting)	☐	☐
Used orienting thoughts		
• Planning (e.g., made specific plans for coping with temptations, set a quit date, practiced self-monitoring of smoking)	☐	☐
• Temporal orientation (e.g., thought about quitting smoking one hour at a time, reminded yourself about getting through day by day, remembered that there would be ups and downs)	☐	☐
Used alternative cognitions		
• Distraction (e.g., pushed thoughts about smoking out of your head, kept your mind busy)	☐	☐
• Relaxation (e.g., took "mental vacations" to manage stress, thought about peaceful memories)	☐	☐
Experienced other cognitions		
• Remorse (e.g., accused yourself of being weak or lacking willpower, told yourself "I'm an idiot")	☐	☐
• Guilt (e.g., felt guilty about slipping or relapsing, told yourself "I haven't really tried hard enough")	☐	☐
• Consequences of slips (e.g., said to yourself "If I have one cigarette, I will relapse; it must be all or nothing"; told yourself "I've gotten this far; it's not worth blowing it now")	☐	☐
• Minimizing slips (e.g., told yourself "One cigarette doesn't mean complete relapse; I don't have to go back to being a smoker")	☐	☐

Note. Adapted from "Behavioral Assessment," by S. Shiffman, 1988, in D. M. Donovan and G. A. Marlatt (Eds.), *Assessment of Addictive Behavior*, New York: Guilford Press. Copyright 1988 by The Guilford Press. Adapted by permission.

throughout treatment as a source of possible adaptive coping responses for high-risk situations.

An additional method for assessing coping skills is to inquire about the smoker's perceived barriers and facilitators to quitting smoking. More specifically, smokers can be asked, "Is there anything that you can identify that would make it more difficult for you to quit smoking?" (barriers) and "Is there anything that will make it easier for you to quit smoking?" (facilitators). In general, individuals who identify a greater number of barriers than facilitators are in need of more intensive coping skills training.

Coping Assessment Option 2

Self-monitoring also can be used to assess coping skills, especially once the smoker has begun the process of changing his/her behavior. Self-monitoring is useful to assess coping because it permits an "on-line" situational and time-dependent analysis of when and where coping occurs as it happens. The concept of self-monitoring is discussed in detail in Chapter 5 and the corresponding self-monitoring forms can be found in Figure 5.1.

Basic Assessment Module 2: Stress, Withdrawal, Cravings, and Urges

Stress

Background and Rationale

Perceived stress is positively related to increased smoking in regular smokers (Cohen, Kamark, & Mermelstein, 1983; Epstein & Perkins, 1988) and is the most frequent reason given by ex-smokers for slipping or for relapse (Baer & Lichtenstein, 1988). Furthermore, field studies of smokers have found that levels of perceived stress increase after relapse (Cohen & Lichtenstein, 1990). Smokers who report high levels of stress would benefit from stress or anxiety management training (see Chapter 5), which should increase their chances of smoking cessation.

Stress Assessment Option

One measure that has demonstrated consistent support as being predictive of relapse is the Perceived Stress Scale (PSS; see Cohen et al., 1983; Cohen & Lichtenstein, 1990). The PSS is available in both a 14-item format and a 4-item format, and both versions have been shown to have good psychometric properties (see Table 2.10). Higher levels of perceived stress, measured via the PSS at the end of treatment, predict a lower chance of cessation following treatment. Given its utility at predicting cessation success when measured at the end of treatment, the PSS is best used after a smoker has made a quit attempt, in order to determine whether more intensive stress management training is necessary. The decision to use either the short or long form of the PSS will depend on the time available to the provider.

TABLE 2.10. Basic Assessment Module 2: Perceived Stress

Perceived Stress Scale

INSTRUCTIONS: *For the following questions, we are interested in how things have been, in general, for the past month. Circle the number that best describes your answer.*

	Never	Almost never	Some-times	Fairly often	Very often
1. In the last month, how often have you felt that you were unable to control the important things in your life?	0	1	2	3	4
2. In the last month, how often have you felt confident about your ability to handle your personal problems?	0	1	2	3	4
3. In the last month, how often have you felt that things were going your way?	0	1	2	3	4
4. In the last month, how often have you felt that difficulties were piling up so high that you could not overcome them?	0	1	2	3	4

SCORING INSTRUCTIONS: Perceived Stress Scale (PSS) scores are obtained by reversing the scores (e.g., 0 = 4, 1 = 3, 2 = 2, 3 = 1, 4 = 0) on the two positive items (Items 2 and 3) and summing across the four items. Higher scores reflect higher levels of perceived stress.

Note. From "A Global Measure of Perceived Stress," by S. Cohen, T. Kamark, and R. Mermelstein, 1983, *Journal of Health and Behavior, 24,* 385–396. Reprinted by permission of the American Sociological Association.

Withdrawal Symptoms

Background and Rationale

The nicotine withdrawal syndrome is well defined and is viewed as a hallmark sign of dependence (J. R. Hughes, 1992). The syndrome includes irritability, frustration, or anger; anxiety; difficulty concentrating; restlessness; decreased heart rate; and increased appetite or weight gain (see DSM-IV; American Psychiatric Association, 1994). The signs and symptoms of the nicotine withdrawal syndrome can appear within 2 hours after the last use of tobacco, usually peak between 24 and 48 hours after cessation, and last from a few days to a few weeks (Hughes, Higgins, & Hatsukami, 1990; Piasecki, Fiore, & Baker, 1997). However, there is a great deal of individual variation in both the symptom pattern and time course of withdrawal symptoms (Piasecki et al., 1997; Piasecki et al., 2000). Withdrawal experiences, especially cravings, can predict lapse and relapse after a cessation attempt (Killen & Fortman, 1997; Shiffman et al., 1997). Smokers who report increased frequency or severity of nicotine withdrawal are candidates for withdrawal management training or perhaps more intensive pharmacotherapy that directly treats withdrawal symptoms (see Chapter 7).

Withdrawal Assessment Option 1

The provider can query the smoker as to his/her experience of withdrawal symptoms during past attempts to quit smoking or when he/she goes without smoking for extended periods of time. Even though past experience of withdrawal is not necessarily predictive of current or future symptoms, this knowledge can serve as a useful index. Table 2.11 provides sample items.

Withdrawal Assessment Option 2

The Shiffman–Jarvik Withdrawal Scale (Shiffman & Jarvik, 1976) is a 25-item scale that taps five dimensions of withdrawal (i.e., craving, psychological symptoms, physical symptoms, arousal disturbance, and appetite disturbance). Smokers respond either "Yes" or "No" to questions about whether they have experienced any of the signs or symptoms that are listed. Higher scores reflect a greater degree of withdrawal experienced. Table 2.11 provides a 15-item version of this measure.

Withdrawal Assessment Option 3

A shorter scale, called the Minnesota Withdrawal Scale (8 items), was developed by J. R. Hughes and Hatsukami (1986) to correspond closely to the DSM-III-R criteria for nicotine withdrawal. Smokers respond to the severity of the symptoms they experienced rather than endorsing which symptoms they experienced, as with the Shiffman-Jarvik scale (Shiffman & Jarvik, 1976). Higher scores indicate greater severity of withdrawal. Table 2.11 provides these items.

Cravings and Urges

Background and Rationale

There is general agreement that cravings for addictive substances are an important part of use and abuse of those substances (American Psychiatric Association, 1994). Cravings are generally accepted as a desire to use a drug. Thus, as a result of the craving, the individual engages in behaviors geared toward using the drug or actually uses the drug (Tiffany, 1990). Smokers who experience greater degrees of craving should be considered for more intensive pharmacotherapy, which can directly reduce cravings (Chapter 4), or instructed more specifically on coping skills that can be used to help them to manage cravings (Chapter 6).

Craving Assessment Option 1

Single-item assessments of craving have been shown to be as reliable and as valid as longer scales and to demonstrate ability to predict smoking behaviors (Kozlowski, Pillitteri, Sweeney, Whitfield, & Graham, 1996). Table 2.12 presents a sample one-item question.

Craving Assessment Option 2

The Questionnaire of Smoking Urges (QSU) is a multi-item self-report scale (Tiffany & Hackenworth, 1991) that purports to measure multiple aspects of craving (e.g., desires for smoking, expectancies about cravings). The scale is available in both a long form (Tiffany & Hackenworth, 1991) and a shorter form (Elash, Tiffany, & Vrana, 1995). Table 2.12 presents the long form of this scale.

TABLE 2.11. Basic Assessment Module 2: Three Options for Withdrawal Symptoms

Option 1. Ask the smoker directly

  a. "When you have quit smoking in the past, how did you feel?"
  b. "Did you experience any unpleasant symptoms when you last quit smoking?"
  c. "When you go without smoking, do you experience any unpleasant symptoms?"

Option 2. Shiffman–Jarvik Withdrawal Scale[a]
Option 3. Minnesota Withdrawal Scale[b]

Shiffman–Jarvik Withdrawal Scale—Short Version

INSTRUCTIONS: Please CIRCLE the number to the right of each question that most accurately reflects how you feel at this moment.

		Definitely not				Definitely		
1.	If you could smoke freely, would you like a cigarette this minute?	1	2	3	4	5	6	7
2.	Is your heart beating faster than usual?	1	2	3	4	5	6	7
3.	Do you feel more calm than usual?	1	2	3	4	5	6	7
4.	Are you able to concentrate as well as usual?	1	2	3	4	5	6	7
5.	Do you feel wide awake?	1	2	3	4	5	6	7
6.	Do you feel content?	1	2	3	4	5	6	7
7.	Are you thinking of cigarettes more than usual?	1	2	3	4	5	6	7
8.	Do you have fluttery feelings in your chest?	1	2	3	4	5	6	7
9.	Do you feel hungrier than usual for this time of day?	1	2	3	4	5	6	7
10.	If you were permitted to smoke, would you refuse a cigarette right now?	1	2	3	4	5	6	7
11.	Do you feel more tense than usual?	1	2	3	4	5	6	7
12.	Do you miss a cigarette?	1	2	3	4	5	6	7
13.	Do you have an urge to smoke a cigarette right now?	1	2	3	4	5	6	7
14.	Are you feeling irritable?	1	2	3	4	5	6	7
15.	Are your hands shaky?	1	2	3	4	5	6	7

SCORING INSTRUCTIONS: The Shiffman–Jarvik Withdrawal Scale yields an overall score and five subscale sores: Craving (items 1, 7, 10, 12, 13), Physical Symptoms (items 2, 8, 15), Stimulation/Sedation (item 5), Psychological Symptoms (items 3, 4, 6, 11, 14), and Appetite (item 9).

Items 3, 4, 5, 6, and 10 are reverse scored (1 = 7, 2 = 6, 3 = 5, etc.). The overall score is obtained by averaging across the 14 items. Subscale scores are obtained by averaging responses to items within each subscale. Higher scores reflect a greater degree of nicotine withdrawal.

(continued)

TABLE 2.11. *(continued)*

<u>Minnesota Withdrawal Scale</u>

INSTRUCTIONS: *For each of the following, rate yourself on how you have been feeling over the past twenty-four hours. Mark the number that applies to you.*

	None	Slight	Mild	Moderate	Severe
1. Anger, irritability, frustration	0	1	2	3	4
2. Anxiety, nervousness	0	1	2	3	4
3. Difficulty concentrating	0	1	2	3	4
4. Impatience, restlessness	0	1	2	3	4
5. Hunger	0	1	2	3	4
6. Awakening at night	0	1	2	3	4
7. Depression	0	1	2	3	4
8. Desire to smoke	0	1	2	3	4

SCORING INSTRUCTIONS: A total withdrawal discomfort score is calculated by adding the scores for individual items. Higher scores reflect higher levels of discomfort. It is important to note that the scale is not labeled a "withdrawal scale" when used as a handout because smokers (1) are confused by filling out a "withdrawal" scale prior to cessation, and (2) will sometimes not report a symptom if they do not believe it is due to withdrawal.

[a]From "Smoking Withdrawal Symptoms in Two Weeks of Abstinence," by S. Shiffman and M. Jarvik, 1976, *Psychopharmacology, 50*, 35–39. Reprinted by permission of Springer-Verlag.
[b]From "Signs and Symptoms of Tobacco Withdrawal," by J. R. Hughes and D. Hatsukami, March 1986, *Archives of General Psychiatry, 43*(3), 289–294. Copyright 1986, American Medical Association.

TABLE 2.12. Basic Assessment Module 2: Two Options for Cravings and Urges

Option 1. Ask the smoker directly
"On a scale from 1 to 10, where 1 is no craving at all, and 10 is extreme cravings, how strong is your smoking craving now?"

Option 2. Questionnaire of Smoking Urges: QSU[a]

<u>Questionnaire of Smoking Urges (QSU)—Long Form</u>

INSTRUCTIONS: *After reading each statement carefully, rate the degree to which the statement describes how you are feeling right now.*

	Strongly disagree						Strongly agree
1. Smoking would make me feel very good right now.	1	2	3	4	5	6	7
2. I would be less irritable now if I could smoke.	1	2	3	4	5	6	7
3. Nothing would be better than smoking a cigarette right now.	1	2	3	4	5	6	7
4. I am not missing smoking right now.	1	2	3	4	5	6	7
5. I will smoke as soon as I get the chance.	1	2	3	4	5	6	7
6. I don't want to smoke now.	1	2	3	4	5	6	7
7. Smoking would make me less depressed.	1	2	3	4	5	6	7
8. Smoking would not help me calm down now.	1	2	3	4	5	6	7
9. If I were offered a cigarette, I would smoke it immediately.	1	2	3	4	5	6	7
10. Starting now, I could go without smoking for a long time.	1	2	3	4	5	6	7
11. Smoking a cigarette would not be pleasant.	1	2	3	4	5	6	7
12. If I were smoking this minute, I would feel less bored.	1	2	3	4	5	6	7
13. All I want right now is a cigarette.	1	2	3	4	5	6	7
14. Smoking right now would make me feel less tired.	1	2	3	4	5	6	7
15. Smoking would make me happier now.	1	2	3	4	5	6	7
16. Even if it were possible, I probably wouldn't smoke now.	1	2	3	4	5	6	7
17. I have no desire for a cigarette right now.	1	2	3	4	5	6	7
18. My desire to smoke seems overpowering.	1	2	3	4	5	6	7
19. Smoking now would make things seem just perfect.	1	2	3	4	5	6	7
20. I crave a cigarette right now.	1	2	3	4	5	6	7
21. I would not enjoy a cigarette right now.	1	2	3	4	5	6	7
22. A cigarette would not taste good right now.	1	2	3	4	5	6	7
23. I have an urge for a cigarette.	1	2	3	4	5	6	7
24. I could control things better right now if I could smoke.	1	2	3	4	5	6	7
25. I am going to smoke as soon as possible.	1	2	3	4	5	6	7
26. I would not feel better physically if I were smoking.	1	2	3	4	5	6	7
27. A cigarette would not be very satisfying now.	1	2	3	4	5	6	7
28. If I had a lit cigarette in my hand, I probably wouldn't smoke it.	1	2	3	4	5	6	7
29. If I were smoking now, I could think more clearly.	1	2	3	4	5	6	7
30. I would do almost anything for a cigarette now.	1	2	3	4	5	6	7
31. I need to smoke now.	1	2	3	4	5	6	7
32. Right now, I am not making plans to smoke.	1	2	3	4	5	6	7

Items 4, 6, 8, 10, 11, 16, 17, 21, 22, 26, 27, 28, and 32 are reverse-scored (1 = 7, 2 = 6, 3 = 5, etc.). An overall score is computed by averaging across the 32 items. Scores for the positive and negative reinforcement subscales are obtained by averaging the responses to items within each subscale. The QSU yields an overall measure of self-reported urge to smoke and two subscale urge scores: positive reinforcement items (4, 5, 6, 9, 11, 16, 17, 20, 21, 22, 23, 25, 27, 28, and 32) and negative reinforcement items (2, 3, 7, 12, 13, 14, 18, 19, 24, 29, and 30). Higher scores suggest greater urge to smoke.

[a]From "The Development and Initial Validation of a Questionnaire of Smoking Urges," by S. T. Tiffany and D. J. Drobes, 1991, *British Journal of Addiction,* 86, 1467–1476. Reprinted by permission of Blackwell Science.

Basic Assessment Module 3: Cognition

Self-Efficacy

Background and Rationale

Self-efficacy is an individual's level of confidence in his/her ability to perform a particular behavior (Bandura, 1997). Self-efficacy is not a global, stable construct that applies to all facets of an individual's life. Rather, self-efficacy encompasses a specific level of confidence about engaging in a specific behavior and may not generalize to other behaviors (Cervone & Scott, 1995). For example, one can have high levels of confidence in obtaining a passing grade in a literature course but have low levels of confidence in obtaining a passing mark in a mathematics course.

Self-efficacy measured at the end of smoking cessation treatment (i.e., confidence in quitting or in remaining abstinent) is a consistently strong predictor of later relapse, though self-efficacy measured at the beginning of treatment does not necessarily predict cessation or relapse (Baer & Lichtenstein, 1988). Moreover, compared with both high and low levels, moderate levels of self-efficacy measured following a slip or lapse may predict increased ability to stay abstinent (Haaga & Stewart, 1992). Measures of self-efficacy and motivation are highly related to one another (Borrelli & Mermelstein, 1994), but it is important to recognize that the constructs are indeed distinct. For example, a given smoker may be highly motivated to quit smoking but may lack the confidence that he/she can do so successfully. Conversely, another smoker may lack the motivation to quit but may have high levels of confidence that he/she can quit when motivated.

In any case, an assessment of self-efficacy near the end of treatment can be a good indicator of how successful the individual will be at staying abstinent from smoking. A person who demonstrates low levels of self-efficacy would benefit from more intensive relapse prevention training (see Chapter 6).

Self-Efficacy Assessment Option 1

A single-item measure of self-efficacy can be obtained. Research has shown that single-item measures of self-efficacy are highly related to such measures as the Confidence Questionnaire (Borrelli & Mermelstein, 1994). Table 2.13 presents the type of question that we typically ask smokers when we are short on time.

Self-Efficacy Assessment Option 2

The Self-Efficacy/Temptations Scale (Velicer, DiClemente, Rossi, & Prochaska, 1990; see Table 2.13) is a measure of self-efficacy. Smokers respond according to their level of temptation in the situations represented by the items. This scale may be reliably divided into subscales that assess self-efficacy in three broad situational domains: Positive Affect/Social Situations, Negative Affect Situations, and Habitual/Craving Situations. The authors of the Self-Efficacy/Temptations Scale suggest that it is best to use the subscales to target problem areas for relapse after a cessation attempt, whereas the total scale score should be used to index general level of confidence in quitting smoking (Velicer et al., 1990).

TABLE 2.13. Basic Assessment Module 3: Two Options for Self-Efficacy

Option 1. Ask the smoker directly
"On a scale from 1 to 10, where 1 is not at all confident, and 10 is extremely confident, how confident are you that you can quit smoking (remain quit) now?"

Option 2. Self-Efficacy/Temptations Scale—Long Form[a]

Self-Efficacy/Temptations Scale—Long Form

INSTRUCTIONS: *Listed below are situations that lead some people to smoke. We would like to know HOW TEMPTED you may be to smoke in each situation. Please answer the following questions using a 5-point scale with 1 = NOT AT ALL TEMPTED and 5 = EXTREMELY TEMPTED.*

How tempted are you to smoke . . .	Not at all tempted	Not very tempted	Moderately tempted	Very tempted	Extremely tempted
1. At a bar or cocktail lounge having a drink.	1	2	3	4	5
2. When I am desiring a cigarette.	1	2	3	4	5
3. When things are just not going the way I want and I am frustrated.	1	2	3	4	5
4. With my spouse or close friend who is smoking.	1	2	3	4	5
5. When there are arguments and conflicts with my family.	1	2	3	4	5
6. When I am happy and celebrating.	1	2	3	4	5
7. When I am very angry about something or someone.	1	2	3	4	5
8. When I would experience an emotional crisis, such as an accident or death in the family.	1	2	3	4	5
9. When I see someone smoking and enjoying it.	1	2	3	4	5
10. Over coffee while talking and relaxing.	1	2	3	4	5
11. When I realize that quitting smoking is an extremely difficult task for me.	1	2	3	4	5
12. When I am craving a cigarette.	1	2	3	4	5
13. When I first get up in the morning.	1	2	3	4	5
14. When I feel I need a lift.	1	2	3	4	5
15. When I begin to let down on my concern about my health and am less physically active.	1	2	3	4	5
16. With friends at a party.	1	2	3	4	5
17. When I wake up in the morning and face a tough day.	1	2	3	4	5
18. When I am extremely depressed.	1	2	3	4	5
19. When I am extremely anxious and stressed.	1	2	3	4	5
20. When I realize I haven't smoked for a while.	1	2	3	4	5

SCORING INSTRUCTIONS: The Self-Efficacy/Temptations Scale (Long Form) provides a measure of confidence in resisting smoking in situations represented by the items. An overall score is computed by averaging across the 20 items. In addition, there are three subscales that measure broad aspects of self-efficacy to resist smoking: Positive Affect/Social Situations (items 1, 4, 6, 9, 10, and 16); Negative Affect Situations (items 3, 5, 7, 8, 18, and 19); Habit/Craving Situations (items 11, 13, 14, 15, and 20). Subscale scores are obtained by averaging the responses to items within each subscale.

[a]From "Relapse Situations and Self-Efficacy: An Integrative Model," by W. F. Velicer, C. C. DiClemente, J. S. Rossi, and J. O. Prochaska, 1990, *Addictive Behaviors, 15,* 271–283. Reprinted by permission of Elsevier Science.

Outcome Expectancies and Beliefs

Background and Rationale

Expectancies and beliefs about smoking and quitting are at the core of many theories of relapse prevention (see Chapter 5; Abrams et al., 1987; Marlatt & Gordon, 1985). Outcome expectancies have been defined in a number of ways in research on smoking, but they are generally thought of as beliefs about the consequences or results that follow both smoking and quitting (e.g., "How much does smoking help you to relax?"; "How much does smoking help you to control your weight?"). Research on outcome expectancies among smokers has focused on developing assessments that tap the multidimensional nature of the consequences of smoking (Brandon & Baker, 1991; Copeland, Brandon, & Quinn, 1995; Wetter et al., 1994) and expectancies for the coping value of smoking (Shadel & Mermelstein, 1993b). Smokers who hold greater positive expectancies for the value of smoking would probably benefit from cognitive restructuring strategies to help change those thoughts and beliefs.

Expectancies Assessment Option 1

One method for assessing expectancies is the Decisional Balance Scale developed by Velicer and colleagues (1985). This measure is based on the concept of decisional balance put forth by Janis and Mann (1977) and can be used in a short form (6 items) or a long form (20 items). This scale assesses factors that are supportive of smoking (pros), as well as the factors that are supportive of change (cons). Table 2.14 presents the long form.

Expectancies Assessment Option 2

Similar to the Decisional Balance Scale, the Smoking Consequences Questionnaire (Brandon & Baker, 1991; Wetter et al., 1994) has received the most empirical attention as a measure of smoking expectancies. This 55-item expectancy assessment (see Table 2.14) taps 10 domains of expectancies that could potentially be important for understanding the positive value that smoking has to the smoker (i.e., Negative Affect Reduction, Stimulation/State Enhancement, Health Risk, Taste/Sensorimotor Manipulation, Social Facilitation, Weight Control, Craving/Addiction, Negative Physical Feelings, Boredom Reduction, and Negative Social Impression). In general, when measured at baseline, the scales independently predict smokers' short-term experience of withdrawal (i.e., greater expectancies for the value of smoking predict increased withdrawal symptoms), and reduction in negative affect predicts end-of-treatment smoking status (i.e., greater expectancies for the negative-affect-reducing potential of smoking predicts decreased chances of cessation success; Wetter et al., 1994).

Self-Concept

Background and Rationale

Smokers believe that they differ from nonsmokers on a number of descriptive attributes (Burton et al., 1989). In general, smokers who see themselves as more similar to nonsmokers than to smokers may have a greater chance of cessation success (Gibbons & Gerrard, 1996). Fur-

TABLE 2.14. Basic Assessment Module 3: Two Options for Outcome Expectancies and Beliefs

Option 1. Decisional Balance Scale (Long Form)[a]
Option 2. Smoking Consequences Questionnaire[b]

Decisional Balance Scale (Long Form)

INSTRUCTIONS: *The following statements represent different opinions about smoking. Please rate HOW IMPORTANT each statement is to your decision to smoke according to the following 5-point scale:*

Not important	Slightly important	Moderately important	Very important	Extremely important
1	2	3	4	5

1. Smoking cigarettes is pleasurable	1	2	3	4	5
2. My smoking affects the health of others	1	2	3	4	5
3. I like the image of a cigarette smoker	1	2	3	4	5
4. Others close to me would suffer if I became ill from smoking	1	2	3	4	5
5. I am relaxed and therefore more pleasant when smoking	1	2	3	4	5
6. Because I continue to smoke, some people I know think I lack the character to quit	1	2	3	4	5
7. If I try to stop smoking I'll be irritable and a pain to be around	1	2	3	4	5
8. Smoking cigarettes is hazardous to my health	1	2	3	4	5
9. My family and friends like me better when I am happily smoking than when I am miserably trying to quit	1	2	3	4	5
10. I'm embarrassed to have to smoke	1	2	3	4	5
11. I like myself better when I smoke	1	2	3	4	5
12. My cigarette smoking bothers other people	1	2	3	4	5
13. Smoking helps me concentrate and do better work	1	2	3	4	5
14. People think I'm foolish for ignoring the warnings about cigarette smoking	1	2	3	4	5
15. Smoking cigarettes relieves tension	1	2	3	4	5
16. People close to me disapprove of my smoking	1	2	3	4	5
17. By continuing to smoke I feel I am making my own decisions	1	2	3	4	5
18. I'm foolish to ignore the warnings about cigarettes	1	2	3	4	5
19. After not smoking for a while a cigarette makes me feel great	1	2	3	4	5
20. I would be more energetic right now if I didn't smoke	1	2	3	4	5

SCORING INSTRUCTIONS: Sum the items that comprise the PROS subscale and the items that comprise the CONS scale.

PROS: 1, 3, 5, 7, 9, 11, 13, 15, 17, 19 (odd numbers)

CONS: 2, 4, 6, 8, 10, 12, 14, 16, 18, 20 (even numbers)

(continued)

TABLE 2.14. *(continued)*

Smoking Consequences Questionnaire

INSTRUCTIONS: Below is a list of statements about smoking. Each statement contains a possible consequence of smoking. For each of the statements listed below, please rate how LIKELY or UNLIKELY you believe each consequence is for you when you smoke. If the consequences seems UNLIKELY to you, mark a number from 0–4. If the consequence seems LIKELY to you, mark a number from 5–9. That is, if you believe that a consequence would never happen, mark the 0; if you believe a consequence would happen every time you smoke, mark the number 9. Use the guide below to aid you further.

0	1	2	3	4	5	6	7	8	9
Completely	Extremely	Very	Somewhat	A little	A little	Somewhat	Very	Extremely	Completely
UNLIKELY					**LIKELY**				

		UNLIKELY					LIKELY			
1. Cigarettes taste good.	0	1	2	3	4	5	6	7	8	9
2. Smoking controls my appetite.	0	1	2	3	4	5	6	7	8	9
3. My throat burns after smoking.	0	1	2	3	4	5	6	7	8	9
4. Cigarettes help me deal with anxiety or worry.	0	1	2	3	4	5	6	7	8	9
5. Nicotine "fits" can be controlled by smoking.	0	1	2	3	4	5	6	7	8	9
6. When I'm angry, a cigarette can calm me down.	0	1	2	3	4	5	6	7	8	9
7. When I'm alone, a cigarette can help me pass the time.	0	1	2	3	4	5	6	7	8	9
8. I become more addicted the more I smoke.	0	1	2	3	4	5	6	7	8	9
9. If I'm tense, a cigarette helps me to relax.	0	1	2	3	4	5	6	7	8	9
10. Cigarettes keep me from overeating.	0	1	2	3	4	5	6	7	8	9
11. Smoking a cigarette energizes me.	0	1	2	3	4	5	6	7	8	9
12. Cigarettes help me deal with anger.	0	1	2	3	4	5	6	7	8	9
13. Smoking calms me down when I feel nervous.	0	1	2	3	4	5	6	7	8	9
14. Cigarettes make my lungs hurt.	0	1	2	3	4	5	6	7	8	9
15. I feel like I do a better job when I am smoking.	0	1	2	3	4	5	6	7	8	9
16. A cigarette can give me energy when I'm bored and tired.	0	1	2	3	4	5	6	7	8	9
17. Cigarettes can really make me feel good.	0	1	2	3	4	5	6	7	8	9
18. When I'm feeling happy, smoking helps keep that feeling.	0	1	2	3	4	5	6	7	8	9
19. I will enjoy the flavor of a cigarette.	0	1	2	3	4	5	6	7	8	9
20. If I have nothing to do, a smoke can help kill time.	0	1	2	3	4	5	6	7	8	9
21. I will enjoy feeling a cigarette on my tongue and lips.	0	1	2	3	4	5	6	7	8	9
22. Smoking will satisfy my nicotine cravings.	0	1	2	3	4	5	6	7	8	9
23. I feel like part of a group when I'm around other smokers.	0	1	2	3	4	5	6	7	8	9
24. Smoking makes me seem less attractive.	0	1	2	3	4	5	6	7	8	9
25. By smoking I risk heart disease and lung cancer.	0	1	2	3	4	5	6	7	8	9
26. Smoking helps me enjoy people more.	0	1	2	3	4	5	6	7	8	9
27. Cigarettes help me reduce tension.	0	1	2	3	4	5	6	7	8	9
28. I feel better physically after having a smoke.	0	1	2	3	4	5	6	7	8	9

(continued)

TABLE 2.14. *(continued)*

29.	I enjoy parties more when I am smoking.	0	1	2	3	4	5	6	7	8	9
30.	People think less of me if they see me smoking.	0	1	2	3	4	5	6	7	8	9
31.	A cigarette can satisfy my urge to smoke.	0	1	2	3	4	5	6	7	8	9
32.	Just handling a cigarette is pleasurable.	0	1	2	3	4	5	6	7	8	9
33.	If I'm feeling irritable, a smoke will help me relax.	0	1	2	3	4	5	6	7	8	9
34.	Smoking irritates my mouth and throat.	0	1	2	3	4	5	6	7	8	9
35.	When I feel bored and tired, a cigarette can really help.	0	1	2	3	4	5	6	7	8	9
36.	I will become more dependent on nicotine if I continue smoking.	0	1	2	3	4	5	6	7	8	9
37.	Smoking helps me control my weight.	0	1	2	3	4	5	6	7	8	9
38.	When I'm upset with someone, a cigarette helps me cope.	0	1	2	3	4	5	6	7	8	9
39.	The more I smoke, the more I risk my health.	0	1	2	3	4	5	6	7	8	9
40.	Cigarettes keep me from eating more than I should.	0	1	2	3	4	5	6	7	8	9
41.	I enjoy the steps I take to light up.	0	1	2	3	4	5	6	7	8	9
42.	Conversations seem more special if we are all smoking.	0	1	2	3	4	5	6	7	8	9
43.	I look ridiculous while smoking.	0	1	2	3	4	5	6	7	8	9
44.	Smoking keeps my weight down.	0	1	2	3	4	5	6	7	8	9
45.	I like the way a cigarette makes me feel physically.	0	1	2	3	4	5	6	7	8	9
46.	Smoking is hazardous to my health.	0	1	2	3	4	5	6	7	8	9
47.	I enjoy feeling the smoke hit my mouth and the back of my throat.	0	1	2	3	4	5	6	7	8	9
48.	When I smoke, the taste is pleasant.	0	1	2	3	4	5	6	7	8	9
49.	I like to watch the smoke from my cigarette.	0	1	2	3	4	5	6	7	8	9
50.	When I am worrying about something, a cigarette is helpful.	0	1	2	3	4	5	6	7	8	9
51.	Smoking temporarily reduces those repeated urges for cigarettes.	0	1	2	3	4	5	6	7	8	9
52.	I enjoy the taste sensations while smoking.	0	1	2	3	4	5	6	7	8	9
53.	I feel more at ease with other people if I have a cigarette.	0	1	2	3	4	5	6	7	8	9
54.	Cigarettes are good for dealing with boredom.	0	1	2	3	4	5	6	7	8	9
55.	Smoking is taking years off my life.	0	1	2	3	4	5	6	7	8	9

SCORING INSTRUCTIONS: Responses on the SCQ can be used to derive 10 subscale scores: Negative Affect Reduction, Stimulation/State Enhancement, Health Risk, Taste/Sensorimotor Manipulation, Social Facilitation, Weight Control, Craving/Addiction, Negative Physical Feelings, Boredom Reduction, and Negative Social Impression.

Negative Affect Reduction items are 4, 6, 9, 12, 13, 27, 33, 38, and 50; Stimulation/State Enhancement items are 11, 15, 16, 17, 18, 28, and 45; Health risk items are 25, 39, 46, and 55; Taste/Sensorimotor Manipulation items are 1, 19, 21, 32, 41, 48, 49, and 52; Social Facilitation items are 23, 26, 29, 42, and 53; Weight Control items are 2, 10, 37, 40, and 44; Craving/Addiction items are 5, 8, 22, 31, 36, and 51; Negative Physical Feelings items are 3, 14, and 34; Boredom Reduction items are 7, 20, 35, and 54; Negative Social Impression items are 24, 30, and 43. Subscale scores are obtained by averaging the responses to items within each subscale. For all subscales, higher scores suggest stronger smoking-related outcome expectancies.

[a]From "A Decisional Balance Measure for Assessing and Predicting Smoking Status," by W. F. Velicer, C. DiClemente, J. O. Prochaska, and N. Brandenburg, 1985, *Journal of Personality and Social Psychology, 48,* 1279–1289. Copyright © 1985 by the American Psychological Association. Adapted with permission.
[b]From "The Smoking Consequences Questionnaire—Adult: Measurement of Smoking Outcome Expectancies of Experienced Smokers," by A. L. Copeland, T. H. Brandon, & E. P. Quinn, 1995, *Psychological Assessment, 7*(4), 484–494. Copyright © 1995 by the American Psychological Association. Adapted with permission.

thermore, smokers who enter treatment with a stronger image of what a nonsmoker is like compared with a smoker are more likely to quit than smokers who do not hold such images (Shadel & Mermelstein, 1996). It also seems as though a maximal-level cognitive-behavioral treatment can be effective in changing these self-concept images (Shadel, Mermelstein, & Borrelli, 1996).

Self-Concept Assessment Option 1

Smokers have been presented with lists of adjectives and asked to indicate which adjectives best describe themselves, the "typical" smoker, and the "typical" nonsmoker. Correspondence between the adjectives in these different self-concept domains are then used to predict similarity between the way smokers see themselves, the typical smoker, and the typical non-smoker (Gibbons & Gerrard, 1996). Table 2.15 presents sample adjectives and questionnaire structure.

Self-Concept Assessment Option 2

Questionnaires that assess smoker self-concept and abstainer self-concept have been validated (Shadel & Mermelstein, 1996; see Table 2.15). When measured at pretreatment, scores on these questionnaires predict posttreatment cessation success; higher scores for an abstainer self-concept relative to a smoker self-concept, are associated with increased chances of abstinence several months after treatment.

Intrinsic and Extrinsic Motivation

Background and Rationale

As we noted previously, motivation, on its face, is one of the core components that is necessary for successful smoking cessation. One theory suggests that motivation to quit is driven in part by the rewards that will result from cessation (Curry, Wagner, & Grothaus, 1990). Two types of motivation have been identified in this regard. *Intrinsic motivation* is defined by rewards that are internal to the person (e.g., quitting smoking for personal control or because of personal concern over illness), whereas *extrinsic motivation* is defined by rewards that are external to the person (e.g., quitting smoking to save money or to get people to "stop nagging").

Intrinsic–Extrinsic Motivation Assessment

A 12-item Reasons for Quitting (RFQ) questionnaire has been developed to tap into the two dimensions of intrinsic and extrinsic motivation (Curry et al., 1990; see Table 2.16). Research has shown that the relationship of intrinsic to extrinsic motivation predicts cessation success. A higher ratio of intrinsic to extrinsic motivation predicts increased chances that the smoker will quit (Curry et al., 1990). In other words, a cessation attempt that is motivated by rewards that are internal to the person is more likely to be successful than a cessation attempt motivated by rewards that are external to the person. The RFQ has shown strong psychometric properties (Curry et al., 1990) and is a good measure of motivation to use if the provider is concerned with measuring the causal aspects of motivation.

TABLE 2.15. Basic Assessment Module 3: Self-Concept

Option 1. Adjective Identification Task[a]
Option 2. Smoker Self-Concept and Abstainer Self-Concept Questionnaire[b]

<u>Adjective Identification Task</u>

INSTRUCTIONS: *Ask smoker directly: "Do you know a typical smoker? Now we would like to get your opinion of other smokers; in other words, the 'typical' smoker. We are not looking for anyone in particular, we just want to know what you think the average person (or most people) who smokes is like."*

	Not at all				Very
1. Considerate	1	2	3	4	5
2. Friendly	1	2	3	4	5
3. Self-centered	1	2	3	4	5
4. Smart	1	2	3	4	5
5. Moody	1	2	3	4	5
6. Attractive	1	2	3	4	5
7. Honest	1	2	3	4	5
8. Dependent	1	2	3	4	5
9. Irrational	1	2	3	4	5
10. Reliable	1	2	3	4	5
11. Weak	1	2	3	4	5

SCORING INSTRUCTIONS: A measure of an individual's perceptions of the typical smoker is derived by averaging responses to the 11 items. Items 3, 5, 8, 9, and 11 are reverse scored (1 = 5, 2 = 4, etc.). Lower scores suggest a more negative perception, or image, of the typical smoker.

<u>Smoker Self-Concept and Abstainer Self-Concept Questionnaire</u>

INSTRUCTIONS: *On a scale of 1 to 10, with 1 = STRONGLY DISAGREE and 10 = STRONGLY AGREE, please mark how you are feeling in each of the statements below.*

Smoker Self-Concept Scale

	STRONGLY DISAGREE						STRONGLY AGREE			
1. Smoking is part of my self-image.	1	2	3	4	5	6	7	8	9	10
2. Smoking is part of "Who I am."	1	2	3	4	5	6	7	8	9	10
3. Smoking is part of my personality.	1	2	3	4	5	6	7	8	9	10
4. Smoking is a large part of my daily life.	1	2	3	4	5	6	7	8	9	10
5. Others view smoking as part of my personality.	1	2	3	4	5	6	7	8	9	10

Abstainer Self-Concept Scale

	STRONGLY DISAGREE						STRONGLY AGREE			
1. I am able to see myself as a nonsmoker.	1	2	3	4	5	6	7	8	9	10
2. It is easy to imagine myself as a nonsmoker.	1	2	3	4	5	6	7	8	9	10
3. Not smoking is "like me."	1	2	3	4	5	6	7	8	9	10
4. I am comfortable with the idea of being a nonsmoker.	1	2	3	4	5	6	7	8	9	10

SCORING INSTRUCTIONS: For both scales, responses to individual items are averaged to provide an assessment of the smoker's view of him- or herself. For the Smoker Self-concept Scale, higher scores reflect greater importance of being a smoker to the individual's self-concept. For the Abstainer Self-concept Scale, higher scores reflect greater importance to the individual of being an abstainer.

---

[a]For additional information, see "Smoker Networks and the Typical Smoker: A Prospective Analysis of Smoking Cessation," by F. X. Gibbons and M. Gerrard, 1996, *Health Psychology, 15,* 469–477.
[b]From "Individual Differences in Self-Concept among Smokers Attempting to Quit: Validation and Predictive Utility of Measures of the Smoker Self-Concept and Abstainer Self-Concept," by W. G. Shadel and R. Mermelstein, 1996, *Annals of Behavioral Medicine, 18,* 151–156.

TABLE 2.16. Basic Assessment Module 3: Intrinsic and Extrinsic Motivation

<u>Reasons for Quitting Questionnaire</u>

INSTRUCTIONS: *This scale is about reasons for quitting smoking. Read each of the following reasons that smokers may have for quitting and decide how true each is for you* right now. *If you are not thinking of quitting* right now, *decide how true each would be for you* if you were to decide to quit. *Please use the following scale to answer each item.*

How true for you is each of the following reasons for quitting?	Not at all true	A little true	Moderately true	Quite true	Extremely true
1. Because I am afraid that I will get very sick if I don't quit smoking.	1	2	3	4	5
2. To prove that I can quit if I really want to.	1	2	3	4	5
3. Because I feel like smoking is hurting my health.	1	2	3	4	5
4. To feel in control of my life.	1	2	3	4	5
5. To show that I can do other things that are important to me.	1	2	3	4	5
6. Because I am afraid that smoking will shorten my life.	1	2	3	4	5
7. So other people will stop nagging me.	1	2	3	4	5
8. To save money that I spend on cigarettes.	1	2	3	4	5
9. Because someone is making me quit.	1	2	3	4	5
10. So I won't burn holes in clothes or furniture.	1	2	3	4	5
11. Because people I am close to will be mad at me if I don't quit.	1	2	3	4	5
12. So my house or car won't smell.	1	2	3	4	5

SCORING INSTRUCTIONS: The RFQ provides measures of intrinsic and extrinsic motivation to quit smoking. The intrinsic subscale is derived from items 1–6, while the extrinsic subscale is derived from items 7–12. For both subscales, responses are averaged to provide a subscale score. Higher scores suggest higher levels of motivation.

Note. For additional information, see "Intrinsic and Extrinsic Motivation for Smoking Cessation," by S. Curry, E. H. Wagner, and L. C. Grothaus, 1990, *Journal of Consulting and Clinical Psychology, 58,* 310–316.

Basic Assessment Module 4: Social Environment

Social Support

Background and Rationale

Social support influences outcome after smoking cessation attempts (Fiore et al., 1996; U.S. Department of Health and Human Services, 1988). A greater amount of support (i.e., encouragement from others, reinforcement from others) that the smoker perceives from important others in the social environment is an important component of success (Mermelstein et al., 1986).

Social Support Assessment Option 1

One method involves simply counting the number of supportive individuals in the smoker's social environment (see R. Murray, Johnston, Dolce, Lee, & O'Hara, 1995). Table 2.17 provides an example of the type of question that can be asked.

TABLE 2.17. Basic Assessment Module 4: Social Environment—Social Support

Option 1. Number of supportive individuals
"How many people in your household currently smoke?"

Option 2. Partner Interaction Questionnaire (PIQ)

<u>Partner Interaction Questionnaire (PIQ)</u>

PART I INSTRUCTIONS: "We are interested in what kind of encouragement or help—if any—you expect from your spouse or friends. We are including a broad range of items. If you are married or living with a romantic partner, please answer with respect to how you expect that person will interact with you. If not, pick the person—friend or relative—who will follow your progress in quitting most closely, and answer in terms of how you expect that person will interact with you."

Whom are you thinking of (circle one)?

| Spouse/partner | Parent | Child | Sibling | Friend |

Does the person you are thinking of smoke?   No   Yes

Are they also trying to quit smoking?   No   Yes

PART II INSTRUCTIONS: For the following questions, think of the person you identified in PART I. Please answer the items using the scale below:

| Never | Almost Never | Sometimes | Fairly Often | Very Often |
| 0 | 1 | 2 | 3 | 4 |

During the first weeks that I'm quitting, how often will _____ do each of the following?	Never	Almost Never	Some-times	Fairly Often	Very Often
1. Compliment you on not smoking.	0	1	2	3	4
2. Comment that smoking is a dirty habit.	0	1	2	3	4
3. Talk you out of smoking a cigarette.	0	1	2	3	4
4. Comment on your lack of willpower.	0	1	2	3	4
5. Comment that the house smells of smoke.	0	1	2	3	4
6. Refuse to let you smoke in the house.	0	1	2	3	4
7. Congratulate you for your decision to quit smoking.	0	1	2	3	4
8. Help you think of substitutes for smoking.	0	1	2	3	4
9. Mention being bothered by smoke.	0	1	2	3	4
10. Celebrate your quitting with you.	0	1	2	3	4
11. Criticize your smoking.	0	1	2	3	4
12. Express doubt about your ability to quit/stay quit.	0	1	2	3	4
13. Refuse to clean up your cigarette butts.	0	1	2	3	4
14. Help to calm you down when you are feeling stressed or irritable.	0	1	2	3	4
15. Tell you to stick with it.	0	1	2	3	4
16. Express confidence in your ability to quit/remain quit.	0	1	2	3	4
17. Help you to use substitutes for cigarettes.	0	1	2	3	4
18. Express pleasure at your efforts to quit.	0	1	2	3	4
19. Participate in an activity with you that keeps you from smoking (e.g., going for a walk instead of smoking).	0	1	2	3	4
20. Ask you to quit smoking.	0	1	2	3	4

SCORING INSTRUCTIONS: The PIQ yields two subscale scores: Negative Behaviors and Positive Behaviors. The Negative Behavior subscale is composed of items 2, 3, 4, 5, 6, 9, 11, 12, 13, and 20, while the positive behavior subscale is composed of items 1, 7, 8, 10, 14, 15, 16, 17, 18, and 19. For each subscale, responses are summed to provide a total subscale score.

Note. For additional information, see "Social Support and Smoking Cessation and Maintenance," by R. J. Mermelstein, S. Cohen, E. Lichtenstein, J. S. Baer, and T. Kamarck, 1986, *Journal of Consulting and Clinical Psychology, 54,* 447–453.

Social Support Assessment Option 2

The Partner Interaction Questionnaire (PIQ; Mermelstein, Lichtenstein, & McIntyre, 1983; see Table 2.17) is a 20-item questionnaire that was designed to assess level of support the smoker perceives from a significant other that contributes to his/her efforts to quit smoking. Pretreatment scores on the PIQ have been found to predict smoking cessation and relapse: High levels of perceived support from a significant other were associated with greater success at quitting smoking (Mermelstein et al., 1986). An important footnote to these findings of increased social support facilitating cessation is that support seems to have the opposite effect if the significant other is a smoker; a significant other who smokes seems to enhance likelihood of relapse (Mermelstein et al., 1986).

SPECIALIZED MODULES

Specialized modules are, by definition, reserved for the "more complicated" smoker, that is, the smoker who exhibits during the triage process signs or symptoms of psychiatric or other substance abuse involvement or who is generally not motivated to quit smoking. These specialized assessments require more provider training to administer and interpret. Thus we recommend that training be conducted with anyone who desires to use specialized assessments in his/her practice. In any case, we provide a brief review of those assessments and guide the clinician in the direction of obtaining the actual assessments and training when necessary.

Specialized Assessment Module 1: Biochemical Markers

A number of biological and biochemical indices can measure strength of smoking habit and level of nicotine in the smoker's body. *Carbon monoxide* (CO) is a crude index of very recent smoking ($\leq$ 12 hours) or exposure to cigarette smoking (Kozlowski & Herlig, 1988), though it is imperfectly associated with actual levels of nicotine in the blood (Kozlowski & Herlig, 1988) and with self-report measures of nicotine dependence (Fagerstrom & Schneider, 1989). Obtaining CO levels requires the use of relatively expensive equipment (e.g., more than $1,200 for some units) that can detect CO up to about 12 hours after smoking (Kozlowski & Herlig, 1988).

The primary nicotinic metabolite cotinine is a more stable measure of recent tobacco smoking (half-life of 11–20 hours) and may be assessed in almost any bodily fluid, most commonly saliva. The cost of having these samples analyzed varies between $30 and $80, depending on the type of biochemical assay used. Some clinicians have used cotinine levels to optimize the degree of nicotine replacement, for example, by measuring steady state levels prior to quitting, starting nicotine replacement, reassessing cotinine, and adjusting the dose of nicotine replacement to achieve levels comparable to those prior to quitting (Lawson et al., 1998). It is thought that more complete replacement results in better control of craving and withdrawal symptoms and greater ease of quitting. This type of ongoing biochemical assessment is quite expensive, both in terms of assay costs and time.

These biochemical indices are most often used in the context of treatment to (1) give the provider an objective sense of the level of the smoker's addiction to cigarettes and (2) provide feedback to the smoker as to the level and seriousness of his/her smoking. Providing this sort of biochemical feedback to smokers can have a beneficial treatment impact. These specific treatment components are reviewed in Chapter 3.

Specialized Assessment Module 2: Psychopathology

It is important to bear in mind that the assessments of psychopathology that we suggest be administered during the triage process are intended only to be screening devices. More intensive assessments of psychopathology should be administered to persons who showed positive signs of psychopathology during the triage process or, alternatively, who develop possible symptoms of psychopathology during treatment.

The Center for Epidemiologic Studies Depression Scale (CES-D; Radloff, 1977) is a 20-item scale that has been used in past research studies to identify level of depressive symptoms among smokers (Anda et al., 1990). We have used it in our own clinical work and have found it to be extremely useful in distinguishing level of depressive symptoms among smokers. Frequency responses are made according to the smoker's feelings during the previous week. A score of 16 is useful in differentiating depressed from nondepressed persons. Smokers who score above a 16 are candidates for more intensive treatment, perhaps involving mood management treatment within the context of smoking treatment (Chapter 6), referral to a provider who specializes in treating depression, or treatment with an antidepressant in the context of the smoking treatment.

Assessing more severe psychopathology requires the use of more intensive assessments. For example, the Structured Clinical Interview for DSM-III-R, Non-Patient Edition (SCID-NP; Spitzer, Williams, Gibbon, & First, 1990) is a structured interview that yields reliable and valid diagnoses of DSM-III-R Axis I disorders. Because the SCID-NP is a complex instrument to administer, a training protocol has been developed (Spitzer et al., 1990), complete with written materials, training manuals, and videotaped role plays of proper diagnostic interviewing using the SCID (please note that the SCID-NP also can be administered to diagnose past and current depressive symptoms). The Schizophrenia and Affective Disorders Schedule (SADS; see Mannuzza, Fryer, Klein, & Endicott, 1986) is a structured interview that can yield reliable and valid psychiatric diagnoses but that also requires some training. Note that the entire interviews need not be administered; for example, you can use only certain modules, such as those for mood or anxiety disorders.

Self-report instruments that yield DSM diagnoses and that may be more easily administered include PRIME-MD (Spitzer et al., 1994) and the Psychiatric Diagnostic Screening Questionnaire (PDSQ; Zimmerman & Mattia, 2001). Other specialized assessments include daily mood monitoring, an inventory of positive and negative thoughts, and a pleasant events schedule (Levinson, Shapiro, Schwartz, & Tursky, 1971). These tools can be used to help tailor treatment for smoking cessation in the presence of comorbid mood disorders. A complete description of the measures and their use is provided in Chapter 6.

Specialized Assessment Module 3: Other Substance Use

As with the triage assessments of psychopathology, the triage assessments of other substance abuse are also intended to be only screening assessments. More intensive assessments of other substance abuse can be administered to any individual whose results from the triage are positive for substance abuse. Alternatively, given that some smokers will be followed for more extended periods of time, it is possible that indications of substance misuse will appear during the course of smoking treatment (e.g., routinely missing appointments with inadequate explanations, demonstrating signs of intoxication during treatment).

CAGE questions provide a relatively straightforward method for assessing whether alcohol is problematic for an individual. CAGE is an acronym for "Cut-down," "Annoyed," "Guilty," and "Eye-opener," which are mnemonics for recalling four questions that assess for potential alcohol problems and that are valid for this use among smokers (Pomerleau, Aubin, & Pomerleau, 1997). (C = Have you ever thought you should CUT DOWN on your drinking?; A = Have you ever felt ANNOYED by others' criticism of your drinking?; G = Have you ever felt GUILTY about your drinking?; E = Do you have a morning EYE OPENER?) The Alcohol Dependence Scale (ADS; Skinner & Allen, 1982) is a relatively brief questionnaire that assesses physical dependence on alcohol—more specifically, the likelihood of experiencing withdrawal symptoms on stopping alcohol use on a continuous scale. It may be an indication that the individual is in need of stepping up to a more intensive level of treatment. The Cocaine Abuse Assessment Profile (CAAP) is a lengthy questionnaire that describes many aspects of cocaine use, but a 38-item subscale assesses the strength of the respondents' dependence on cocaine (Washton et al., 1988). Individuals who score above a 10 on this subscale are probably more dependent on cocaine and may have more difficulty in stopping smoking. The CAAP also has a set of items that assess frequency of use of other drugs (e.g., heroin, hallucinogens). Individuals who have higher scores on any of these assessments probably have substance abuse problems that should be addressed. The SCID-NP and SADS also contain modules that assess other substance abuse and dependence across a wide array of substances.

TREATMENT ASSESSMENTS: CASE EXAMPLES

We have devoted lengthy sections of this chapter to reviewing the assessments that you can administer to smokers under your care with an eye toward delivering the most effective treatment possible to them. Indeed, conducting a triage assessment and administering even one or two basic-module brief assessments to smokers have the potential to provide you with a wealth of information that you can use to help that smoker quit smoking. The difficulty with treatment assessments, as with triage assessments, is that so much information is available to you that it can seem nearly impossible to know what to do with it; for example, how do you weigh the different information from the different modules to help guide treatment? Which information do you present to smokers? When does the information dictate that you refer the patient out? As a guide, we provide some case examples that include both triage and treatment information.

CASE EXAMPLES

CASE EXAMPLE 1: MRS. D.

Background Information

Mrs. D. is a 48-year-old married woman who was admitted to an inpatient general hospital for a lower left lobe pneumonia and exacerbation of chronic obstructive pulmonary disease (COPD). As a clinical social worker assigned to manage her case, you are preparing her discharge papers and placing them in her medical record when you notice that her admission note stated that she smokes a pack of cigarettes per day. You telephone her physician to ask him about her smoking, and he replies that he's "been after her for years to stop" and that she often tries, but relapses after only a few days, even with nicotine replacement. He sounds exasperated and ends the conversation by stating that he has "pretty much given up on her quitting." You ask if he would mind if you spoke with her about quitting, to which he replies "Good luck."

Triage and Disposition

You have very little time to see the smoker (by your estimates, about 10 minutes), as her daughter has arrived to take her home. You have none of the triage assessments with you on paper but decide to proceed by asking her the questions before she leaves.

You approach her and reintroduce yourself to her (you met her before to discuss discharge planning). You ask if she could answer a few more questions for you before she leaves, specifically about her smoking. She replies, "I don't smoke anymore, I can't even breathe, but ask away." She appears motivated (she reports that she never wants to smoke again), so you decide not to ask about her motivation. However, you decide to ask the following triage assessments and get the following results:

Dependence: Smokes when she gets to work (about 2 hours after waking)
   Smokes 10 cigarettes per day
Past quit attempts: Quit five times in the past
   Most recent time was 9 months ago for 2 weeks
Substance abuse: None reported
Psychiatric history: None reported

You congratulate Mrs. D. for not smoking and indicate to her that it seems as though she is on her way to success. Privately, however, you question the degree of success that she will have with cessation; given your limited time with her, you decide to ask her a few additional questions and, based on those results, conduct a brief smoking intervention with her that focuses on relapse prevention (see Chapter 5).

Treatment Assessments

The briefer assessments from Basic Module 1 are your target, and your desire is to assess her ability to cope with high-risk situations. You first ask about three occasions on which she is sure to smoke and how she might prevent smoking in those situations. She is able to identify (1) work, (2) stress, and (3) after dinnertime as three sure triggers, and when asked how she would cope, she replies "I just won't smoke." This response indicates to you that she is lacking in coping skills that could potentially help her to not smoke. Therefore, you engage in brief coping skills training with her (see Chapter 4) for 5 minutes and give her your card should she need help with smoking cessation issues in the future.

Comment

Mrs. D. presents an interesting case. She had essentially a "forced abstinence" due to her hospitalization and as a result apparently decided that she would not smoke again. Her past history suggested that she had experience with quitting but that something was continually preventing her from maintaining abstinence. The assessment had to be brief and to the point and to focus on those issues that were relevant to treatment. Despite the fact that you had no real prior relationship with Mrs. D., your brief assessment of coping revealed that she apparently had not tried any other coping strategies to help her aside from "not smoking." This information allowed a focused brief intervention to take place.

CASE EXAMPLE 2: MR. S.

Background Information

Mr. S. is a 45-year-old married man whom you have seen on a regular basis in your internal medicine practice for the past 15 years. You generally see him once per year for his annual physical, and he is generally in good health (except for the occasional common cold). However, you know that he smokes about two packs of cigarettes per day; you have discussed quitting smoking with him in the past and have administered smoking triage assessments to him during the past two years; however, he has never expressed any interest in quitting and, in fact, seems to ignore you when you have attempted to do some brief motivational interviewing with him (see Chapter 3). Thus you have typically given any talk of smoking cessation a lower health priority than other issues (e.g., Mr. S.'s hypertension). During this most recent visit, however, you notice something different about his triage assessment results (compared with last year's results):

Ladder:　8 (an increase of 5 points)

FTQ score:　10 (same)

Most recent quit attempts:　Made one attempt to quit smoking in the past year (previously had no quit attempts), which lasted for about 24 hours.

Substance use:　Answers "no" to all questions (same as before)

Psychiatric history:　Reports feeling acutely depressed for about 1 month during the past year after his father died; no treatment sought (none previously reported)

You weigh two key factors in thinking about what type of treatment would be most appropriate for Mr. S. First, you note that he is highly nicotine dependent and, second, that he has no real history of not smoking. Although it was significant for the time during which it occurred, you decide not to weigh his apparently grief-related depressed moods heavily in your decision (you have known Mr. S. for 15 years and have never known him to be depressed and know that he has no significant psychiatric or substance abuse history). In any case, you decide that a more intensive treatment is appropriate for Mr. S., one that particularly involves some form of pharmacotherapy (see Chapter 4). Your initial plan (without taking Mr. S.'s preferences into account) is to refer him to a formalized clinic-based smoking cessation program (see Chapter 5).

Treatment Assessments

After examining Mr. S., you ask him about his motivation to quit smoking and share the results of the triage assessments. He says that he finds the results interesting and asks about options for treatment, which you subsequently discuss with him, emphasizing that a more intensive approach is probably a good option for him. However, he is hesitant to take on the responsibility of attending weekly smoking cessation sessions due to the cost and his work schedule. He asks whether you, as his physician, could help him particularly by providing him with the nicotine patch. You discuss the pros and cons of each form of treatment again, though he is insistent that he does not want any more formalized treatment. You agree to help him quit smoking but want to find out a bit more about his smoking habit so that you can better tailor your brief treatment (see Chapter 4). You have about 20 minutes in which to conduct an assessment and deliver your treatment. You decide to administer orally the shortest assessment (Option 1) from Module 1 (Smoking Triggers; see Table 2.8).

He reports that three consistent triggers for his smoking are: "first thing in the morning"; "with coffee in the morning"; and "in the car on the way to work." You find out from him that he smokes primarily in these situations because of an intense craving and that he would hate to give up the first cigarette of the day. Given that he stated that "intense cravings" are the reasons that he invariably smokes in these situations, you ask him to compare other cravings during the day to the cravings he experiences in these situations (Module 2, Craving Assessment Option 1, Table 2.12). He reports that his cravings in these situations are "an 11" on the 10-point scale, but that his cravings during other times of the day rate between 3 and 6.

This information suggests to you that Mr. S. is probably experiencing intense cravings in the morning due, in part, to the fact that he is depriving his body of nicotine while he sleeps (i.e., he has to "load up" on nicotine in the morning), whereas his cigarettes during the rest of the day are more externally stimulus bound. Based on this information and his high score on the FTQ, you recommend to him that he use some form of nicotine replacement (Chapter 7). You also mention to him that the nicotine patch will not necessarily prevent his cravings in all situations and that he must execute coping strategies in order to successfully manage other cravings and situations (see Chapter 5). At the end of your session with him, you contract to a quit date 1 week later.

Comment

The case of Mr. S. illustrates how repeated assessments over time can benefit smokers who may initially not want to quit. It also demonstrates the manner in which treatment options can be negotiated with the smoker's preferences in mind and how the triage assessments and smoking trigger assessments led to a more in-depth assessment of cravings as triggers and ultimately led to treatment recommendations.

CONCLUDING REMARKS

A critical factor to remember when treating smokers is that no two are alike and that no two smokers' experiences with quitting will be the same. The key to successful treatment is to find out which factors are important to a smoker's chances of success and to use those factors to inform treatment planning and delivery. Our goal in this chapter was to provide you with guidance in assessing factors that are important to smoking cessation and with a flexible set of decision rules to apply when determining what sorts of treatments are appropriate for your patients who are smokers. Figure 2.2 depicts a general triage and assessment decision tree.

Note that triage begins with assessment of motivation, which then triggers a decision to deal with motivational issues or, if the smoker is ready, to plan for action. Triage and assessment intensity is stepped up, although still brief. Out of necessity or desire, questions concerning past quit attempts, nicotine dependence, other substance use, and psychiatric disorders may then be used to guide preliminary decisions concerning the intensity of behavioral treatment (brief vs. intensive) and whether to consider adding some form of pharmacotherapy. If time permits, assessment intensity should be increased, with the addi-

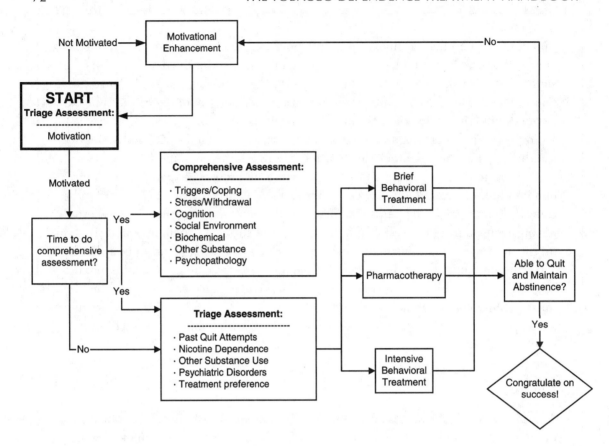

FIGURE 2.2. Assessment and treatment planning.

tion of basic modules that assess triggers/coping, stress/withdrawal, cognition, and the social environment. These assessments should be used to determine not only the intensity of behavioral therapy but also certain components of therapy. The assessments may also point to options for pharmacotherapy. The triage assessments of nicotine dependence, other substance use, and psychiatric disorders can also be thought of as brief screening instruments that, when positive, indicate further assessment, including biochemical measures and assessment of comorbid conditions, other substance use, and psychopathology. Comorbid drug use and psychiatric conditions potentially complicate smoking cessation treatment and may require referral for treatment of these conditions and coordination of care with other health care providers.

We encourage you, however, to use the algorithms and decision trees as a starting point for your work with smokers. Your clinical judgment, knowledge of the smoker, unique relationship with that smoker, and capacity to have extended contact with the smoker all are equally important in the treatment services you deliver to that individual. An ideal setting is one in which there is an interactive blend of the information in this chapter and your unique treatment situation. Such a marriage does not necessarily mean that the smoker will stop smoking for good on the first try, but it does mean that his/her chances of stopping successfully the next time have improved significantly.

3

Increasing Motivation to Stop Smoking

Karen M. Emmons

For many years, smoking interventions were designed exclusively to target smoking cessation, and little emphasis was placed on helping individuals who did not have short-term plans to quit smoking (e.g., within the next month). Although 90% of smokers state that they want to quit smoking, the vast majority (70%) are not ready to quit in the next 6 months, and even fewer (20%) would actually be willing to quit in the next 30 days (Abrams & Biener, 1992; Velicer et al., 1995). Instructing smokers who are not interested in quitting about how to quit smoking can lead to resistance from the smoker and frustration for both you and the smoker. This mismatch between smoker readiness to change and treatment strategies has led to new motivation-based intervention approaches, which are the focus of this chapter.

As outlined in Chapter 1, smoking is a chronic refractory condition requiring a long-term and consistent treatment plan. Over time, a smoker's motivation can be thought of as his/her "readiness to change," ranging from the low extreme (i.e., no interest in quitting at any time in the future because the smoker has made an informed choice to smoke and wants to be respected for that decision and left alone) to the high extreme (i.e., ready to quit immediately and willing to persist until successful) of the range. The treatment plan allows for the waxing and waning of motivation and also permits "recycling" and multiple quit attempts as smokers learn the skills they need to master all the steps along the pathway to permanent cessation. Maintaining high levels of motivation can encourage a smoker to consider making a quit attempt sooner rather than later and can improve adherence during cessation treatment.

As a treatment provider, your key goals are to move smokers along the continuum of readiness to change and to increase or maintain their motivation to actively engage in the change process. Many researchers believe that motivation can be best enhanced through interpersonal relationships such as counseling strategies delivered by a provider within a trusting, empathic, and "smoker-centered" (i.e., client- or patient-centered) treatment philosophy. The way you approach a smoker can have a significant impact on his/her receptivity to treatment. In today's climate, in which smokers face substantial antismoking social pressure, it is important to approach the issue of smoking respectfully and sensitively. Smokers' unique past experiences with being pressured to quit, failure to quit despite their best efforts, and personality styles (e.g., how they respond to others' requests that they change; their guilt, shame, or fear of letting themselves or others down) must be gently elicited, empathetically understood, and taken into account. Smokers may try to avoid, deny, or minimize the need to consider smoking cessation. In particular, it may be more productive to gently address smoking on an ongoing basis than to try to convince smokers who are not ready that they need to quit smoking. Throughout this chapter, I provide suggestions for counseling styles and strategies that can be effective with smokers of varying levels of motivation to quit smoking and that are based on an individual assessment of the smokers' knowledge, beliefs, and attitudes.

Over the past several years, there has been increased attention to the role that motivation plays in an individual's likelihood of trying to quit smoking and in their ultimate success in doing so. It is now widely recognized that smoking interventions must build motivation for cessation first and then provide individuals with skills needed to quit when they are ready. Moreover, maintaining motivation throughout the entire treatment process is critical, because motivation can influence adherence to coping skills treatments, can increase the likelihood of proper medication use, and can encourage rapid recycling (e.g., new quit attempts) should the smoker have a temporary "slip" back into smoking after he/she has quit.

ASSESSMENT OF MOTIVATION

There are several reasons that smokers may not be interested in or willing to make a commitment to quit smoking. These individuals may be less convinced or concerned about the impact of smoking on their own health. Further, they may be concerned about the effects of quitting (e.g., withdrawal, weight gain, irritability, difficulty handling stress), demoralized, or afraid of failing again because of previous relapse; or they may have other concerns and priorities that are more pressing (e.g., stress at work or home, domestic or neighborhood violence, poverty, unstable housing situation). It is important to assess a smoker's motivational status, as well as the factors that may be affecting his/her readiness to quit smoking.

Several brief motivational assessments can be used in a variety of settings. This discussion is limited to those strategies that are most practical for time-limited counseling (e.g., in a busy medical office) and those that have been most rigorously evaluated, including the readiness ladder, stages of change, locus (intrinsic vs. extrinsic) of motivation to quit, and barriers to change.

It is important to note that a nonjudgmental, open dialogue is important to minimize the social pressure smokers can feel when discussing their smoking behavior (see Table 3.1 for examples of questions that can be used for this purpose). Smokers who feel "lectured at" are less likely to ask for help when they are ready to quit, or, worse, they may not tell you that they smoke. Counseling will be most effective if you can be a good listener and meet the smoker where he/she is and adjust your strategy to be sensitive to the smokers' current beliefs and needs.

TABLE 3.1. Suggested Questions for Creating a Nonjudgmental Approach When Addressing Smoking

"More and more of my smoking clients/patients tell me that they get a lot of pressure about smoking from their family and friends. How about you? If so, how does that make you feel? I can understand those feelings."

"There's a lot of pressure on smokers these days. But sometimes people who smoke have other pressures that make it difficult to think about quitting. How about you, where does quitting fit into your priorities?"

"Smokers hear a lot about how much smoking hurts their health. But there are lots of other factors to consider when you think about smoking. What are some of the things that you think about regarding your smoking or quitting?"

[Pros of smoking] "What do you like about smoking?" [Cons of smoking] "What do you not like about smoking?"

The following tools can help you conceptualize and assess your patients' positions on the continuum of motivation and the beliefs and expectations they have that could be the focus of treatment to increase motivation.

CONCEPTUAL MODELS OF MOTIVATION

Stages of Change

The *Stages of Change* or *Transtheoretical Model* (Prochaska & DiClemente, 1983; Prochaska et al., 1997) hypothesizes that change occurs in distinct steps or stages. This model can be used to assess motivational level. Five different stages of readiness to quit smoking have been identified. Table 3.2 demonstrates assessment of the following stages.

TABLE 3.2. Stages of Change Algorithm for Assessing Readiness to Change

Smokers

Are you seriously thinking about quitting smoking in the next 6 months?

    Yes   No ⟶ Precontemplator (stop questioning)
    ↓

Are you planning to quit smoking in the next 30 days?

    Yes   No ⟶ Contemplator (stop questioning)
    ↓

Have you quit smoking for at least 24 hours in the past year?

    Yes   No ⟶ Contemplator (stop questioning)
    ↓

Preparation stage

Ex-smokers

Did you quit:

    within the last 6 months? ⟶ Action
    more than 6 months ago? ⟶ Maintenance

Precontemplation

Individuals in precontemplation are not at all interested in quitting smoking and have no specific plans to change their behavior in the foreseeable future. Individuals who state that they are not planning to quit smoking within the *next 6 months* are in the precontemplation stage. Your main task is to understand the smoker's reasons for smoking and his/her fears about quitting. Over time, you can begin to raise doubt in the precontemplator's mind about the perceived benefits of smoking and increase his/her perception of the risks associated with smoking. Within the category of precontemplation are those smokers who have made an active decision to remain smokers. These individuals are likely to resist motivational strategies, and their decision to remain smokers may have to be respected. Precontemplators are the least ready to change and may take the longest time to quit. A strong provider–smoker relationship forms the basis for continuity of care and thus permits the long-term goals to be achieved.

Contemplation

Individuals in contemplation are considering quitting smoking in the next 6 months but not in the next 30 days. As with precontemplation, the primary intervention goal is to enhance motivation for change. However, because the contemplator has at least started to consider smoking cessation as an option, your tasks can be focused on tipping the balance toward change by eliciting reasons to change and strengthening the smoker's self-efficacy for change (W. R. Miller & Rollnick, 2002).

Preparation

Individuals in preparation are planning to quit smoking in the next 30 days, have tried to quit in the past year, and they may have already taken some steps to change their smoking patterns, such as cutting down on the number of cigarettes they smoke each day. The primary intervention focus for these individuals is helping them to make a sustained quit attempt that will lead to long-term abstinence. They are ready to quit (see Chapters 4–7).

Action

Individuals in the action stage have recently quit smoking (within the past 6 months), and the primary focus is on relapse prevention. Your efforts are focused on identifying barriers to sustained abstinence and helping smokers to develop coping strategies that will be effective in a wide variety of situations (see Chapters 4–7).

Maintenance

Individuals in the maintenance stage have quit smoking for more than 6 months. Although less effort is usually required than in the action stage, individuals in maintenance need to be vigilant to prevent relapse.

Precaution Adoption Process

The stages of change model has received considerable research attention and applied interest. Recent research suggests that this model may be a good strategy for structuring interventions but that it may have some weaknesses (Fiore et al., 2000) related to the ability of the model's components to predict change in smoking status via stage-based mechanisms (A. Farkas, Pierce, Gilpin, et al., 1996; Herzog, Abrams, Emmons, Linnan, & Shadel, 1999; Sutton, 1996; N. D. Weinstein, 1993). There are other stage-based motivational models that make important contributions to understanding the change process.

The precaution adoption model (PAM; N. Weinstein, 1988) comprises a series of six distinct stages in which people process information related to risks. Within these six stages, the first three are related to awareness and personal assessment of risk and the last three are related to the decision to act. These stages are described as follows (questions to assess the steps are provided in Table 3.3):

Stage 1. Unaware of the risk
Stage 2. Acknowledges the risk to others, but not to the self
Stage 3. Acknowledges the risk to the self and considers changing to reduce risk
Stage 4. Decides to act or to not act (if decisions is not to act, the process ends here)
Stage 5. Adopts the behavior change
Stage 6. Maintains behavior change over time.

Unlike the stages of change model, PAM does not utilize a time domain in categorizing stages; it has been suggested that the time domain adds an artificial dimension to the process of change and is not appropriate for stage-based models (Sutton, 1996; N. Weinstein, Rothman, & Sutton, 1998). An important aspect of this model is that it takes into account the notion that individuals do not judge each risk factor independently but rather in the context

---

TABLE 3.3. Questions to Elicit Stage of Precaution Adoption

STAGE 1: Unaware of the Risk
- Have you heard anything about the effect of smoking on health? What have you heard?
- Have you heard anything about the effect of being exposed to smoke on nonsmokers' and children's health? What have you heard?

STAGE 2: Acknowledges Risk to Others
- Who (or what kind of people) do you think would be most likely to be affected by smoking?
- Has smoking affected your life in any way? Do you think it will?

STAGE 3: Acknowledges Risk to Self
- What do you think are the greatest risks to your health? Are you considering changing any of these risks?
- Has smoking affected your life in any way? Do you think it will?

STAGE 4: Decides to Act
- What are the steps you are planning to take to change your smoking?

STAGE 5: Adopts the Behavior Change

STAGE 6: Maintains the Behavior Change

of their other life risks. Individuals who know about a hazard tend to deny their own suscepti-bility to that risk factor (N. Weinstein, 1980, 1984, 1987). This denial can lead to selective at-tention to information that supports these faulty beliefs and to optimistic bias or the incorrect assumption that personal risk is less than that faced by others (e.g., "Smokers who are over-weight are at risk, but I'm not at risk because I am physically fit"). Further, positive beliefs that quitting smoking can achieve a desired goal can strengthen a smoker's perseverance in the quitting process (N. Weinstein, 1988). Provision of personalized physiological or risk in-formation, along with information addressing effectiveness of change on reducing risk, can be an important strategy for targeting the beliefs and biases that maintain risk behaviors (these issues are addressed in a later section).

Readiness Ladder

Another strategy for assessing motivation to quit smoking is the readiness ladder (Biener & Abrams, 1991). This tool uses a visual representation of the continuum of change and has some advantages over other motivational screening tools in terms of its conceptual, practical, and statistical properties (see Figure 2.1). Its primary advantage from a practical perspective is that it visually represents the change process as "climbing a ladder" and can serve as a use-ful means of discussing with smokers how they can move from lower rungs of the ladder to the higher ones that represent higher levels of motivation. Thus it is easily understood by people with varying levels of education and cognitive ability and from different cultural back-grounds. It also does not exclusively utilize a time-based conceptualization of readiness and thus may more closely match the change process than those that impose time constraints (Sutton, 1996).

Inspection of the readiness ladder (Figure 2.1) shows that it incorporates the stages of change classification system but goes into more fine-grained gradations within stages. These gradations can be helpful to you the provider in planning and tailoring a motivational inter-vention. For example, a rating of 1 on the ladder corresponds to the most recalcitrant smoker. About 8–12% of smokers endorse rung 1, and generally they are so resistant to considering cessation that they may not be willing to engage in such a dialogue even if you use the most extreme neutral, nonjudgmental stance. In brief, they have made up their minds to smoke, and they are willing to take the risks. They want to be left alone. Those who endorse rungs 2 through 5 are all precontemplators, but clearly a smoker who endorses a 4 or 5 rung is closer to a contemplator and is more motivated than a smoker who rates 2 or 3. Approximately 30–40% of smokers will endorse rungs 2 through 5. Rung 6 is equivalent to the contemplation stage. About 30–40% of smokers endorse this rung of the readiness ladder. Rung 7 and higher indicates that the smoker is ready to quit (preparation stage) in the next 30 days, is in the pro-cess of quitting, has recently quit, or is in long-term maintenance. Rung 10 represents those who have become permanent nonsmokers and who have little concern that they will relapse. Consider any smoker or ex-smoker with less than 12 months of continuous abstinence at risk for relapse. Ideally, your treatment plan should remain active to ensure that the smoker or re-cent quitter continues to receive your support and encouragement. Thus any smoker in the maintenance stage (less than 6 months since quitting) or any smoker who scores 9 or less on the readiness ladder should remain in active treatment or follow-up.

Internal versus External Locus of Motivation to Quit

In addition to the level of motivation for smoking cessation, some researchers have noted the importance of the locus or types of motivation an individual has (Curry, Wagner, & Grothaus, 1991). Two primary types of motivation have been noted: (1) internal motivation, in which the impetus for change is driven by internal factors such as health concerns and self-control; and (2) external motivation, in which factors such as anticipation of immediate rewards and social pressure are the impetus for change. It has been found that individuals with high levels of internal motivation are more successful at long-term cessation. Assessing type of motivation allows providers to identify patients with whom an emphasis on internal sources of motivation might be helpful (see Table 2.16). Smokers who have high internal motivation to quit may need less assistance throughout the process, whereas smokers with higher external motivation may be more vulnerable to relapse, as they are more influenced in quitting by external and perhaps unstable factors. Helping smokers who have high external motivation to identify internal sources may be an effective way of helping these individuals stay abstinent.

Barriers to Quitting Smoking

Several key theoretical perspectives on health behavior change emphasize the importance of removing barriers to change (Curry & Emmons, 1994). Barriers not only can reduce an individual's motivation to change but also can increase the risk of relapse following a quit attempt. Thus it may be first necessary to address some of these barriers as a prerequisite to focusing on smoking. Barriers to change often fall into one of four categories: (1) physical and/or social barriers (e.g., living with a smoker; working in an environment in which smoking is allowed); (2) psychological or emotional barriers that make the smoker feel he/she cannot survive or live without cigarettes (e.g., stress; depression, anxiety, or substance use comorbidity; concern about weight gain); (3) barriers to access (e.g., to health education campaigns; to the ability to purchase nicotine replacement therapy; to the availability and cost of smoking cessation programs); or (4) social contextual or life circumstances barriers that may result in a smoker giving smoking cessation a low priority (e.g., poverty; living in an unsafe neighborhood; social isolation). The specific barriers may vary by population. Table 3.4 provides an example of a barriers checklist that can be used to help assess these factors. Focusing on removing these barriers to change can be an important way to enhance motivation and start the behavior change process.

The Decisional Balance Scale is another method of assessing barriers to change. As discussed in Chapter 2, this scale assesses factors that are supportive of smoking (pros), as well as the factors that are supportive of change (cons; see Table 2.14). In precontemplation, the pros of smoking outweigh the cons. It has been hypothesized that, as individuals move through the stages of readiness to change, the balance of pros to cons shifts, with more emphasis being placed on the cons of the target behavior (Velicer et al., 1985). For smoking, that means that you can help smokers who have higher scores on the pros of smoking subscale to begin to talk about things they do not like about smoking (e.g., the cost, the smell, social pressure).

TABLE 3.4. Barriers to Smoking Cessation Checklist

INSTRUCTIONS: *Please indicate the extent to which each of the following factors influences your thoughts about quitting smoking.*

	Not at all	Somewhat	A lot
There are too many difficult things going on in my life right now.	1	2	3
Without cigarettes, I would feel too anxious or worried about things.	1	2	3
Without cigarettes, I would feel too down or sad.	1	2	3
Without cigarettes, I would feel too irritable to be around.	1	2	3
I enjoy smoking too much to give it up.	1	2	3
It would be too hard to control my weight without smoking.	1	2	3
Smoking helps me control other behaviors that I have already changed.	1	2	3
My family and friends don't think it is important to quit smoking.	1	2	3
I don't know how to go about quitting smoking.	1	2	3
I have tried to quit smoking in the past so many times, I've given up.	1	2	3
I can't afford or find a smoking cessation program.	1	2	3

OPPORTUNITIES FOR ENHANCING MOTIVATION

Several naturally occurring opportunities often rise within a counseling relationship for enhancing smokers' motivation to quit smoking.

Review of Personal Life Goals

Participation in other forms of health-related counseling often offers the opportunity to review one's long-term life goals and to consider how current lifestyle behaviors may affect one's ability to eventually reach those goals. For example, a smoker who is in mental health or alcohol counseling may be considering reasons for reducing his drinking, including his desire to be a more active grandparent. Smoking may also get in the way of his goal of being a good role model as a grandparent. Review of how smoking may affect the ability to reach one's goals can be a useful strategy for starting the process of thinking about smoking cessation.

Provision of Routine Medical Care and Presentation of the Results of Medical Tests

Physical exams and regular medical care visits offer an important opportunity for demonstrating to smokers the role that smoking plays in their general health functioning and well-being. For example, when smokers have an echocardiogram or pulmonary function test, health care providers have an opportunity to place the results in the context of the patient's smoking status. For patients whose results are in the normal range but could still be improved, these results can be presented as an "early warning" of the impact of smoking on health. Sometimes even long-term, heavy smokers will receive excellent test results; with these patients, providers should emphasize the importance of smoking cessation as a strategy to prevent future deterioration. It is important for health care providers to realize that if they do *not* mention smoking to their smoking patients, it will be interpreted as tacit approval of smoking and/or as evidence that smoking has not and will not affect the patient's health (see later section on "Feedback" for further examples and illustrations).

For providers of smoking cessation counseling in nonmedical settings, a treatment plan could include referral and working with a health care provider to enhance motivation. Moreover, during counseling, the smokers' report of physical symptoms (shortness of breath, persistent cough, lowering of sexual performance, etc.) can be used to suggest a referral to a physician and inclusion of the physician in the treatment. In addition, as smokers who are in substance abuse or alcohol treatment programs achieve success on these behavioral targets, it is important to point out that many of the skills needed to stop substance or alcohol abuse are similar to those needed to stop smoking. More substance abusers or alcoholics die of smoking-related causes than of their substance abuse. When smokers realize that they can apply these skills to other behaviors, it can have a positive impact on their self-efficacy. There is also evidence that smoking cessation may prevent relapse to alcohol or substance abuse (Abrams et al., 1995).

Treatment of Acute Illnesses

When smokers present with acute illnesses, health care providers have another opportunity to build motivation for smoking cessation. A large proportion of pulmonary and cardiovascular illnesses and cancers are directly related to smoking, and many other illnesses are exacerbated by smoking (see Table 1.1). However, there are some barriers to providing counseling during sick visits, most notably the limited time available during these visits. However, even a very brief discussion about the impact of smoking on the development and treatment of the presenting illness and provision of written materials about smoking can help smokers begin to reevaluate their smoking status and can set the stage for continued counseling at subsequent visits.

Hospitalization

Hospitalization provides a very important opportunity for building motivation for smoking cessation. First, because all accredited hospitals in the United States are required by the Joint Commission on Accreditation of Healthcare Organizations (JCAHO) to be smoke free, hospitalization provides smokers with experience in smoking cessation. For those who find cessation during their hospital stay relatively easy, motivation for trying to stay abstinent after hospitalization may be increased. For those who find it more difficult, providing support for refraining from smoking during hospitalization is an important way to enhance patients' ability to quit in the short term, as well as to enhance their confidence in their ability to quit smoking. Many hospitals now have smoking cessation counseling services. In addition, nicotine replacement therapy (NRT) offers an important strategy for helping nicotine-dependent smokers refrain from smoking during hospitalization and following discharge (see Chapter 7 for more details on NRT). Unfortunately, NRT is greatly underutilized in hospital settings, with only 7% of hospitalized smokers being prescribed nicotine gum or a transdermal nicotine patch during hospitalization (Emmons et al., 2000). In addition to these opportunities for enhancing motivation in the context of general medical care delivery, other motivational opportunities exist with specific target groups.

Patients with Alcohol and Substance Abuse Susceptibility

Although many providers in the substance abuse and alcohol treatment communities believe that smoking cessation places recovering alcoholics and addicts at risk for relapse, there is little evidence in the literature to suggest that this is actually the case. On the contrary, providing former alcoholics, for example, with a supported opportunity to consider smoking cessation may be an important way to enhance their sense of self-efficacy and motivation to change. In addition, many of the skills needed to change one addictive behavior can transfer to another, such as smoking. Consideration of cosobriety is important in both the assessment and counseling of smokers.

Women of Childbearing Age

The context of gynecological care for women of childbearing age is an important opportunity to educate women who smoke and plan to have children about the importance of quitting smoking *before* conception (Jack, Campanile, McQuade, & Kogan, 1995). Smokers who become pregnant require special counseling efforts because of the impact of their smoking on the pregnancy outcome. Many women reduce their smoking rate during pregnancy, which can provide a great start toward quitting smoking. Women who live with smokers may have a particularly difficult time quitting smoking during pregnancy and may need extra support. It should also be noted that health care providers have become much more diligent about asking pregnant women about their smoking status. Although this is excellent from a health care delivery perspective, some investigators have noted that women may feel undue pressure and judgment about smoking during pregnancy and therefore may be more likely to misreport their smoking status. Health care providers and smoking cessation counselors can minimize the likelihood of false reporting by fostering a sense of trust and support and by reassuring women that they will work together on whatever goals the smoker sets, no matter what her smoking status is. Table 3.5 includes a list of resources that have been developed for special populations, including pregnant women.

Parents of Young Children

Knowledge of the impact of their smoking on family members, particularly children, is an important motivational factor for many smokers. The detrimental health consequences of environmental tobacco smoke are well established (Environmental Protection Agency, 1992; see Table 3.6), although many smokers may either be unaware of these concerns or may not fully believe them (Pirie, Murray, & Luepker, 1991). Therefore, discussion of a parent's smoking within the context of their child's medical care, for example, has been found to be an important strategy for increasing the likelihood of smoking cessation (Emmons & Wall, 1999; Hovell et al., 2000; Wall, Severson, Andrews, & Lichtenstein, 1995). This strategy can be

TABLE 3.5. Selected Cessation Resources

Title	Audience		Focus
Language	Source	Cost	
"Healthy Moms, Healthy Kids"	Pregnant women		Motivation
English/Spanish	TECC[a]	$.20	
"Hey Girlfriend: Let's Talk About Smoking and You"	Pregnant Afr-Am Women		Cessation
English	TECC[a]	$.30	
"Your Family Needs a Healthy Mother"	Pregnant Afr-Am Women		Motivation
English	TECC[a]	$.10	
"Smoke Signals"	Parents		Motivation
English/Spanish/Cambodian	TECC[a]	$.10	
"Passive Smoke: Protect Your Baby & Your Loved Ones"	American Indian Women		Motivation
English	TECC[a]	$.10	
"Not Smoking Makes Your Family Healthier"	Hmong Parents		Motivation
Hmong	TECC[a]	$.10	
"Freedom From Smoking for You and Your Family"	General		Cessation
English	ALA[b]	$10.00	
"Pathways to Freedom"	African Americans		Motivation/
English	TECC[a]	$.90	Cessation
"It's All About Us"	African American Women		Motivation/
English	TECC[a]	$1.50	Cessation
"Free At Last"	African Americans		Motivation
English	TECC[a]	$.20	
"It's Your Life—It's Our Future"	American Indians		Cessation
English	TECC[a]	$.45	
"Lam The Nao De Bo Hut Thuoc"	Vietnamese Men		Cessation
Vietnamese	TECC[a]	$2.05	
"Victory Over Smoking"	Chinese Americans		Cessation
Chinese	TECC[a]	$3.40	

[a]TECC: Tobacco Education Clearinghouse of California, P.O. Box 1830, Santa Cruz, CA 95061-1830, (831)438-4822. Prices based on those listed in Sept. 1997 TECC Catalog of Tobacco Education Materials. For complete listing of resources, see TECC Catalogue or call 1-800-4CANCER for information about resources available from the National Cancer Institute.
[b]ALA: American Lung Association. Contact local ALA affiliates.

TABLE 3.6. Impact of Environmental Tobacco Smoke

Environmental tobacco smoke exposure:
1. Is a group A carcinogen
2. Increases risk for lung cancer
3. Increases risk for coronary heart disease
4. Increases children's risk of
   - developing coughs, colds
   - tonsillectomy and adenoidectomy
   - otitis media
   - sudden infant death syndrome
   - developing and exacerbating asthma
   - lower respiratory infections
   - hospitalization during first 3 years of life due to respiratory illness
   - having reduced lung function

used in the context of prevention of disease (e.g., "Your child is healthy—let's work together to keep it that way") and is particularly important in the context of treatment of family members for asthma and other respiratory disease, otitis media, and cancer. Information about the constituents of environmental tobacco smoke can also be helpful to parents as they reconsider the impact of smoking on their families (see Table 3.7).

Older and Elderly Populations

Although recent data suggest that the longer an individual smokes, the less benefit is conferred from cessation in terms of lung cancer risk (Hanrahan, Sherman, & Emmons, 1996), there are still substantial data to suggest that smoking cessation at any age provides important health benefits (Orleans, Rimer, Cristinzio, Keintz, & Fleisher, 1991). However, many older smokers may feel that it is too late for them to quit, even if they are very interested in quitting. It is important for providers to emphasize the health, financial, and social benefits of quitting smoking in the later years of life (see Tables 3.8 and 1.1).

MOTIVATIONAL INTERVIEWING

One way to integrate these intervention strategies for enhancing motivation for smoking cessation into routine care is motivational interviewing, a series of counseling strategies developed by Miller and colleagues (W. R. Miller & Rollnick, 1991) to enhance readiness to change. Motivational interviewing is an interpersonal process that places heavy emphasis on the relationship between you, the provider, and the smoker. Further, motivational interviewing is based on the premise that it is the individual smoker who has primary responsibility for change, not the provider. Therefore, your role is not to convince the smoker that he/she should change but rather to present objective information to the smoker and allow him/her to decide for him/herself. The characteristics of motivational interviewing and of the more traditional directed or confrontational approaches are outlined in Table 3.9.

Motivational interviewing and other strategies for motivational enhancement have been used effectively to address factors that can increase the likelihood of smoking cessation, such as self-efficacy (Colby et al., 1998). Motivational interviewing has also been found to influ-

---

TABLE 3.7. Constituents of Environmental Tobacco Smoke

Compared with cigarette (mainstream) smoke, environmental tobacco smoke contains
- 2 to 3 times the amount of nicotine
- 3 to 5 times the amount of carbon monoxide
- 8 to 11 times the amount of carbon dioxide
- 5 to 10 times the amount of benzene[a]
- 13 to 30 times the amount of nickel[a]
- 30 times the amount of 2-naphthylamine[a]
- 31 times the amount of 4-aminobiphenyl[a]

[a]Known animal or human carcinogen.

TABLE 3.8. Benefits of Smoking Cessation for All Smokers

Short-term benefits

- Improved circulation
- Improved sleep, taste, and smell
- Less shortness of breath
- Reduced risk of home fires
- Improved effectiveness of medications that are affected by smoking (e.g., propranolol, theophylline, insulin, phenylbutazone, as well as medications for pain, depression, anxiety, and insomnia)
- Availability of money that was previously spent on cigarettes

Longer-term benefits

- Risk of dying from a heart attack is cut by half within 1 year of quitting
- Risk of developing emphysema and bronchitis is greatly reduced
- Improved memory, compared with those who continue to smoke
- Reduced risk of osteoporosis and cervical cancer
- Increased life expectancy and quality of life

ence decision making about health behaviors. Most of the studies available that support motivational interviewing have applied this approach to problem drinking and alcohol use (W. R. Miller & Rollnick, 2002; Monti et al., 1999). Relatively few empirical studies have applied motivational interviewing to smoking (Colby et al., 1998; Emmons, 1994; Ershoff et al., 1999), but several large-scale studies are currently under way. Those studies that have been done provide considerable evidence that motivational interviewing leads to higher levels of patient satisfaction and improved patient–provider relationships. Some studies have also shown improved rates of behavior change (Emmons et al., 2001; Hovell et al., 2000).

TABLE 3.9. Characteristics of Directed/Confrontational vs. Motivational Interviewing Approaches

Counseling strategy	Confrontational approach	Motivational interviewing approach
Labeling	Heavily emphasized	Not used
Locus of decision making	Provider	Patient
Evidence for change	Presented and interpreted by provider	Presented by provider, interpreted by patient
Problem solving	Driven by provider	Guided by provider, but driven by patient
Interpretation of resistance	Denial that must be altered through confrontation	In part due to a provider's behavior; resistance can be altered by changing provider's approach and use of reflection
Goals for treatment	Set by provider	Negotiated between patient and provider
Strategies for change	Prescribed by provider	Negotiated between patient and provider

Note. Adapted from *Motivational Interviewing: Preparing People to Change Addictive Behaviors*, by W. R. Miller and S. Rollnick, 1991, New York: Guilford Press. Copyright 1991 by The Guilford Press. Adapted by permission.

Many providers are reluctant to counsel smokers about risk behaviors because they are concerned that smokers will become upset or offended. Motivational interviewing focuses on the smokers' needs or concerns and gives them the responsibility for change, while also providing a set of alternative strategies for change, each of which are effective for some individuals. In this way, motivational interviewing functions to minimize smokers' resistance. There are several key components to motivational interviewing, as outlined here. A motivational interviewing approach can be particularly useful in the context of an ongoing or established relationship, in which the repeated visits provide good opportunities to explore motivation for change on an ongoing basis. The six "active ingredients," or building blocks, of motivational interviewing are summarized in the acronym FRAMES (for more detailed discussion of motivational interviewing strategies, see W. R. Miller & Rollnick, 2002).

F—Feedback

Effective motivational interventions typically include a structured assessment, from which the smoker is given feedback on his/her current status. Motivational assessment can include a review of the smoker's readiness (on the readiness ladder; see Figure 2.1) and stage in the PAM process and an assessment of their primary sources of motivation (e.g., internal vs. external; see Table 2.16). In the context of smoking cessation treatment, feedback about carbon monoxide level, pulmonary function tests, smoking rate, level of nicotine dependence, status of other health measures that are affected by smoking, and levels of nicotine in the air of the smoker's home can be utilized to demonstrate the impact of smoking on the smoker and his/her family (Emmons & Wall, 1999; Risser & Belcher, 1990; see Figures 3.1 and 3.2 for examples). In the context of brief alcohol counseling, for example, feedback has included measures such as level of alcohol consumption, liver function tests, cognitive function tests, and indices of occupational and social functioning and impairment (cf. W. R. Miller & Rollnick, 2002). Corrective feedback regarding inaccurate information can also be provided. For example, the PHS guideline (Fiore et al., 2000) recommends that providers emphasize that smoking low-tar, low-nicotine cigarettes or using other forms of tobacco (e.g., smokeless tobacco, cigars, pipes) do not eliminate the health risks of smoking (see Table 3.10 for a list of the health consequences of smoking).

Providing objective information about health or other factors that are affected by smoking is an important component of a motivational intervention. Presentation of the feedback in graphic form can help smokers to understand their results and how they compare with others and can provide them with tangible and personalized information that they can share with other family members. For example, studies that have utilized pulmonary-function or carbon-monoxide feedback (Emmons et al., 2001; Emmons, Weidner, Foster, & Collins, 1992; Hovell et al., 2000; Risser & Belcher, 1990) have provided information about the smokers' results relative to nonsmokers. Information about lung age can be particularly motivating and may be more easily understood than information about percent-predicted values of forced expiratory volume, or other standard pulmonary-function test results (see Figure 3.1). Similar charts can be prepared as templates for providing feedback on the positive health impact of cessation on blood pressure, cholesterol level, carbon monoxide levels, blood sugar levels for diabetics, and a wide variety of other health tests commonly conducted on an out-

TABLE 3.10. The Health and Social Consequences of Smoking

Acute risks

Health risks
- Shortness of breath
- Exacerbation of asthma
- Impotence
- Infertility
- Increased levels of carbon monoxide, carbon dioxide, benzene,[a] nickel,[a] 2-naphthylamine,[a] and 4-aminobiphenyl[a]

Social risks
- Expensive
- Bad breath
- Less accepted socially
- Family's exposure to environmental tobacco smoke

Long-term risks

Health risks
- Myocardial infarction
- Stroke
- Chronic obstructive pulmonary disease
- Emphysema
- Cancer, including cancer of the
  - lung
  - cervix
  - bladder
  - oral cavity
  - pharynx
  - esophagus
  - pancreas
  - colon

Social risks
- Wrinkles
- Children are more likely to smoke
- Some employers may not hire smokers

[a]Known animal or human carcinogen.

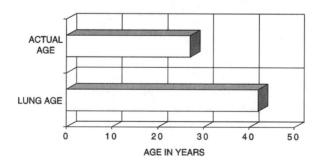

SPIROMETRIC LUNG AGE ESTIMATION
FOR: Mary Smith

You have a lung age of 42 even though you are only 27 years old

ACTUAL AGE

LUNG AGE

0   10   20   30   40   50
AGE IN YEARS

FIGURE 3.1. Spirometric lung age estimation.

patient basis (see Table 3.11). Recent developments in early detection of lung cancer via computed tomography (CT) scanning, as well as the ability to detect very early signs of emphysema (e.g., via spiral CT or electron beam CT), provide additional and powerful tools for smokers to be given information to motivate them to quit (Henschke et al., 1999; Henschke et al., 2001).

When available, environmental measures such as levels of nicotine in household air (see Figure 3.2) can also provide very powerful information to help motivate smokers to consider quitting, especially if they have loved ones and young children in the house (Hovell et al., 1994; Risser & Belcher, 1990).

R—Responsibility

An important element of a motivational interviewing approach is the emphasis on the smoker's personal responsibility for change. This is often stated explicitly, so that the smoker understands that what he/she decides to do with the objective health feedback and other information given by the provider is his/her choice. For example, you might say, "Based on

---

TABLE 3.11. The Positive Impact of Smoking Cessation on Health

Within 20 minutes of quitting smoking, a quitter's body begins a series of long-term changes, including:

20 minutes:	Blood pressure drops to normal. Pulse rate drops to normal. Body temperature of hands and feet increases to normal.
8 hours:	Carbon monoxide level in blood drops to normal. Oxygen level in blood increases to normal.
24 hours:	Chance of heart attack decreases.
48 hours:	Nerve endings start regrowing. Ability to smell and taste is enhanced.
2 weeks to 3 months:	Circulation improves. Walking becomes easier. Lung function increases as much as 30%.
1 to 9 months:	Coughing, sinus congestion, fatigue, shortness of breath decrease. Cilia regrow in lungs, increasing ability to handle mucus, clean the lungs, reduce infection. Energy level increases.
1 year:	Excess risk of coronary heart disease is half that of a smoker.
5 years:	Stroke risk is reduced to that of a nonsmoker within 5–15 years after quitting. Risk of cancer of the mouth, throat, and esophagus is half that of a smoker.
10 years:	Precancerous cells are replaced. Risk of cancer of the mouth, throat, esophagus, bladder, kidney, and pancreas decreases.
15 years:	Risk of coronary heart disease is equal to that of a nonsmoker.

Source. American Cancer Society, Centers for Disease Control and Prevention.

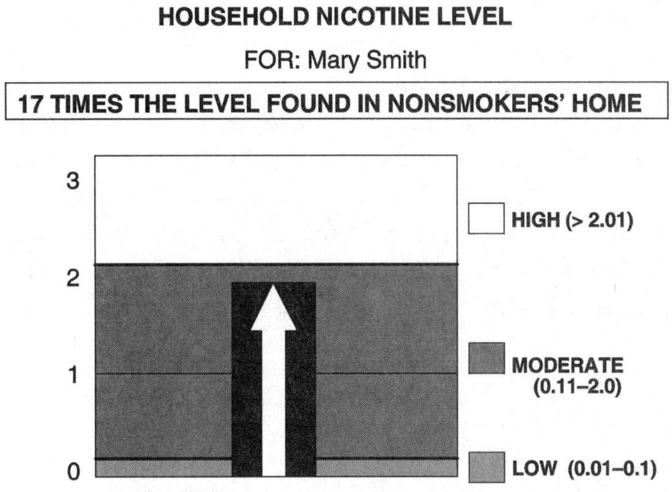

HOUSEHOLD NICOTINE LEVEL

FOR: Mary Smith

17 TIMES THE LEVEL FOUND IN NONSMOKERS' HOME

FIGURE 3.2. Household nicotine levels.

your blood pressure and the results of your lung-function test, the best thing you could do for your health is to quit smoking. However, I understand that it may be more complicated than that, and what you decide to do about your smoking is up to you." Ideally, you would also offer to provide support and encouragement to the smoker as he/she thinks about quitting and when he/she decides to quit. In the alcohol and substance abuse treatment setting, the provider might say something like:

> "I know one of the reasons that you quit drinking was to feel physically better, and that you were hoping to feel more improvement by now. Maybe there are other reasons why you're not feeling better. For example, it is likely that smoking is continuing to take a toll on your body and is masking some of the benefit you've gained from quitting drinking. I know it's hard to consider, but one of the best things you could do for your health now that you've quit drinking may be to quit smoking. However, what you decide to do about that is up to you."

This component of a motivational intervention differs from traditional approaches, in which smokers are told they must quit smoking, which in essence puts them in the position of disobeying the provider if they are unwilling or unable to quit.

A—Advice

Although smokers are given responsibility for change, it is important that providers clearly state their recommendations regarding smoking cessation. Rather than stating "You have to quit smoking" as a command that the smoker is obliged to follow, a motivational style would focus on the provider's *recommendation* for change: "In my opinion, it would really help your health if you quit smoking. But what you decide to do is up to you." This approach allows the smoker to retain control, yet still benefit from a clear message of support in quitting.

M—Menu

Many smokers have unsuccessfully tried to quit smoking in the past. Therefore, providing a menu of strategies for quitting can help individuals select the strategies that were the most helpful in the past and can provide an opportunity for identifying new strategies that are most appropriate for the present circumstances. For example, if a smoker is ready to consider cutting down on his/her daily smoking rate, the provider could suggest a number of ways to accomplish that goal (e.g., smoke on a set time interval, preset the number of cigarettes per day that he/she will smoke, smoke only in certain situations, do not smoke after dinner, etc.).

E—Empathy

The provider's style is an important predictor of patient motivation and change (S. M. Miller, 1995; Valle, 1981). An empathic style is one in which the provider shares an understanding of the smoker's experience and meaning through reflective listening strategies. Reflective listening is the process of hearing what the smoker is saying, making a guess at what the smoker means, and communicating this understanding in the form of a statement. This process serves to convey the provider's genuine desire to understand the smoker's predicament, while encouraging the smoker to clarify his/her thoughts, values, and beliefs. A brief conversation using reflective listening might go like this:

PROVIDER: The most important thing you can do for your health right now is to quit smoking. How do you feel about this?

SMOKER: I just have too much stress in my life. I can't imagine how I would get by without my cigarettes.

PROVIDER: So life is pretty hectic for you.

SMOKER: Yes, I work long hours, have a wife and three young kids, and smoking is my only outlet.

PROVIDER: So smoking helps you deal with daily stressors, but it is also putting you at high risk for having a heart attack.

SMOKER: Yeah, and that scares me. I really want to be around for my family.

PROVIDER: And you're worried that smoking might shorten your life.

SMOKER: Yeah, my father died of a heart attack when I was a teenager.

PROVIDER: And you don't want this for your kids.

SMOKER: No. I really do want to quit, but I think I'll need help.

PROVIDER: Would you like to talk about some options that might work for you?

In this example, the provider is able to use reflective statements to help the client explore his conflicting feelings about smoking and articulate the values that are most important to him. This empathic style of communication helps to reduce client defensiveness and creates an environment that is conducive to self-discovery.

A complete review of how to utilize reflective listening is beyond the scope of this chapter but is well presented in W. R. Miller and Rollnick (2002); the reader is referred to that volume for details about this important strategy.

S—Self-Efficacy

Self-efficacy is a smoker's belief (or self-confidence) in his/her ability to successfully carry out a specific task. A substantial body of literature has shown self-efficacy to be a critical factor in the change process (Bandura, 1997). You as provider play an important role in helping the smoker recognize his/her potential for change and in reinforcing beliefs about his/her ability to successfully initiate and sustain change. The goal is to enhance self-efficacy for making an attempt to quit. One strategy for building efficacy, especially among those who are less ready to quit, is to focus on the smoker's self-efficacy or confidence about his/her ability to handle specific circumstances without smoking (e.g., having an argument, relaxing after dinner, having the first cup of coffee in the morning). By troubleshooting alternative strategies for handling these situations, smokers' confidence in their ability to function without cigarettes will increase.

Although motivational interviewing requires significant training and skill, several of its components are quite easy to incorporate into your clinical style and are likely to be helpful in building smokers' motivation for change. Underlying the components of motivational interviewing are five *general principles* that guide motivational interactions.

Express Empathy

Research has shown that providers who are most effective at enhancing patients' motivation for change have a very empathic style that accepts patients' feelings without criticism or blame. Studies have found that ambivalence about change is normal (W. R. Miller & Rollnick, 2002), even in situations in which there seems to be tremendous reason to change (e.g., birth of a child, diagnosis of cancer). Expression of empathy, and the acceptance that it reflects, facilitates change. For example, you might express empathy about a new mother's stress by stating, "I understand how difficult it must be having a new baby in the house and dealing with all of the other stressors you face. It must seem pretty overwhelming at times." Empathy for a recovering alcoholic who is also struggling to quit smoking might be expressed by stating, "I know it can be very difficult to face two major life changes at once. Even though you feel it's the best approach for you at this time, it must feel pretty overwhelming at times."

Develop Discrepancy

Smokers can become more motivated to quit if they can be helped to develop a discrepancy between their current situation and the one in which they would like to be. Traditional approaches would advocate use of confrontation in order to develop such discrepancy. However, within the context of motivational interviewing, it is believed that motivation for change is created when people come to their own conclusions about the discrepancy between their current situation and important personal goals (W. Miller, 1985). Clarifying important future goals for the smoker and exploring the consequences of smoking that conflict with those goals can help the smoker to see the discrepancy without feeling pressured or confronted. When smokers present their own reasons for change, rather than being told by others what their reasons *should* be, they are more likely to personalize and internalize the need for change.

In order to help smokers explore their ambivalence about change, it is helpful to have them explicitly evaluate the factors that are associated with their smoking behavior. The decisional worksheet (Figure 3.3) allows smokers to consider things that they like about smoking, as well as those things that they do not like. Many smokers find that there are more things they do *not* like about smoking than things that they *do* like. The surprise associated with this revelation can serve as an "aha" experience for many people in that they start to seriously reconsider the role that smoking plays in their lives. The decisional worksheet also allows individuals to explore things that they think they will like about quitting smoking, as well as things they will find to be difficult; as a result, smokers can then go on to explore strategies for smoking cessation that will minimize the difficulties and build on the things they have identified as positive.

THINGS I LIKE ABOUT SMOKING	THINGS I DON'T LIKE ABOUT SMOKING

THINGS I WOULD DISLIKE ABOUT QUITTING	THINGS I WOULD LIKE ABOUT QUITTING

REASONS TO STAY THE SAME	REASONS FOR MAKING A CHANGE

FIGURE 3.3. Decisional worksheet.

Avoid Argumentation

While working with smokers to develop discrepancy, you should recognize the importance of avoiding argumentation. Confrontation and argumentation are counterproductive; when they do occur, the smoker is typically backed into a corner, and his/her most likely response is to do the *opposite* of what is being proposed. As W. R. Miller and Rollnick (2002) point out, the more you tell someone, "You can't," the more likely they are to respond, "I will." By strongly defending a particular position on the need for change, you are likely to generate opposition and defensiveness from the smoker. Resistance is an important sign that you are being too confrontational and should shift strategies.

Roll with Resistance

A key principle in motivational interviewing is that the smoker is the ultimate decision maker regarding what to do about a problem. Rather than imposing your own opinion on the smoker, your role is to offer new perspectives and to encourage the smoker to consider new points of view. If you place the smoker in the role of being the active leader of the problem-solving process, then he/she is more likely to find solutions that are most appropriate for his/her own circumstances.

Support Self-Efficacy

The final principle of motivational interviewing involves interacting with smokers so that their confidence in their ability to change is maximized. As mentioned previously, a large number of studies have found that self-efficacy is a critical element in the change process (Baranowski, Lin, Wetter, Resnicow, & Hearn, 2001; Glanz, Lewis, & Rimer, 1997). Self-efficacy is such an important factor that it is also considered one of the key building blocks of motivational interviewing, as noted previously. There are a number of ways to enhance self-efficacy regarding smoking cessation. For example, by giving the individual responsibility for change, the provider's belief in the smoker's ability to change is highlighted. Providing examples of other smokers who were in similar situations and who were able to quit smoking can help smokers to recognize that: (1) They are not alone—there are many others who have had similar problems; (2) There is hope for being able to change; and (3) The provider has had experience helping other smokers and is both persistent and supportive of the change process. Self-help materials often provide examples of individuals who have successfully quit smoking and can help smokers to identify strategies that may work well for themselves. Helping smokers to break the goal of "smoking cessation" down into smaller steps (proximal goal setting) can provide success experiences that build up a smoker's self-confidence regarding the bigger step of actually quitting. For example, one proximal goal might be to cut down and make small changes in smoking patterns by not smoking in the car for 1 week. Finally, by providing a menu of change strategies, individuals can select those that are best matched to their own needs and interests.

Summary

In order to accomplish the goals of a motivational interview, a relationship must be developed that respects the smoker's readiness to quit. The process of motivating behavior change is then based on personalized feedback regarding psychosocial, neuropsychological, occupational, and health factors. Feedback takes the form of a dialogue between you and the smoker that is designed to increase motivation for change by increasing awareness and creating dissonance between an individual's current expectations, beliefs, and behavior and the target or desired future behavior. Outcome studies using motivational interviewing provide growing empirical support for the utility of this motivational strategy in the context of brief interventions (Emmons, Marcus, Linnan, Rossi, & Abrams, 1994; Hall et al., 1992; Martinez, McPherson, Annegers, & Levin, 1995). Brief motivational interventions are currently considered to be a viable outpatient treatment approach to alcoholism (Janz & Becker, 1984; Pirie et al., 1992; Unger, 1996). The Institute of Medicine has identified motivational interventions as a high-priority area for future research on the treatment of alcohol-related problems (Syme, 2000). Recent work in the area of smoking suggests that motivational interviewing may be effective for increasing behavior change related to smoking (e.g., cigarette consumption, household exposure to environmental tobacco smoke, adoption of household smoking bans) but that further work may be needed to increase smoking cessation rates (Colby et al., 1998; Emmons, 1994; Emmons et al., 2001; Ershoff et al., 1999; Hovell et al., 2000). Motivational techniques are also an effective strategy for improving communication and adherence, as well as persistence, all of which are important along the pathway to smoking cessation.

ADDITIONAL TOOLS THAT CAN ENHANCE MOTIVATION

Motivational interviewing offers some very useful approaches to improving motivation for behavior change. In addition, other strategies that should be considered with smokers include the following:

Assessment of Nicotine Dependence

Even smokers who are not ready to quit can benefit from information about nicotine dependence. About 60–80% of smokers are dependent on nicotine, which means that they may experience significant withdrawal symptoms during the quitting process. An evaluation of the smoker's level of nicotine dependence is an important step in helping him/her select the best strategies for quitting. For example, smokers who are not as strongly nicotine dependent (biologically) may need to focus more on their psychological dependence on cigarettes. In contrast, smokers who are more strongly biologically nicotine dependent may first need to understand that their body has become used to a certain level of nicotine and that they may experience some physical discomfort on a short-term basis as they quit. The latter group of smokers may gain significant benefit and relief from nicotine replacement (see Chapter 7 and Table 2.2). It may also be useful to provide patients with information about common withdrawal symptoms so they understand that these are characteristic of short-term withdrawal and will pass with time. For many nicotine-dependent smokers, fear of withdrawal may be a significant barrier to quitting, and knowledge that withdrawal symptoms can be addressed may increase interest in cessation.

Goal Setting

Even when smokers are not interested in quitting smoking, it can be very helpful to set some small goals related to their smoking and to discuss them during the subsequent visit. A goal-setting worksheet (see Figure 3.4) can be a way for smokers to identify their goals and to remind themselves in between appointments about addressing these issues. The goal-setting worksheet can easily be tailored to the motivational level of the participant. For example, for smokers who are not interested in quitting smoking, a goal could be to think about and list the ways in which smoking might affect their families or their own personal goals. For smokers who are being pressured by others but who have low levels of internal motivation to quit, a goal may be to work on identifying internal, personal reasons for quitting. In addition, smokers who are not yet ready to quit might set goals to reduce their barriers to change (e.g.,

The changes I want to make are:

GOAL #1:	GOAL #2:
To smoke less at work	To stop smoking in my house

The steps I plan to take in meeting my goals are:

To smoke less at work . . .	To stop smoking in my house . . .
• Ask my friends who smoke to not offer me any cigarettes • Take a walk on breaks instead of smoking	• Set up a chair outside to smoke on the porch • Ask my family to remind me if I slip and smoke in the house

Other people can help me by:

Person who can help:	Possible ways to help:
• Joe and Steve at work • Kids • Mary, my wife	• Not offer me cigarettes • Remind me to go outside to smoke • To watch the kids while I go outside to smoke

Some things that I could do if problems get in the way of my plan are:

Problems:	Things I can do:
• My friends who smoke at work teasing me • Wife not helping me get out of the house to smoke	• Ignore them • Spend my breaks with other friends • Take the kids with me

FIGURE 3.4. Goals worksheet.

too busy because of accepting too many new projects at work), so that it will be easier to quit once they are ready.

Smokers who are seriously considering quitting smoking but have not yet committed to a quit date might consider goals that represent small steps toward quitting. For example, appropriate goals might be to delay the first cigarette in the morning by 15 or 20 minutes, to start cutting down on the number of cigarettes smoked each day, to participate in the Great American Smokeout and quit for one day, or to extend the time between cigarettes each day.

Social Support

Social support is a very important part of the smoking cessation process. Many smokers live with other smokers, which may be a significant barrier to quitting. Many smokers may not have resources to help them through the quitting process. Therefore, helping smokers to identify strategies for building their social support networks before they quit smoking can be very important. A "buddy contract" can be a helpful tool to help smokers identify (1) who would be most supportive to them as they try to change their smoking and (2) in what ways others can be supportive (Figure 3.5). As a first step, smokers should consider what types of support they would find most helpful. This may include (1) help with problem solving, (2) moral or emotional support, (3) help with specific tasks (e.g., household chores, child care) that will facilitate the smoker's efforts at quitting smoking, and (4) information and resources about quitting and staying abstinent from those who have been through the process. Social support can be critical to sustaining motivation to quit or to sustain a smoke-free life. According to the PHS guideline (Fiore et al., 2000), both intratreatment support from you the provider and extratreatment support can improve success rates.

MY BUDDY CONTRACT

My goal(s) are to:

1. <u>Increase my level of physical activity</u>
2. <u>Reduce my stress level at home</u>

My buddy <u>MARY</u> has agreed to help me meet these goals in the following ways:

1. <u>Take a walk together every night after dinner.</u>
2. <u>Give me 15 minutes of quiet time every night after I come home from work.</u>

If I need additional help, I can call on my buddy at any time!

_____   _____
My Signature   Buddy's Signature

FIGURE 3.5. Sample buddy contract to increase social support for smoking cessation.

Stress Management Strategies

Many smokers identify stress as a key reason that they are unwilling or unable to quit smoking. For these smokers, it may be more productive to talk directly about stress management first and to approach smoking cessation later. Helping smokers to identify the sources of their stress, as well as any direct ways of reducing it, is an important place to start. For example, some smokers may report that the morning rush of getting children and themselves ready for school and work is very stressful and that these unpleasant feelings stay with them for much of the day. Helping these smokers identify strategies for reducing morning stress (e.g., pick out children's clothes and pack lunches the night before, get up 15 minutes earlier, set rules for children about not watching TV or reading before they are completely ready for school, etc.) may be one way to directly address an important stressor in their lives. However, other types of stress (e.g., having a limited income, living in an unsafe neighborhood, job instability) may be more difficult to manage. Although strategies such as relaxation exercises or deep breathing will not remove the source of the stress, they may help to reduce the impact of these stressors on the smoker. A sample relaxation exercise that may be useful for some patients is provided in Figure 3.6. More detailed instructions for relaxation coping skills may be found in Chapter 5.

WHAT MOTIVATIONAL STRATEGIES TO USE AND WHEN TO USE THEM

Several motivational strategies have been recommended in this chapter. It is not expected nor desired that you would use all of these tools with any one individual. The decision about what tools are best with a particular individual will be determined in part by your relationship with that smoker and your growing knowledge of the smoker's style and personal charac-

---

The goal of this relaxation exercise is to learn the difference between muscle tension and relaxation. Once that distinction is mastered, it's much easier to evoke a feeling of relaxation, even in stressful settings!

Here's how to get started:

1. Find a quiet, darkened room. Lie on your back or sit in a comfortable, straight-backed chair.
2. Slowly draw as much air as you can into your chest and release it. Do this three or four times. Then let your breathing go back to its normal rhythm. Listen to it.
3. Starting with your face, you are going to tighten and relax groups of muscles as you move down the body. Scrunch your face up tightly for 5 seconds, then relax it. Do this for each of these muscle groups: the neck and shoulders, the arms, the stomach and chest, the legs, and the feet. As each part of your body relaxes, let it go limp. Feel the tension leave your body. You should feel like you are floating in space.

FIGURE 3.6. Sample relaxation exercise.

teristics. Some general guidelines that can also help to determine which tools are best, based on motivational level, include the following.

Smokers Not Considering Cessation

As noted earlier, your main tasks with smokers who are not ready to quit are to raise doubt in their minds about their smoking, to increase their perception of the benefits of stopping and of the risks associated with smoking, and to make these images as strong as possible. For example, use guided imagery to project into the future an image of all the wonderful benefits of a long, healthy life, together with beloved family and friends, that awaits the smoker who quits. Objective feedback related to the health effects of smoking is another good strategy to start this process with less motivated individuals. Review of one's life goals and how stopping smoking can enhance and continuing smoking can impede progress toward reaching those goals can also be a helpful strategy toward considering quitting. Smokers who are afraid they will not be able to manage their lives (e.g., stress, frustration, boredom, depression, social anxiety, weight gain) without the help of smoking may first need to obtain better coping skills or alternative strategies to get through life without smoking before they can "let go."

Smokers Who Are Starting to Consider Quitting

As smokers begin to think about quitting, your main task is to tip the balance toward change by eliciting reasons to change and strengthening the smoker's belief and self-efficacy that he/she can change (W. R. Miller & Rollnick, 2002). The decisional worksheet and social support strategies are very helpful with such individuals.

Smokers Who Are Ready to Quit

When smokers are ready to actively engage in a quit attempt, the provider's role is to help them determine the best strategies for starting and maintaining the cessation process. Assessment of nicotine dependence is very important; in addition, the goal-setting worksheet can be very useful. Providers should also offer a menu of different cessation strategies.

Smokers Who Have Quit

With individuals who have already quit smoking, the main task is to maintain their motivation for continued long-term abstinence. Providing feedback and information about the health improvements that have occurred since quitting and focusing on self-efficacy for continued cessation can help accomplish this goal. Reminders about the health risks of smoking that have now been reduced may be more powerful once a smoker has stopped than before they quit. Fear can trigger denial and avoidance if one is not sure one can quit, whereas fear can motivate one to keep going once some success has already been achieved.

Regardless of the smoker's level of motivation to quit, an intervention form can serve as a reminder for providers about the possible motivational steps to cover. This form should be placed in the chart and used as a reference regarding the patient's smoking status at the time of the previous visit. A sample of a form that was developed for an intervention targeting smoking cessation among pregnant women is presented in Figure 3.7.

SUMMARY

The majority of smokers express a desire to quit smoking yet have relatively low levels of motivation regarding cessation. You have an opportunity to help build smokers' motivation to quit and sustain that motivation for long-term cessation. In particular, the nature of repeated contacts facilitates both exploration of motivation over an extended period of time and the of-

Client Name: <u>Mary Smith</u>   Chart ID#: <u>7120</u>

Visit Date: <u>September 1, 1996</u>   Type of Visit: <u>Annual physical</u>

Nurse Name: <u>Sue Johnson</u>

Currently smoking?   Yes   ☐ No

   If yes, # cigarettes/day: <u>15 cigs/day</u>

   If no, quit date: _____

Decisional worksheet completed/reviewed?   Yes   ☐ No

Health-related feedback given?   Yes   ☐ No

Motivational readiness for *Cutting Back* (circle one):

1	2	3
Not thinking about it	Thinking about it	(Ready for change)

Motivational readiness for *Quitting* (circle one):

1	2	3
Not thinking about it	(Thinking about it)	Ready for change

Goal Setting and Plans to Achieve Goal(s):

   Goal #1: <u>To cut down to 5 cigs/day</u>   Goal #2: <u>To reduce baby's exposure to smoke</u>

   Plan #1: <u>Taper slowly</u>   Plan #2: <u>Smoke outside</u>

Materials given: <u>American Academy of Pediatrics ETS Booklet</u>

Comments: <u>Follow-up at next visit</u>

FIGURE 3.7. Healthy baby secondhand smoke study, smoking intervention form.

fer of support and assistance when the individual is ready to quit. The treatment planning process offers an excellent model for incorporating motivational enhancement into ongoing care (see Chapter 1). Providers and smokers alike must remember that smoking cessation is a process that can occur over a period of months to years. Every time you ask about a smoker's status and interest in cessation and offer assistance, small but critical steps are being taken that will increase readiness to quit smoking in the long term. And when smoking is placed on the agenda for regular care in other settings (e.g., primary care office, hospital, mental health clinic, substance abuse program, worksite wellness program), everyone becomes aware of the need for smokers to quit. This also gives providers the opportunity to keep smokers who relapse from becoming demoralized by encouraging them to keep trying to quit.

Assessment of motivational level, either in the context of a clinical interview or via written materials or visual aids such as the readiness-to-quit ladder (Figure 2.1), is an important part of any treatment encounter. Tailoring intervention strategies to the level of motivation will help you maximize your counseling time and will help the smoker feel that you understand his/her special needs and interests, have truly listened to his/her concerns, and are on his/her side with support, empathy, encouragement, and confidence in his/her own ability to succeed. Providers who wish to further enhance their motivational interviewing skills are encouraged to take a formal training workshop and to obtain the excellent guidebook on the subject by W. R. Miller and Rollnick (2002).

4

Brief Behavioral Treatment

William G. Shadel
Raymond Niaura

The goal of this chapter is to review brief smoking cessation treatments and the way in which these treatments may be applied to help smokers to quit smoking. The results obtained during a triage assessment of the individual smoker (e.g., motivation, nicotine dependence, psychiatric and substance abuse comorbidity, past quit attempts; see Table 2.1) help you and the smoker to determine together the most appropriate level of treatment (see also Chapter 1). Although brief treatments can be delivered in many community settings (medical, mental health, or public health), they are most commonly provided in medical office, community health centers, outpatient, and inpatient hospital settings.

WHAT ARE BRIEF TREATMENTS AND WHO CAN DELIVER THEM?

Brief treatments can be defined as those cessation interventions that can be delivered by a provider in fewer than 10 minutes (Fiore et al., 2000). The basic smoking cessation message that we review in depth in this chapter consists of the "5 A's": Ask about smoking; Advise the smoker to quit; Assess willingness to quit; Assist the smoker to quit; and Arrange follow-up. Features such as pharmacotherapy or skills training can be added or combined, depending on the needs of the smoker and the constraints of your practice. Figure 4.1 illustrates the components of brief treatment.

The term "brief" does not imply that the quality of care is in some way minimal or that the effectiveness of the intervention per se is small. Although more intensive treatments have greater success rates (see Fiore et al., 2000), the effectiveness of brief treatments cannot be underestimated. For example, given that the current population of smokers in the United States is

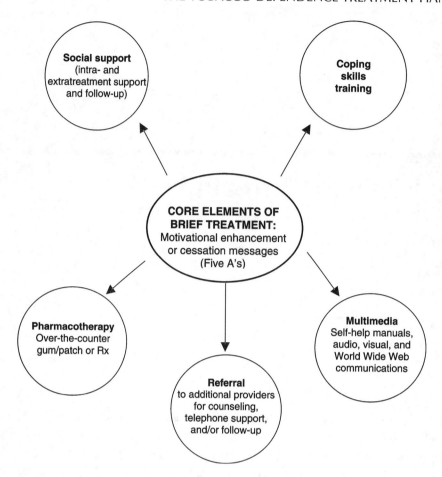

FIGURE 4.1. Core and specialized components of brief treatment.

roughly 50 million, if we assume that 70% (35 million) of smokers routinely visit a physician or health care provider at least once a year and that up to 13% of smokers are able to quit with a single, 3-minute intervention delivered by that provider, then 4.6 million individuals will have quit smoking. There is nothing modest about brief treatments with broad reach.

A "more is better" philosophy applies to brief treatments as well. Interventions lasting less than 3 minutes produce quit rates of 13.4%; interventions between 3 and 10 minutes produce quit rates of 16%; and those greater than 10 minutes produce quit rates of 22.1% (Fiore et al., 2000). On a public health level, spending the extra 7 minutes with each smoker could help an additional 1 million smokers to quit. Providers who deliver brief cessation treatment should spend as much time as possible with each smoker to achieve maximal benefits. There is also evidence from the PHS guideline (Fiore et al., 2000) that a greater number of shorter visits is more effective than a small number of treatment sessions of longer duration. The addition of other providers (e.g., physician assistants, nurses, respiratory therapists) and other treatment modalities such as NRT can boost the efficacy of brief treatments even further (see Chapter 7).

TABLE 4.1. Providers Who Can Deliver Brief Behavioral Treatments

All physicians and all medical specialties	Psychologists
All trainees, interns, residents, and fellows	Psychiatric nurse specialists
Physician assistants	Substance abuse counselors
Dentists	Social workers
Dental assistants	Exercise physiologists
Pharmacists	Occupational therapists
Career counselors	Respiratory therapists
Family/marital counselors	Public health practitioners
Guidance counselors	Nurses
Lay counselors	Nurse educators
Pastoral counselors	Nurse practitioners
Health educators	Specialists in addiction medicine

Provider Training

Almost anyone in any setting can deliver brief treatment (see Table 4.1). However, there can be no substitute for formalized training and practice in delivering brief smoking cessation interventions. Provider training can be completed in a short period of time. In this section, we briefly highlight some of the issues that are typically considered in training providers to deliver such treatments.

Many training programs are based on the National Cancer Institute's (NCI) 5 A's model (Fiore et al., 2000; Goldstein & Niaura, 1998), and this chapter, in many ways, mirrors this general training approach. For example, more formal training for providers who deliver brief smoking cessation treatment has generally included the following components (Glynn & Manley, 1989; Lindsay et al., 1987): (1) a didactic presentation that includes an overview of nicotine dependence, NRT, and the 5 A's approach to counseling; (2) a demonstration role play or training video to demonstrate the 5 A's counseling technique and a viewing of a training videotape; and (3) an opportunity for providers to practice the intervention using scripted role plays. Other manuals also are available for providers and are either free or available for a nominal fee (e.g., *How to Help Your Patients Stop Smoking*, Glynn & Manley, 1989; see also Fiore et al., 2000). This type of training is effective in enhancing provider skills and in increasing their ability to execute brief smoking cessation interventions (Ockene et al., 1994). Recently, a more formal training program has been established by the University of Massachusetts Medical Center in Worcester, Massachusetts.[1] This program confers certification as a smoking cessation counselor, a designation that is now used in many states as a prerequisite for reimbursement.

---

[1]Massachusetts Tobacco Treatment Specialist Training Program, University of Massachusetts Medical School, Division of Preventive and Behavioral Medicine, Center for Tobacco Prevention and Control, 55 Lake Avenue North, Worcester MA 01655; phone: 508-856-4099; fax: 508-856-3840.

WHERE CAN BRIEF BEHAVIORAL TREATMENTS BE DELIVERED?

The short answer to this question is: everywhere. Just as assessment can occur in any treatment context and at any point or level in a given service delivery system, so too can brief treatments. Indeed, a greater number of occasions on which a smoker hears brief advice to quit smoking from many members of his/her service provider network can have a lasting impact on his/her ability to quit smoking (Kottke, Battista, DeFriese, & Brekke, 1988). Chapter 8 reviews system strategies for incorporating treatments into community settings. Here we focus on health care settings.

Health care settings, broadly defined, provide ideal opportunities to deliver brief smoking cessation treatments. First, more than 70% of individuals who smoke see their physicians each year (Prochaska & Goldstein, 1991), low-income and minority smokers present for cessation services in health care settings most frequently (U.S. Department of Health and Human Services, 1990), and more than 85% of alcohol and other substance abusers smoke (Burling & Ziff, 1988). Health care settings provide access to a large population of smokers. Second, office visits are teachable moments in which the provider has a unique opportunity to discuss smoking cessation in the context of other health concerns. Third, in the age of managed care, brief smoking cessation treatments are a viable, cost-effective disease prevention option that can reduce the costs of more serious smoking-related illnesses and expensive repeated visits over the long term.

Brief *physician-delivered* smoking cessation counseling is effective and can significantly increase 1-year smoking abstinence rates up to 16% (Fiore et al., 2000). Furthermore, research has demonstrated that physician training, reminders to intervene with smokers, pharmacological agents, follow-up visits, and supplemental educational materials all increase the effectiveness of physician-delivered interventions (see Chapter 8).

Other allied health care providers (e.g., social workers, health educators, psychologists) can easily deliver brief smoking cessation treatments. In fact, the percentage of smokers who are able to quit with advice from nonphysician health care providers is about the same as with physicians (16%; see Fiore et al., 2000). *Dental offices* are another setting within which brief smoking cessation treatments can be delivered, given the high risk of developing oral and throat cancers among smokers. Brief interventions in the context of routine dental visits can increase smoking cessation rates (MacGregor, 1996).

WHO SHOULD RECEIVE BRIEF BEHAVIORAL TREATMENTS?

Brief treatments are most appropriate for relatively "uncomplicated" smokers—individuals who are motivated to quit, have low levels of nicotine dependence, exhibit no psychiatric or other substance abuse comorbidity, and have lengthy and/or recent prior quit attempts with few or no withdrawal symptoms (see Table 4.2; also see Chapters 1 and 2). Those who have little or no previous experience with cessation attempts may also be good candidates, as it will not be known if indeed they will have difficulty quitting, will have severe withdrawal symptoms, or both. These relatively uncomplicated smokers may also prefer treatments that are of shorter duration (see Chapter 2). Smokers who are low in motivation (not ready to quit

TABLE 4.2. Characteristics of Patients for Whom Brief Behavioral Treatments Are Appropriate

Assessment construct	Level
Motivation	High
Nicotine dependence	Low
Past quit attempts	None or few
Withdrawal (if quit attempts made)	None/mild
Length of abstinence (if quit attempts made)	Several months
Substance abuse	None
Psychiatric comorbidity	None

Note. A review of assessment instruments that measure these constructs can be found in Chapter 2.

within the next 6 months—see readiness ladder, Table 2.1) can be given brief motivation counseling and followed up (see Chapter 3). In addition, brief treatments can be considered first-line treatments with smokers for whom specific assessment information is not available; that is, brief treatments should at a minimum be offered to all smokers if nothing else is possible (recognizing that some smokers may respond more or less well).

WHAT ABOUT SMOKERS WHO WANT TO QUIT ON THEIR OWN?

A majority of smokers have attempted to quit on their own (Cohen et al., 1989). In fact, when given a choice, most smokers would prefer to quit on their own without any formal advice or guidance (Lichtenstein & Hollis, 1992). This method is sometimes referred to as "self-change," or the "cold turkey" approach—the smoker awakens one morning, seemingly spontaneously makes the decision to quit, and throws his/her cigarettes in the trash. It is important to note, though, that despite the fact that the actual quit-smoking effort and strategies used are initiated by the smoker him/herself, the so-called "unaided" quit attempt may be prompted by prior experiences with health care providers or other sources of treatment information (Lichtenstein & Glasgow, 1992). Studies have indicated that less than 5% of smokers are able to quit successfully on their own (Cohen et al., 1989). This percentage is lower among smokers who are highly dependent (Cohen et al., 1989). Thus many smokers can make repeated unsuccessful attempts to quit on their own (Cohen et al., 1989), become discouraged by multiple failure experiences (Shadel & Mermelstein, 1993a), and frequently feel like giving up (Shiffman et al., 1997). Such undesirable consequences of repeated failures to quit compose a compelling argument in favor of coordinated efforts among all of a smoker's providers and the need to consider a stepped-care approach. Smokers can be given self-help materials (e.g., manuals, booklets, video, audio) or informed about quality services on the World Wide Web (e.g., QuitNet: *www.quitnet.com*) as additional supports for your brief treatment efforts (see Tables 4.8 and 4.9).

SETTING THE STAGE FOR BRIEF BEHAVIORAL TREATMENT

Preliminary Remarks to Smokers

Several concerns are important to keep in mind as you discuss brief cessation treatments with smokers under your care. Most smokers you see for brief treatment may have made unsuccessful attempts to quit in the past. It is crucial to recognize that these smokers may exhibit strong feelings of ambivalence about stopping smoking, may feel discouraged or pessimistic about their chances of quitting, or may even become resistant to attempts to encourage them to seek help with cessation. They may feel they have "tried that" and it did not work. For smokers who say they are pessimistic, you will need to conduct client-centered motivational counseling and explain that trying techniques as part of a more structured program may produce better results (e.g., using nicotine replacement together with brief counseling and support, as opposed to simply using the patch over the counter without any structure or support). Chapter 3 describes in detail several strategies that can be utilized to treat these unmotivated smokers. If smokers are motivated to consider cessation, then a more active approach, described herein, can be taken.

Preparing to Quit Smoking

Smokers need to know that self-change and cold turkey work only for a small minority of persons and that most smokers attempt to quit numerous times before they are ultimately successful. In fact, they should be made to recognize that these past attempts are not indicative of failure but rather of their motivation and determination to stop smoking for good. In short, the take-home message for these individuals is that most smokers need some sort of cessation treatment and will try multiple times to quit over periods of many years before they are eventually successful. Table 4.3 provides sample statements that we have used often with smokers.

As we noted, quitting smoking is a process, and many smokers have had numerous experiences with attempting to quit. Those past experiences have shaped the way that the smoker

---

TABLE 4.3. Sample Provider Statement That Can Be Used to Place Brief Treatment in Context

"I realize that it must be hard for you to think about quitting smoking again. I notice that you've tried to quit _____ times before. The prospect of attempting to quit again must seem overwhelming to you right now.

"Quitting smoking is hard. Most smokers will try nearly half a dozen times and use different methods to quit each time before they eventually are able to stay off of cigarettes for good. You've been smoking for _____ years at about _____ packs per day. Basically, you've gotten very good at being a smoker. In fact, its probably difficult for you to remember a time when you didn't smoke. This doesn't mean that it is or will be impossible to quit; it just means that it took a lot of time and a lot of cigarettes for you to get to be very good at smoking. It will take some time for you to unlearn smoking and to learn to be a nonsmoker.

"Consider also that each time that you quit is different. You are a different person than you were during your last quit attempt, primarily because you learned a little more each time about what it is like to be a nonsmoker. You're not starting from scratch. The more times that you try to quit, and the longer that you are able to stay quit, means that you are more likely to remain a nonsmoker on your next attempt."

is looking at this current attempt and his/her receptivity to your intervention. One of your first goals is to set positive expectations for the smoker about what this attempt at quitting could be like and about the intervention components that will follow. Table 4.4 presents sample statements that we have used in our clinical experience.

CORE ELEMENTS OF BRIEF BEHAVIORAL TREATMENT

The current recommendation and standard of care for all health care providers is to advise smokers to quit smoking at every contact (Fiore et al., 2000; Goldstein & Niaura, 1998). Brief advice to quit smoking typically consists of some variation on the 5 A's initially developed by the NCI (see Fiore et al., 2000; Goldstein & Niaura, 1998). This message is a brief counseling strategy with five discrete components:

1. Ask the smoker about smoking at every treatment contact. Studies have indicated that a majority of health care providers do not ask about smoking status nor provide advice to quit (Goldstein et al., 1997).

2. Advise the smoker to quit smoking in a strong fashion, taking into account any individualized assessment information available about the smoker. You are likely to have available to you information about the smoker's physical or emotional health, depending on your

---

TABLE 4.4. Sample Provider Statement That Sets the Stage for Smoking Cessation

"I'm very pleased that you've made the decision to quit. I know that it was not an easy decision to come to, and the fact that you've decided that this is the route that you'd like to take speaks very highly about your commitment to make positive changes in your life.

"I'm here to help you in any way I can to make your experience with quitting a successful one. You should feel free to ask me any questions you have about quitting, and about smoking for that matter. My only goal here is make sure that I can help you in any way I can.

"Quitting smoking is like driving across the country, for example, like taking a drive from Rhode Island to Los Angeles. You have a specific destination in mind and know sort of the direction you have to go to get there, but you might be unsure as to the specific roads, highways, and exits you would take to get there. Most people probably would not just jump in their car and head off in any direction in driving across the country like this—there are too many unknowns, too many chances for getting lost.

"Most people would look at a map ahead of time, carefully plan out their route of travel—roads and highways they might take, states and cities they would cross through—and places along the way where they will stop for gas and food to recharge their batteries so to speak. Importantly, if two people were making the same trip in two separate cars, each of them might take different roads to get there, and each of them might take different amounts of time. Despite their best planning, though, some people may get unexpectedly lost, held up in traffic due to construction, or stop to ask for directions, but if they keep driving with the goal of getting to LA, they will eventually get there.

"Quitting smoking is a lot like taking a long trip across the country. We know that people who are successful at quitting spend a lot of time planning what they'll do to help them quit—a unique menu of coping strategies that will help them to manage their smoking urges and situations in which they would smoke. Think of it as a personal road map to becoming a nonsmoker. Just like taking a trip, though, and despite the best plans, sometimes some people encounter tough situations that they did not anticipate in which they end up having a cigarette or two. This doesn't mean that they don't still go on to quit; it just means that they have to look for alternative routes or coping strategies to help them to not smoke."

practice, service setting, or specialty. You should have available the results of triage smoking cessation assessments and treatment assessments that were discussed in Chapter 2.

3. Assess the smoker's willingness to make a quit attempt. If the smoker is ready to make a quit attempt, then you can proceed to Step 4. If he/she is not willing to make an attempt, you may be able to increase his/her motivation to quit by using brief motivational interviewing techniques (Chapter 3).

4. Assist the smoker to quit by setting a specific target quit day with him/her and providing support and coping skills training. Collaboratively deciding on a date on which the smoker is to attempt cessation is important to his/her overall success (Fiore et al., 2000). A specific date provides a clear goal for the smoker to achieve, and it also serves as a useful guide to gauge progress toward cessation or to complete smaller steps or subgoals (e.g., reducing the number of cigarettes smoked) that may help with quitting (Borrelli & Mermelstein, 1994). We will discuss the ways in which you can provide social support and coping skills training to smokers in a brief format in the next sections.

5. Arrange follow-up to discuss the smoker's progress toward smoking cessation. Smokers should be made to feel that they are accountable for their actions and that they may contact you if they have questions as they move through the process of quitting.

Table 4.5 presents a sample smoking cessation message that may be used by any provider.

SPECIALIZED ELEMENTS OF BRIEF BEHAVIORAL TREATMENT

Social Support

Smokers who perceive that they have positive support for stopping smoking are more likely to be successful than smokers who do not perceive such support (Fiore et al., 2000). One way to ensure that smokers receive adequate support is for you to communicate to the smoker that you support his/her quitting efforts. Specific strategies to support the smoker include providing basic information, encouraging the smoker to quit, noting that effective methods are available, and conveying your confidence that the smoker can succeed. Also, be caring, express concern, and encourage the smoker to talk about the process. Table 4.6 presents these elements of supportive counseling, and Chapter 3 details additional strategies that you can use.

Coping Skills Training

Coping skills training is an essential component of helping smokers quit successfully (Marlatt & Gordon, 1985). The basic principle behind coping skills training is that smokers need to be able to manage (i.e., cope with) various life circumstances without smoking. You should convey to smokers that learning to use coping skills successfully will help them learn to be non-smokers again. Typically, coping skill execution is more intense and frequent within the first few weeks of cessation and gradually diminishes in frequency as the individual becomes more comfortable with not smoking.

TABLE 4.5. Sample Brief Intervention Model Using the 5 A's

1. *Ask about smoking status.*
   Do you currently smoke?

2. *Assess past quit attempts.*
   Have you tried to quit smoking before? What was it like for you?

3. *Assess willingness to make a quit attempt.*
   How would you feel about quitting smoking right now?

4. *Advise patient to quit in a strong, clear, and personalized manner.*

   Quitting smoking is one of the most important things you can do for yourself. It will improve your current health because you will feel better and have more energy. Not smoking will also protect you from developing any number of health problems like cancer and lung diseases in the future. As your _____, I can recommend a few things to you to help you out.
   a. *Set a specific quit day.*
   b. *Use nicotine replacement therapies.* The nicotine skin patches and nicotine gum, or other pharmacological treatments like Zyban, are available to you for about as much as it costs to purchase a pack of cigarettes. These medicines can help you to manage withdrawal symptoms and urges to smoke after you quit. If you're interested in the OTC medications, I can help you to locate a place where you can purchase them. If you're interested in the prescription medicines, I can help you with that by talking to you about your options or referring you to someone who can talk to you about your options.
   c. *Read about quitting.* There are a number of different materials you can read. Here is something to get you started. I can tell you how to get access to other materials.
   d. *Get support from family and friends for quitting smoking.* There are also other resources in your community for getting help with quitting. Here is a list that you can use whenever you like.

5. *Arrange for a follow-up.*
   Here is your appointment for next time. I'll be curious to see how you're doing with your smoking then, but if you have any questions in the meantime, please call me.

TABLE 4.6. Examples of Supportive Counseling Techniques

1. Encourage the patient in his/her quit attempt.
   - Note that effective cessation treatments are available.
   - Communicate your belief in the patient's ability to quit.

2. Communicate caring and concern.
   - Ask how the patient feels about quitting.
   - Directly express concern and a willingness to help.
   - Be open to the patient's expression of fears of quitting, difficulties experienced, and ambivalence about quitting and/or continuing to smoke.

3. Encourage the patient to talk about the process of quitting.
   - Ask about the patient's reasons for quitting, difficulties with stopping, and concerns.

4. Provide basic information about smoking and quitting.
   - The nature of withdrawal
   - The addictive nature of smoking
   - The relapsing nature of smoking

Coping skills training can be very intensive and may take several practice sessions to master. Chapter 6 focuses on this more intensive aspect of training. However, coping skills training can also be completed within the context of brief treatment. In essence, you want to communicate to smokers the basics of self-management training (problem solving)—that they can control their smoking and change their environment to reduce the likelihood that they will want to smoke. This training is based on the assumptions that smoking is a behavior that has distinct triggers and consequences and that the job of coping is to control those triggers and their consequences by substituting alternative behaviors instead of smoking. This is called a functional analysis and involves identifying the ABC's (Antecedent triggers, Behavior [i.e., smoking], and Consequences) of any high-risk situations in which there is a danger that smoking will occur. As recommended in Chapter 2 (Module 1), you should assess each individual smoker's triggers and have this information readily available. Also, you should have information regarding each smoker's level of coping skill based on a Module 1 assessment (Chapter 2). Using this information, you can help the smoker develop a problem-solving strategy that consists of (1) identifying the high-risk situations that could trigger an urge or craving to smoke; (2) substituting an alternative coping skill to prevent smoking; and (3) evaluating how well that alternative worked. If it worked, congratulate the smoker on his/her success. If not, assist him/her in identifying new alternatives to try. Once a high-risk situation is identified using the ABC analysis and a coping skill is found that works, then that particular problem is solved and the next high-risk situation is tackled. It is important to encourage the smoker to brainstorm potential future high-risk situations in addition to current problem areas.

Four broad categories of coping strategies are available:

1. *Avoiding* triggers or trigger situations.
2. *Altering* triggers or trigger situations.
3. *Substituting* some alternative behavior (rather than smoking) when confronted with a trigger.
4. *Thinking differently* about the trigger and about smoking.

Table 4.7 provides sample statements of how these three skills may be introduced to smokers. The information provided in this table could also be adapted for use as a smoker handout.

Written Manuals, Audiotapes, Videotapes, and the World Wide Web

Written manuals generally provide instruction on preparing for quit day; what to expect following quit day; coping with withdrawal, urges, and cravings; securing social support; and ways in which to deal with stress and negative mood. These written materials also may provide information on the use of nicotine replacement products, above and beyond what is provided with the package inserts to these medications. For the most part, all materials are written in easily understandable language (at about the seventh-grade level) and can be given

TABLE 4.7. Brief Coping Skills Training

Smoking doesn't just happen automatically, though it might seem like it sometimes. There are usually triggers or events that cause you to have an urge and then to smoke. These triggers can be feelings, thoughts, or situations. There are three types of *behavioral* or habit changing strategies you can use to cope with these triggers, to break up the chain of events that lead to smoking:

1. *Avoid the trigger.* Avoiding the trigger obviously can be the most powerful strategy. If you are not around the trigger, you will not have an urge and you will not smoke. For example, if you know that having a cup of coffee is a big trigger for you, then not having a cup of coffee will decrease your desire for a cigarette. However, sometimes avoiding a trigger is not always the most practical strategy; if waking up in the morning is a trigger, you can't simply avoid waking up, as much as you might like to sometimes. That's why there are two additional types of strategies to help you manage your smoking triggers.

2. *Alter the trigger situation.* Think of your triggers to smoke as very fixed parts of your daily routine—anything that you can do to alter that routine can help you to manage your smoking urges. What you're doing is essentially taking control of your environment so that you can control your smoking. For example, let's take that cup of coffee as a trigger. If you always drink that cup of coffee in the same place using the same cup at the same time of the day, change any one or all of those parts of the routine: change the cup you use, drink your coffee in a different chair or part of the house. The key with altering a trigger is to be creative. Use it as an opportunity to challenge yourself to outsmart the environment to give you control of your smoking.

3. *Substitute* something else for the cigarette when you encounter the trigger. This can be as simple as putting a piece of gum or hard candy in your mouth when you want a cigarette. Again, think of this as an opportunity to be creative.

Another type of coping strategy is a *cognitive* strategy that involves changing your thoughts or telling yourself things so that you will not want to smoke. These self-statements can include:

   a. Reasons you want to quit
   b. Benefits of quitting
   c. Statements of determination (e.g., "I can do it")
   d. Delay statements (e.g., "only five more minutes").

Other types of self-statements include getting a new perspective on the situation. Take a step back when you feel the urge to smoke and ask yourself a simple question: "Do I really want to smoke here?" Then redefine the situation and your reaction (e.g., "I don't really want to smoke, I really just want to relax here"), and use other coping strategies (e.g., substitute a piece of gum for the cigarette).

   Practice these strategies before you quit. Imagine yourself successfully coping with these trigger situations. Think of this as your road map to becoming a successful nonsmoker.

   You may have to try different types of strategies to cope with your triggers. It can be discouraging if you try things, but they just do not work, and you still feel the need for a cigarette. Don't give up! Have fun with it! It just means you haven't found the right strategy or combinations of strategies to use yet. Although it is important to get advice on some possible strategies, it is equally important to remember that what works for someone else may not necessarily work for you.

to persons of most educational backgrounds. Moreover, many of these materials come in non-English languages (Spanish, primarily) or can easily be translated into the appropriate language. Finally, most of these materials are free or inexpensive and are readily available from the publishing source. A listing of the cost and availability of some of the more popular manuals is provided in Tables 4.8 and 4.9.

For example, the NCI publishes focused manuals for the smoker with specific needs (e.g., *Why Do You Smoke?* and *Smoking Facts and Tips for Quitting*). The American Lung Association (ALA) offers a self-help program that publishes a preparatory manual, complete with motivational exercises and self-monitoring forms, entitled *Freedom from Smoking*. The ALA also publishes a companion relapse prevention manual, *A Lifetime of Freedom from Smoking*, that provides specific strategies to help the recent ex-smoker cope with high-risk situations, other smokers, stress, weight gain, and slips and relapse. The Public Health Service (PHS), on whose guidelines this treatment manual is based, provides a brief consumer guide (*You Can Quit Smoking*) that includes information on use of the nicotine patch and nicotine gum, as well as guidance about setting quit days and increasing motivation to quit smoking. Similar written materials have been developed for specialized populations. For example, *Clear Horizons* is a stop-smoking manual, published by the NCI, specifically designed for smokers who are over the age of 55 (see Orleans et al., 1991). Self-help materials also have been published by the NCI for non-English-speaking individuals. *Guia para Dejar de Fumar* is a manual that is similar in scope and content to other NCI publications.

Although there is a proliferation of smoking cessation information on the World Wide Web, very little of it has been evaluated for efficacy or credibility. Although there may be other credible Web-based resources, we recommend those websites sponsored by the National Institutes of Health or the Centers for Disease Control and Prevention (National Cancer Institute: *www.cancer.gov*; Centers for Disease Control: *www.cdc.gov;* National Institute on Drug Abuse: *www.nida.nih.gov;* Cancer Information Service: *http://cis.nci.nih.gov*; see Table 4.9 for a summary). One promising self-help website is QuitNet (*www.quitnet.com*). Launched in 1995, QuitNet is a commercial website designed to provide the information, help, and social support that people need to successfully quit smoking. It is a Web-based implementation of the PHS guidelines that provides (1) highly tailored individualized information; (2) diagnostic and quitting tools that facilitate setting a quit date; (3) heavy doses of support delivered around the clock through "buddies," chat rooms, and e-mail; (4) counseling delivered online by a smoking cessation expert; and (5) FDA-approved smoking cessation pharmacotherapies. QuitNet resources and services include "quitting tools" such as an evidence-based quitting guide that addresses barriers to quitting, such as concern about weight gain, stress, depression, and alcohol use; a "Quit Date Wizard" that assists users in selecting an appropriate quit date; a customized quitting calendar; assessments and tailored feedback regarding readiness to quit, nicotine dependence, and reasons for smoking; a pharmaceutical guide that provides comprehensive information about approved pharmacotherapies, as well as herbal and other products; the "Q-Gadget," which calculates the amount of money saved after quitting; e-mail support from a trained smoking cessation counselor; and a database of local smoking cessation programs.

TABLE 4.8. Written and Online Self-Help Resources

Publisher	Resource	Approximate cost	Ordering information
		For consumers	
National Cancer Institute	*Why Do You Smoke?*	First 20 are free; $.10 for each additional copy (70 copies for $5.00)	1-800-4CANCER *www.cancer.gov*
National Cancer Institute	*Smoking Facts and Tips for Quitting*[a]	First 20 are free; $.10 for each additional copy (70 copies for $5.00)	1-800-4CANCER *www.cancer.gov*
National Cancer Institute	*Clear Horizons*	Free	1-800-4CANCER (this publication is not currently available online)
National Cancer Institute	*Guia para Dejar de Fumar: No lo deje para manana, deje de fumar hoy*	First 20 are free; $.10 for each additional copy (70 copies for $5.00)	1-800-4CANCER *www.cancer.gov*
	QuitNet	Basic membership free with registration; 3-month premium membership $39.95; 1-year premium membership $99.95	*www.quitnet.com*
American Lung Association	*Freedom from Smoking*[a] *A Lifetime of Freedom from Smoking*[a]	$10.00 for both manuals	1-800-LUNG-USA
Agency for Health Research and Quality	*Consumer Guide: You Can Quit Smoking*[a]	First three are free to public; $.15 for each additional copy	1-800-358-9295
		For providers	
Agency for Health Research and Quality	*Treating Tobacco Use and Dependence*	First 100 free for health professionals	1-800-358-9295 *www.surgeongeneral.gov/tobacco*
American Academy of Family Physicians	*AAFP Stop Smoking Kit*	$60.00 for members; $90 for nonmembers	1-800-944-0000
National Heart, Lung and Blood Institute	*Nurses: Help Your Patients Stop Smoking*	Free	301-592-8573 *http://www.nhlbi.nih.gov/health/prof/lung/other/nurssmok.txt*
National Cancer Institute	*How to Help Your Patients Stop Smoking: NCI Manual for Physicians*	Free	1-800-4CANCER *www.cancer.gov*

Note. [a]Available in Spanish.

TABLE 4.9. Internet Sites with Links to Online Tobacco Control Resources

CDC Office on Smoking and Health
  - can be used for ordering materials published by U.S. Public Health Service, including the Agency for Health Research and Quality consumer guide

www.cdc.gov/tobacco/edumat.htm
e-mail: *tobaccoinfo@cdc.gov*

Massachusetts Tobacco Education Clearinghouse
  - contains a catalog of resources used in the Massachusetts Tobacco Control Program

www.jsi.com/health/mtec
e-mail: *mtec@jsi.com*
617-482-9485

California Youth Media Network
  - has good links to other state and national and international sites for tobacco control resources

www.ymn.org/tobacco/orgs

More Tobacco Stinks!
  - has good links to local (Florida), national, and international resources

www.state.fl.us/team/links2.html

We would like to offer a word of caution, however. Despite the proliferation of written materials on how to stop smoking, written manuals when used alone are not effective in helping smokers to quit (Fiore et al., 2000). Audio and visual materials have not been as extensively tested for their effectiveness at helping smokers quit, though the reason may be these materials are not as readily available as self-help materials. Nonetheless, at this point, when used alone, audio and visual materials are not particularly effective at increasing smoking cessation rates (Fiore et al., 2000). Thus simply providing access to such materials or giving a smoker a manual without the benefit of brief counseling is not a sufficient brief treatment. However, when written and audio materials are combined with the 5 A's counseling strategy, a smoker's chances of stopping smoking may be further increased (Goldstein & Niaura, 1998).

Pharmacotherapy

Pharmacotherapies, especially nicotine replacement therapies such as the nicotine patch or nicotine gum, can be quite compatible with brief treatments (more in-depth attention to their effectiveness and guidelines for use are provided in Chapter 7). Until the mid-1990s, the nicotine transdermal patches and nicotine polacrilex (i.e., gum) had been prescription items, available only through a physician. However, as of this writing, two of the three nicotine patches (i.e., Nicoderm, Nicotrol) and nicotine gum (i.e., Nicorette®) have become available over the counter (OTC). The transition to OTC status of these nicotine replacement products is partly in recognition of the relatively safe side-effect profile, ease of use, and relative effectiveness at helping smokers manage withdrawal and cravings during cessation (Transdermal Nicotine Study Group, 1991). The important point from a brief treatment perspective is that the medications, whether OTC or prescription, are prepackaged with self-help pamphlets and audiotapes to aid the smoker in his/her quit attempt. Inclusion of these materials with the nicotine replacement products is indicative of the general recognition that some form of nonpharmacological treatment (i.e., behavioral therapy) is an important adjunct if a nicotine replacement therapy is to be effective.

For example, Nicorette is packaged with the Committed Quitters Program®, and Zyban® (i.e., the FDA-approved smoking cessation form of the antidepressant Wellbutrin SR) is packaged with the Zyban Advantage Plan (ZAP)®. Upon purchase of either of these medications, the smoker is instructed to call a toll-free telephone number for further instruction and advice on smoking cessation. Smokers then can respond to various brief questions about their reasons for smoking, as well as other smoking habit and cessation items. Based on the information provided, a tailored report is mailed to smokers that details factors that they may wish to consider in their cessation efforts (e.g., how to cope with stress). Standardized self-help treatment materials are also provided. Proactive telephone calls from the medication's sponsor company that are designed to help the smoker with quitting may follow if the smoker so desires. Comprehensive self-help materials such as those provided with Nicorette and Zyban and the tailoring components they provide are important parts of the cessation process. However, it is important to recognize that even though components of the Committed Quitters Program and ZAP have been evaluated (e.g., setting a specific quit day), the specific programs themselves have not been scientifically evaluated as adjuncts to the specific pharmacotherapy treatments per se.

Telephone Hotlines and Telephone Counseling

Brief treatment can take many forms via a telephone hotline. First, the hotline can be used as a central referral source for smokers to find out where many different types of smoking treatments (i.e., from brief to intensive) are offered. If properly promoted and advertised (e.g., via multimedia campaigns), substantial use of this service can be expected (Jaen et al., 1991; cf. Kinne, Thompson, & Wooldridge, 1991). However, it does not appear as though referrals alone are sufficient to increase chances of smoking cessation (Fiore et al., 2000). Second, hotlines can provide smoking cessation information. Use of such services can be high and can produce reasonable rates of smoking cessation for a minimal treatment (11%; Fiore et al., 2000), especially if the callers are highly motivated and have a supportive home environment (Jaen, Cummings, Zielenzy, & O'Shea, 1993). Supportive and reinforcing messages and information, especially once the smoker has quit (Durbren, 1977), seem to be more helpful to smokers than other types of information (e.g., health information, coping information; see Shapiro, Ossip-Klein, & Gerrity, 1985). Thus telephone hotlines can be helpful as adjuncts to brief treatment. Supportive messages and any encouragement that a message can provide regarding use of social support would seem to be particularly helpful as a service. One toll-free resource that can provide information and smoking cessation advice to the smoker is the NCI Cancer Information Line (1-800-4 CANCER). At the very least, the provider can offer this free service to smokers if the smoker is not interested in treatment.

RELAPSE PREVENTION

Most smokers who attempt to quit smoking will relapse within a very short period of time. In fact, it is very possible that smokers will relapse between your visits with them. You can reduce the probability that a smoker will relapse by devoting some time to relapse prevention training. More intensive relapse prevention techniques are discussed in Chapters 5 and 6. However, short versions of this training can be delivered in 10 minutes. Relapse prevention training can be delivered either before the smoker quits (i.e., as he/she plans for a target quit day) or as soon as possible after he/she quits. Our experience has suggested that a good strategy is to "preview" relapse prevention training with the smoker prior to quitting (i.e., so that he/she knows what to expect), then cover it in more detail on quit day or as soon as possible after quit day.

Three key components are useful when delivering relapse prevention training in a brief format. First, the individual should be informed about the nature and time course of nicotine withdrawal, even if he/she is using some sort of pharmacotherapy designed to combat withdrawal. Second, smokers should be informed that their smoking triggers will become high-risk situations after they quit. High-risk situations are those situations in which the individual's risk of slipping or relapsing to smoking is very high (Marlatt & Gordon, 1985). In order to manage and negotiate high-risk situations, individuals should be advised to use some of the same coping strategies that they used before they quit (see Table 4.7) and to develop and practice new ones as they "get better" at becoming nonsmokers. Third, smokers should be counseled to use any slips or relapses as learning experiences for the next time that they quit. The abstinence violation effect (AVE; Marlatt & Gordon, 1985) is an important phenomenon for which smokers need to prepare and with which they need to cope. The AVE refers to feelings of dejection and failure following a slip or relapse after a period of abstinence that are associated with thoughts of giving up their attempts to quit. A sample relapse prevention handout appears in Table 4.10.

TABLE 4.10. A Sample Relapse Prevention Handout

A. *Withdrawal symptoms*. Common withdrawal symptoms include: irritability, increased tension and frustration, trouble concentrating, cravings, trouble sleeping, and increased hunger.

B. *Withdrawal symptom duration*. Not everybody will have the same withdrawal symptoms for the same amount of time. Generally speaking, though, your symptoms will gradually decrease over the 2 to 3 weeks after you've quit. Many people feel better within 2 to 3 days. You may find that you hit some peaks and valleys along the way. Many people report their withdrawal symptoms get worse during the evening hours. In any case, you may not feel like yourself for a few days and that's okay. This will not be a permanent change.

C. *High-risk situations*. The situations that triggered a cigarette before you quit are your high-risk situations now. These are times that you are at most risk for going back to smoking. Understanding these connections gives you the ability to develop a coping plan for those high-risk times.

D. *Abstinence violation effect* (AVE). How do you think you would feel if you did smoke a cigarette? It would be perfectly natural for you to feel guilty, frustrated, or angry, like you've failed. Recognize that these feelings are natural and do not use them as an excuse to start smoking again. Are you really a failure? A failure might be someone who gives up and never thinks of quitting again. If you slip and have a cigarette, use it as a source of information; take a step back and analyze the situation that just occurred. Use it as a learning experience. Find out what happened by asking yourself the following questions: What did you feel like when you smoked? Where were you? Who were you with? Use this information to plan coping strategies for the next time this set of circumstances presents itself so that you can decrease the chances that you'll smoke the next time around.

WHEN IS IT APPROPRIATE TO REFER TO MORE INTENSIVE TREATMENTS?

What should a provider do when, despite his or her best efforts at coordinating and delivering brief treatments, a smoker fails to quit? The answer is reassess and, if necessary, discuss with the smoker the possibility of referral to a more intensive level of treatment (Chapter 2). By definition, smoking behavior and smoking cessation are changing, dynamic processes (Prochaska et al., 1997; W. Shadel, Niaura, & Abrams, 2000). The provider should not assume that a smoker will "look the same" as he/she initially did 1 year, 6 months, or even 2 weeks after an initial assessment. A careful and close monitoring of the smoker is required throughout the quitting process, and the provider needs to be alert to any changes in the smoker's profile along dimensions of nicotine dependence, quit attempts, co-occurrence of psychiatric disorder, and motivation. Moreover, if the smoker does not exhibit a major change along these dimensions yet continues to have difficulty quitting with brief treatment, the provider should initiate the process of referring the smoker to the next level of treatment.

CONCLUSION

Especially for brief treatments, smoking cessation will be a process fraught with frequent stops and false starts, successes and failures, and emotions that swing from very optimistic to very discouraged. The important point for both provider and smoker alike is not to give up after repeated failures to stop smoking. For despite multiple, exhausting attempts at smoking cessation, the more accurate the assessment, the more times minimal advice is provided, and the greater number of resources that the smoker has available, the greater the likelihood is that the next quit attempt will be a lasting one.

5

Intensive Behavioral Treatment

Richard A. Brown

Although some smokers are able to quit successfully without the aid of intensive smoking cessation treatment, a substantial number require more intensive cessation intervention over an extended time frame. These smokers are likely to benefit from a combination of pharmacological (see Chapter 7) and group or individual treatment. The focus of this chapter is on the delivery of the cognitive behavioral components of these intensive interventions. The combination of intensive behavioral treatment and pharmacotherapy is strongly recommended, as it significantly increases success (see Chapter 1). Furthermore, one or more comorbid factors may warrant additional tailored intervention for a subgroup of smokers. This chapter presents a core intensive cessation treatment framework that is applicable to all smokers in need of intensive treatment. Chapter 6 focuses on smokers with comorbidity, on those who need longer or more intensive coping skills training, or both. The specialized interventions provided in Chapter 6 are designed to be added to the core treatment described in this chapter.

This chapter begins with an overview of the various components that are recommended as part of the intensive smoking cessation program and refers to the related assessment strategies described in Chapter 2. This general discussion is followed by a more detailed, session-by-session outline that serves as a guide in the delivery of an intensive smoking cessation intervention. This program is presented as a group intervention, but the components can be used with individual smokers as well. Because the intervention is being presented in a group format, I use the term "facilitator" to describe the provider who is delivering the intervention.

The core intervention consists of eight sessions that can be delivered over a 7-week period, with two sessions being conducted on the week of quit day. This core intervention assumes a relative lack of comorbid, complicating factors among the smoker group and delivers the last group session 2 weeks after quit day. In Chapter 6, intervention components to address comorbid factors such as depression are presented. Addressing these comorbid factors may also warrant extending the length of the group treatment, which is also discussed.

In order to provide a self-contained group intervention approach without inclusion of pharmacological treatment, the intervention described in this chapter includes a nicotine-fading component. In our view, nicotine fading represents an alternative to NRT for smokers who prefer not to use pharmacotherapy or in cases in which NRT is contraindicated. Our research group at Brown Medical School has evaluated the behavioral treatment used in this intensive treatment protocol (Brown et al., 2001) and the use of combined pharmacological and behavioral treatment (Goldstein et al., 1989) and found results that are comparable to the most efficacious outcomes reported in the PHS guideline (Fiore et al., 2000). Facilitators who combine this intensive treatment protocol with pharmacotherapy can use a "cold turkey" quit day rather than nicotine fading. The reason is that nicotine replacement and other pharmacological therapies for smoking cessation start on quit day. Chapter 7 of this volume describes the selection, dosage, and tapering schedule for the various pharmacotherapies. Combined nicotine replacement and behavioral coping skills outperform either treatment alone and are recommended in the PHS guideline (Fiore et al., 2000).

COGNITIVE SOCIAL LEARNING MODEL

As outlined in Chapter 1, the cognitive social learning approach (Bandura, 1997) provides the best framework for conceptualizing smoking cessation interventions. The social learning model views smoking as a learned behavior acquired through classical and operant conditioning principles and cognitive (symbolic) processes, including modeling others' behavior, self-control mechanisms (goal setting, self-monitoring, self-evaluation, self-correction), beliefs, self-efficacy, and outcome expectations. Various environmental and cognitive cues trigger a craving or desire to smoke and are termed "antecedents." Once the smoker smokes a cigarette (the "behavior"), he/she experiences the rewarding "consequences." Symbolic cognitive processes—thoughts, feelings, emotions, expectations—are readily incorporated within this framework, providing they can be reliably self-monitored by the smoker. The general rationale for treatment is that with practice and alternative skills training, the automatic chain of events (A → B → C; Antecedent → Behavior → Consequences) can be broken, and smoking behavior can be "unlearned" and replaced with more adaptive patterns. The new learning involves actual practice of skills that are ideally taught through a series of small success experiences (proximal goal setting) practiced in the group or in individual sessions (role playing) and then practiced outside of the group in the smoker's own natural environment.

Efficacy expectations, or self-efficacy, refers to one's perceived ability to meet a particular challenge or perform a particular task (Bandura, 1997). As the smoker in treatment sets goals, implements new problem-solving coping skills, evaluates how the skills are working, gains self-correcting feedback, and strengthens the necessary skills to quit smoking and resist relapse, his/her self-efficacy is enhanced and the likelihood of success is increased. Measures for assessing smoker self-efficacy are described and can be found within the basic assessment module on cognition in Chapter 2.

MULTICOMPONENT TREATMENT PROGRAMS

Multicomponent approaches have generally achieved long-term (12-month follow up) abstinence rates of approximately 25–30% (Fiore et al., 2000), although rates of 50% or better also have been reported (Schwartz, 1987) . It is useful to think of multicomponent cessation programs as composed of three interrelated phases: preparation, quitting, and maintenance of cessation, or preventing relapse. They are interrelated in the sense that they overlap in time and that some principles and methods are useful in more than one phase.

Phase 1: Preparation

Some programs urge smokers to quit immediately. We strongly recommend, however, that there be a "preparation" period prior to quitting, the length of which can vary according to program needs. During the preparation period, the smokers' motivation to quit and commitment to the program should be reviewed and strengthened. Two objectives are particularly important during this period. First, there should be a clearly established target quit day that allows smokers the time to "mentally prepare" and to develop the coping strategies needed to quit smoking. Second, smokers should self-monitor their daily smoking in order to establish baseline levels and to begin to pay close attention to their smoking triggers or antecedents and consequences. The target quit day is generally set between 14 and 28 days after the program begins and can be approached by gradual reductions in nicotine (fading) or "cold turkey" with initiation of pharmacological therapy.

Target Quit Day

We strongly recommend the establishment of a target quit day at the very beginning of a program. This gives smokers a specific date to work toward and should be established so as to allow sufficient time for the acquisition of coping skills needed to maintain cessation and prevent relapse. The time may also be used to reduce nicotine consumption by changing brands, by reducing the number of cigarettes prior to quitting, or both. In the treatment model described in this chapter, the quit day occurs at the end of the 4th week of treatment.

Self-Monitoring of Smoking Behavior

Keeping a written record of the number of cigarettes smoked is a standard behavioral procedure. A key principle in the initial cessation process is that, in order for smokers to effectively change their smoking habits, they must first gain an understanding of their own unique habit patterns through self-monitoring of their daily cigarette smoking. The enhancement of self-awareness of every cigarette smoked is in fact the beginning of an intervention (Abrams & Wilson, 1979a). Self-monitoring interrupts the automatic habit and gets the smoker to think about every cigarette he/she smokes and why he/she smokes it. Usually, this reduces the number of cigarettes smoked per day. Thus, self-monitoring is an assessment strategy; it is discussed in the smoking triggers and coping skills assessment module in Chapter 2.

A preprinted card or sheet (often called a "Wrap Sheet" or "Pack Wrap"; see Figure 5.1)

WRAP SHEET

CIGARETTES	TIME	HOW DO YOU FEEL?								WHAT ARE YOU DOING?
		Happy	Sad or depressed	Relaxed	Bored	Anxious	Angry	Tired	Frustrated	
1	6:30 am							X		Morning cup of coffee
2	8:00 am					X			X	Driving to work, stuck in traffic
3	10:00 am			X						Morning cigarette break with coworker
4	12:30 pm					X				After lunch on an errand
5	2:00 pm				X					Waiting for computer problem to be solved
6	2:30 pm						X			Argument with vendor
7	3:30 pm					X				Afternoon coffee break
8	5:30 pm								X	Driving home from work
9	6:00 pm							X		In car, after grocery shopping
10	7:15 pm			X						Home, preparing dinner
11	8:30 pm	X								Getting kids washed up and in bed
12	9:00 pm			X				X		Watching TV
13	9:45 pm							X		Folding laundry
14	10:30 pm			X				X		Reading in bed

FIGURE 5.1. Wrap Sheet (or Pack Wrap).

that can be attached to the cigarette pack facilitates self-monitoring. Smokers are instructed to record each cigarette prior to smoking it and to record the time of day and the situation in which the cigarette was smoked (e.g., with coffee, talking with friends who smoked). Assessment of mood at the time of each cigarette (e.g., tense, relaxed, etc.) is also useful. The situational notations allow an opportunity for a smoker to analyze each smoking episode, revealing the antecedent influences that trigger smoking. These events or triggers that are associated with smoking need to be delineated, as they may become future high-risk situations for relapse. Smokers are instructed at this point not to make any changes in their smoking habits but merely to observe and gain an increased awareness of their smoking behaviors.

Phase 2: Quitting

We have conceptualized "quitting" strategies as those that are important and direct prerequisites to quitting successfully on the quit day. This section discusses two major types of social learning–based approaches that are frequently included in multicomponent programs: self-management and nicotine fading.

Self-Management

Self-management (sometimes termed self-control or stimulus control) refers to strategies intended to rearrange environmental cues that trigger smoking behavior or alter the consequences of smoking. As previously presented in the ABC model, the term "trigger" is synonymous with the A—antecedent. The importance of triggers is highlighted by the likelihood that, on quitting, triggers may become high-risk situations for relapse. Therefore, the goal is for smokers to systematically practice using coping strategies to keep from smoking in identified trigger situations prior to quit day. Consistent with the assessment of trigger situations discussed in Chapter 2, the first step in self-management is for smokers to use information from the Wrap Sheets they have completed to develop a list of their various trigger situations. Once triggers have been identified, smokers begin to intervene actively in their natural environment to break up the smoking behavior chain by utilizing one of three general strategies: (1) avoid the trigger situation; (2) alter or change the trigger situation; and (3) use an alternative or substitute in place of the cigarette.

Examples of avoiding trigger situations include forgoing a coffee break at work with other smokers, leaving the table after dinner, and avoiding social situations involving alcohol. Altering a trigger situation might involve drinking tea or juice in the morning instead of coffee, watching TV in the bedroom (a nonsmoking room) rather than in the living room, and putting cigarettes in the trunk of the car before driving. Alternatives or substitutes can be used in conjunction with avoiding or altering trigger situations or in situations that cannot be avoided or altered. Possible alternatives include sugarless candy or gum, raw cut vegetables such as carrot or celery sticks, chewing on toothpicks, using a relaxation technique in a stressful situation, or doing needlework or something else to keep hands busy. There are many other examples of these strategies, and the group can be used to brainstorm and share different possibilities. Smokers should decide on strategies they think will work for them and then try out different approaches, rejecting those that are not useful until they have been able to successfully manage all or most trigger situations without smoking (see Table 4.7).

Relaxation techniques are a logical choice for self-management, because smokers frequently report that they smoke to cope with stress and because relapses frequently occur in negative-affect situations. Smokers can be assessed on the degree to which they perceive stress in their lives, as described in the stress and withdrawal assessment module in Chapter 2. The Benson relaxation response (see Figure 5.4) is a meditative, breathing-based technique that can be easily taught to smokers and readily mastered by them with a moderate amount of practice (Benson, 1975). Progressive muscular relaxation and imagery-based relaxation approaches are also viable alternatives (Jacobson, 1938).

Nicotine Fading

Nicotine fading is a nonaversive procedure that addresses both pharmacological and psychological factors. The rationale for nicotine fading is that cigarette smoking is physically addicting for many smokers and that gradually reducing their dependence on nicotine will reduce the intensity of their withdrawal symptoms at quit day, thus making quitting less difficult. Smokers work toward a target quit day by switching to cigarettes that have progressively lower nicotine content over a period of several weeks. Smokers frequently report mild withdrawal symptoms throughout the brand-switching phase, suggesting a diffusion of the definite withdrawal effects that would ordinarily be experienced had they quit smoking their regular brands cold turkey. Information on the nicotine yields of current cigarette brands is available from the Federal Trade Commission (1997). More details of these procedures are available in Foxx and Brown (1979).

One drawback of nicotine fading is that it may not work for smokers who are already smoking brands with the lowest nicotine content, although they can be encouraged to make any possible switches to a brand with even lower nicotine. Furthermore, some prospective quitters may find smoking reduced-nicotine cigarettes to be aversive or may have a strong desire to quit right away without undergoing a fading process over several weeks. For those smokers, the treatment described in this chapter can be modified to eliminate the fading component; however, treatment should still utilize stimulus control (or self-control) procedures in conjunction with rate fading (i.e., reducing the number of cigarettes) by specifically targeting trigger situations in which to avoid or eliminate smoking. During nicotine fading, smokers may compensate by smoking more cigarettes or changing the topography of their smoking behavior (e.g., inhaling more deeply, smoking more of each cigarette, blocking filter holes). Smokers should be cautioned about this possibility and advised to keep such changes to a minimum.

As nicotine fading may address the physical dependence component of smoking, it can serve as an alternative to nicotine replacement or other pharmacological approaches for smokers who desire a nonpharmacological approach or for whom nicotine replacement or medication usage are otherwise contraindicated. Alternatively, the nicotine-fading component can be deleted for those smokers who wish to avoid lower levels of protracted nicotine withdrawal and would prefer to quit cold turkey. A third option is to incorporate NRT as described in Chapter 7 into this treatment.

Phase 3: Maintenance

Because the majority of smokers who initially quit resume smoking within several months of treatment termination (Hunt & Bespalec, 1974), maintenance is a critical issue for smoking cessation programs. In this section, we focus on several of the more frequently employed maintenance strategies, including relapse prevention, lifestyle modification, physical activity, and social support.

Relapse Prevention/Coping Skills

The coping skills approach assumes that the individual lacks the behavioral and cognitive skills necessary to become a permanent nonsmoker. Marlatt and Gordon (1985) have proposed a cognitive-behavioral model of relapse that has played a major role in current thinking on cessation treatment techniques and has stimulated a considerable amount of research. Relapse prevention theory proposes that the ability to cope with high-risk situations determines an individual's probability of maintaining abstinence. Successful coping in high-risk situations leads to an increased sense of self-efficacy (Bandura, 1997), but failure to cope initiates a chain of events in which diminished self-efficacy may lead to a slip and perhaps to a full-blown relapse. In these instances, smokers are taught to avoid self-defeating attributions and resulting negative emotional reactions (i.e., the abstinence violation effect; see Session 4 later in this chapter) that promote continued smoking (Marlatt & Gordon, 1985). The assessment of coping strategies is more fully described in the basic assessment module on smoking triggers and coping in Chapter 2.

Lifestyle Change

Marlatt and Gordon (1985) discuss the concept of replacing a negative addiction (such as smoking) with a "positive addiction." The idea is that smoking may be due, in part, to the fact that the many demands on an individual from work, family, and other commitments are experienced as "shoulds" that must be done (Type A activities) and do not leave enough time to engage in relaxing, pleasurable activities (Type B activities). Smokers are thus instructed to set aside 45 to 60 minutes as often as possible (ideally, on a daily basis) to engage in a relaxing, enjoyable activity. In this context, we suggest the continued use of relaxation techniques that have been introduced and taught prior to quit day. However, the idea is for the smoker to decide on the types of activities that he or she would find enjoyable and stress relieving; we recognize that not everyone may choose to do a formal relaxation technique during this time.

Physical Activity

We strongly encourage smokers to engage in some type of regular exercise throughout the quitting process. There has been considerable interest recently in the role that physical activity may play in preventing relapse. Because vigorous exercise is incompatible with simultaneous smoking, exercise can serve as a substitute behavior following cessation. Vigorous exercise has recently been shown to enhance smoking cessation and maintenance in women (Marcus et al., 1999). Exercise may also be a good alternative to restrained eating or dieting for individuals who are concerned about postcessation weight gain. In addition, exercise may moderate mood changes such as depression and anxiety, and therefore it may serve to attenuate nicotine withdrawal (Abrams et al., 1987). Ideally, supervised vigorous exercise of the type used in the Commit to Quit trial (see Chapter 1; Marcus et al., 1999) is recommended. If this exercise regimen is too demanding, a self-help or home-based guide to increasing physical activity can be recommended after insuring that the smoker has been cleared by his/her physician (Blair et al., 2001).

Social Support

The role of family and peer influences in successful smoking cessation has been well documented (Fiore et al., 2000; Lichtenstein et al., 1986). Social support can be a source of motivation for quitting and of positive reinforcement for successfully maintaining abstinence. Social support might also provide a buffer against the stress of quitting or other stressful events that might precipitate a relapse. We suggest that smokers identify sources of social support in their environment and make active efforts to harness that support. The Partner Interaction Questionnaire (PIQ; Mermelstein et al., 1986), discussed in Chapter 2, assesses the role of perceived level of support by a significant other in quitting smoking and may be a useful clinical adjunct to help smokers identify areas of support and nonsupport and to intervene accordingly. Special attention must be prov   is married to, lives with, or is otherwise in clo   or work environment. In order to quit success   ration of his/her spouse, coworkers, or friend   es (discussed in Chapter 6) to request that they   port his/her cessation effort in some other i

PROGRAM STRUCTURE

In designing an intensive treatment program   the nature of the treatment program they are developing and the   that are inheren   ent program designs. Intensive treatment prog   ge from 5 or 6 sessions to as many as 12 to 20 sessions and can span anywhere fr   ks to 3 to 6 months in length (Cooper & Clayton, 1993). Group sessions can range in length between 1 and 2 hours, with 90 minutes representing a reasonable compromise. Programs can be structured to devote considerable time prior to quit day to teaching skills, can devote extended time following quit day to managing acute withdrawal and relapse prevention, or can do both. Of course, spending considerable time both before and after quit day results in a 12- to 14-session program. The trade-off here is that many smokers may not be interested in or willing to participate in a program this lengthy. In developing a shorter program (6–10 weeks) that is likely to appeal to a broader group of smokers, one must decide the relative merits of "front-loading" skills training prior to quitting, with relatively fewer sessions devoted to maintenance, versus having smokers quit within the first several sessions and providing extensive skills training and support during the maintenance period.

Another important consideration is, of course, the nature of the treatment interventions. If pharmacotherapy is included in the treatment protocol, the nature of the medication may affect the treatment schedule. Thus, although nicotine replacement products can be started concurrent with quitting, medications such as bupropion SR (Zyban) require that sessions occur for a period of time prior to quit day to allow a buildup of drug levels in the body prior to quitting. Similarly, nonpharmacological interventions such as nicotine fading require that brands and smoking rate be faded over a period of weeks prior to quitting, whereas a program incorporating "cold turkey" quitting (perhaps following several aversion sessions) may not require as much time prior to quit day.

Finally, the provider must consider the schedule by which sessions will be phased out at the end of the treatment program. It is not uncommon for programs to move from weekly sessions to sessions every other week, and possibly to a final session that takes place 1 month after the penultimate session. This type of sequence has the advantage of giving smokers the opportunity to remain connected with the treatment and their support group while navigating their way through the period of greatest risk for relapse (the first 3 months after quit day). However, despite the urgings of group facilitators, a common experience in smoking cessation programs is that smokers who have relapsed often feel embarrassed or otherwise no longer motivated, and they do not continue to attend group treatment sessions. Therefore, the longer the group continues after quit day, the greater the attrition within the group.

The intensive behavioral treatment program presented in this chapter consists of eight sessions over a 7-week time period (see Table 5.1). Sessions are 90 minutes in length. Sessions occur weekly for 7 consecutive weeks with quit day at Session 5. Only Session 6 is not part of the weekly schedule, taking place 3 or 4 days after Session 5. Therefore, there are two sessions during the week of quit day, and Sessions 5, 6, and 7 all occur within a span of 8 days. This schedule is designed to provide a shorter time period between sessions for added support during this acute period of highest risk for relapse. The group ends at Session 8, which occurs 2 weeks after quit day.

SESSION 1: INTRODUCTORY SESSION

Smokers generally come to the initial session with considerable trepidation. Frequently, they have made unsuccessful quit attempts in the past. Many have never attended a formal treatment program in the past and may feel embarrassed or ashamed at having to resort to such an option in order to quit smoking. If they are beginning a group treatment, they may feel more anxiety about who the other people in the group are, and how comfortable they will feel sharing potentially intimate information regarding their past efforts (i.e., "failures") to quit smoking.

Thus the facilitator must keep several objectives in mind for the first session, which in many ways is the most critical session of the entire treatment.

Session 1 Objectives

1. To introduce the group facilitators, the structural details of the treatment program, and the ground rules for the conduct of the group sessions.
2. To conduct a warm-up exercise to help smokers get acquainted with other group members in a way that sets the tone for a supportive and positive group experience.
3. To present a positive focus and framework for quitting smoking, emphasizing the learning gained in past quit attempts, the advantages of learning specific coping skills to aid in quitting, and the benefits of participating in a group program with the support of other group members.
4. To present the cognitive social learning theory rationale for smoking cessation treatment.
5. To introduce self-monitoring of smoking behavior and to give out Wrap Sheets for completion between first and second sessions.
6. To introduce and define the concept of triggers for smoking.
7. To provide a rationale and an explanation of the use of nicotine fading.
8. To preview the homework assignments to be completed prior to Session 2.

TABLE 5.1. Treatment Schedule and Session Content

Phase of treatment	Preparation/cessation				Quit day	Maintenance		
Timeline (Days)	−28	−21	−14	−7	0	+3	+7	+14
Week no.	One	Two	Three	Four	Five	Five	Six	Seven
Session no.	1	2	3	4	5	6	7	8
Focus content of session	Introduction/ground rules Cognitive social learning rationale Self-monitoring Identifying triggers for smoking Nicotine fading	Self-management Deep breathing relaxation	Lifestyle changes	Identifying and coping with high-risk situations Abstinence Violation Effect (AVE) Preparation for quit day	Discussion of quit day experiences Social support for nonsmoking Plan for maintaining abstinence	Discussion of quitting experiences Strategies for coping with urges Plan for maintaining abstinence	Discussion of quitting experiences Strategies for managing thoughts Plan for maintaining abstinence	Discussion of quitting experiences Planning for the future
Review	Cognitive social learning rationale Self-monitoring Identifying triggers Nicotine fading Homework	Self-management Deep breathing relaxation Self-monitoring Nicotine fading Homework	Self-management Deep breathing relaxation Self-monitoring Lifestyle changes Nicotine fading Homework	Self-management Deep breathing relaxation Self-monitoring Lifestyle changes Nicotine fading Homework	Identifying and coping with high-risk situations Lifestyle changes Social support for nonsmoking Abstinence Violation Effect (AVE) Nicotine fading Homework	Identifying and coping with high-risk situations Lifestyle changes Social support for nonsmoking Abstinence Violation Effect (AVE) Homework	Identifying and coping with high-risk situations Abstinence Violation Effect (AVE) Strategies for coping with urges Social support for nonsmoking Homework	Identifying and coping with high-risk situations Abstinence Violation Effect (AVE) Strategies for coping with urges Lifestyle changes Strategies for managing thoughts Homework

Session 1 Handouts and Worksheets

1. Written Program Schedule
2. Wrap Sheets
3. Triggers for Smoking Worksheet

Session 1 Content

1. *Introduce facilitators, structural details of program, and ground rules.*
   a. Welcome smokers to the program. Express enthusiasm about their participation ("Congratulations for taking this first important step toward quitting smoking").
   b. Introduce group facilitators. Provide brief details about facilitators' background and qualifications. Be prepared for questions about the smoking status of facilitators. The most commonly asked question is whether the facilitator previously smoked. It is often a controversial topic as to whether facilitators need to possess certain characteristics in order to conduct certain types of therapy (e.g., whether an unmarried facilitator can provide marital therapy). If facilitators have never smoked, we suggest that they respond nondefensively while accentuating the extent of their experience in counseling smokers. We recommend that group or individual treatment not be conducted by facilitators who are current smokers.
   c. Describe structure of program. Inform smokers of the number of group sessions and how they are scheduled (e.g., weekly, twice weekly, etc.), including dates and starting times. It is generally helpful to provide a written program schedule with this information. A specific "quit day" should be designated for each group and should be indicated clearly on the program schedule. Smokers are informed that the few weeks before the quit day are designed to provide sufficient time for learning and practicing coping skills for quitting smoking and for medication levels (e.g., Zyban) to build up in their bodies. The time from quit day to the end of the program is needed to focus on successfully maintaining abstinence and preventing relapse through the use of coping skills and group support.
   d. Introduction of ground rules for the group treatment.
      i. Indicate to smokers the importance of establishing a sense of group cohesion and caring within the group. Make it clear that supportive, helpful, non-negative comments will be valued in the group and that this is not an "encounter group" or a place to be critical of fellow group members.
      ii. Remind smokers that, during any discussion topic within the group, they always have the option not to participate.
      iii. Ask smokers to assist in providing equal time for everyone to speak. This "equal time" rule involves making an effort not to monopolize conversations in the group.
      iv. Inform smokers that maintaining confidentiality is critical to having a successful group experience. Urge them to maintain the confidentiality of fellow group members' identities and of the content of what is said in the group sessions.
      v. Ask smokers to please call in advance if they cannot make a session as a courtesy to

group leaders, as well as to other group members. Provide them with a phone number at which they can reach a staff member or leave a message.

    vi. Finally, inform smokers that no smoking is allowed during the sessions.

2. *Conduct warm-up exercise to help smokers get acquainted.* We suggest a simple exercise as a great icebreaker during the first 20 minutes of the initial session. We ask participants to pair up with someone in the group, to take about 10 minutes to get acquainted, and then to introduce their partner to the rest of the group. We ask smokers to get to know each other by sharing information about themselves, with a particular focus on how the smoker enjoys spending his or her recreational or leisure time. Smokers generally end up talking a bit about their smoking and quitting histories, which is to be expected although it is not intended. Once the group has had sufficient time to talk, each smoker is asked to introduce the other person to the rest of the group and tell a little bit about him or her.

3. *Present a focus and framework for smoking cessation efforts.*

    a. *Quitting is a process that can be learned.* It is important to set a positive tone for the group efforts that will follow. Facilitators should provide smokers with the perspective that quitting smoking is a long-term process of learning what will and will not work to help them successfully abstain from smoking. Smokers should be provided with a framework that considers prior failed quit attempts to be learning experiences that have assisted them in differentiating which approaches will help them to succeed at quitting smoking and which will not. Inform them that quitting smoking is a process that takes place over a period of years and that multiple quit attempts are commonly required for smokers to finally achieve lasting abstinence (Schachter, 1982).

    b. *Acknowledge mixed feelings about quitting.* Facilitators should acknowledge that they understand that some smokers may enter into this process with considerable mixed feelings, recognizing that smokers may feel anxious or fearful and have doubts about their ability or motivations to quit smoking. On the one hand, they may recognize that they "need" (more about this idea later) or "want" (a preferable perspective) to quit smoking but may also still enjoy smoking and/or be fearful of changes that quitting smoking may bring (e.g., weight gain, irritability).

    c. *Benefits of participating in a group program.* Smokers should be informed that the group treatment will involve learning and applying specific coping skills in a supportive group atmosphere. The coping-skills component of the treatment is critical to their success and will involve certain readings and practice exercises that they will need to accomplish between sessions. The coping skills they learn will help them identify critical aspects of their smoking patterns and develop the means to deal with situations and circumstances that previously might have triggered them to smoke. Also, by participating in a group, they will have the benefit of the group members' collective wisdom and emotional support. Smokers are told that many important suggestions that they will receive will come from other group members (not just from the group facilitators) and that they should also share their own ideas and suggestions freely with others in the group.

    d. *Motivational ups and downs.* Finally, facilitators should remind smokers that there is no substitute for their own motivation and commitment to quit smoking. Quitting smoking is hard work, and facilitators should indicate to smokers that they need to be committed to putting in the effort to succeed. The combination of their own effort and commitment and a quality treatment program should provide smokers with the best chance of success. Motivation can wax and wane as smokers go through the quitting process, and facilitators should carefully monitor each smoker's motivation. Counseling strategies from Chapter 3 may need to be used from time to time to keep motivation and adherence at a high level.

4. *Present the cognitive social learning theory rationale.*

a. Facilitators should explain to smokers that smoking consists of the following three components:

i. *Learned habit.* Cigarette smoking is a behavior pattern (or habit) that is overlearned through years of repetition. It is critical for smokers to learn about their particular smoking patterns, to identify events, situations, and behaviors that prompt them to smoke, and to learn ways to cope without smoking.

ii. *Physical addiction.* The physically addicting ingredient in cigarettes is the drug nicotine. Physical addiction is explained in terms of tolerance and withdrawal. Smokers are reminded of how their bodies gradually acquired tolerance to nicotine when they first began smoking, requiring increasingly greater amounts (i.e., greater numbers of cigarettes) to achieve the same physiological effects. Smokers generally need no reminding about the occurrence of withdrawal symptoms when quitting smoking, as most of them have experienced these symptoms during past quit attempts.

iii. *Means of managing negative mood.* For many people, cigarette smoking serves as a means of helping to manage negative moods. People may learn to rely on cigarettes to cope with upsetting situations and to combat negative feelings such as depression, anxiety, anger, and frustration. Smokers are therefore asked to consider the extent to which cigarettes are, for them, a way of coping with unpleasant feelings. Smokers are also informed about possible psychoactive properties of nicotine and the prospect that the drug itself may serve to change mood by acting like an antidepressant or, in some other physiological manner, reduce negative mood. In this context, smokers are reminded that nicotine is a stimulant and may thus provide some type of "pick-me-up" for smokers. Similarly, smoking may sometimes be used for pleasure or enhancement of an already positive experience, such as in an enjoyable or celebratory context (e.g., at a party, watching a sporting event, at a wedding, etc.).

b. *Treatment rationale.* Smokers should be told that effective treatment must address each aspect of smoking that is relevant to them. At a minimum, treatment must address the first two aspects described (learned habit and physical addiction). The third aspect (managing negative mood) should also be addressed for many smokers who feel that their smoking serves as a means of coping with negative moods or for whom cessation from smoking might trigger depressive symptoms. Treatment must also focus both on initial quitting and on helping to maintain abstinence and prevent relapse. Smokers should be told that this treatment will help them:

i. to understand the *learned habit* aspect of their smoking so they can anticipate and develop nonsmoking habits in former smoking situations

ii. to gradually reduce their *physical addiction* (dependence) on nicotine through a procedure called nicotine fading. (In treatment employing nicotine replacement or other pharmacological means of addressing nicotine dependence [see Chapter 7], the rationale will, of course, reflect the approach taken.)

iii. to learn skills to manage negative moods and cope with negative mood situations more effectively

5. *Introduce self-monitoring of smoking behavior.* Smokers should be provided with a rationale for the importance of self-monitoring their smoking behavior prior to making changes in their smoking habits. Facilitators should indicate that every smoker has his/her own unique learned habit pattern that has been developed over years of smoking and that the first step in changing this habit pattern is to understand it. Learning about one's smoking behavior by self-monitoring (writing down each cigarette smoked) leads to learning effective ways of changing that behavior.

Smokers are told to smoke "normally" between now and the next session (i.e., not to make any changes in their smoking), because they are just trying to learn about their usual smoking habits. Smokers are provided with a sheet or a card (often called a "Wrap Sheet") on which to self-monitor their daily smoking (Figure 5.1). The Wrap Sheet is carried with the pack of cigarettes by "wrapping" it around the pack or folding it and placing it in the cellophane of the pack. Each time the smoker takes out a cigarette to smoke, a self-monitoring entry is made on the Wrap Sheet *before* the smoker lights up the cigarette. The following information is generally recorded:

a. Date and time of day of each cigarette
b. Activity or situation at the time of lighting up (this could include thoughts)
c. Mood experienced at the time of lighting up

One Wrap Sheet has enough space to record 20 cigarettes. Smokers should start a new Wrap Sheet each day and continue onto a subsequent sheet or sheets if they smoke more than 20 cigarettes per day. Starting a new sheet each day allows smokers to easily obtain a count of their daily number of cigarettes. Figure 5.1 shows a sample completed Wrap Sheet.

At the next session, smokers will bring in and review their completed self-monitoring records. Facilitators will be able to discuss the behavior patterns that emerge in terms of times of day when smoking occurs, situations, or activities commonly associated with smoking behavior. Knowledge gained through self-monitoring begins to guide smokers' thinking about the types of changes they may need to accomplish in order to quit smoking. This knowledge then leads to discussions of triggers for smoking and the acquisition of self-management skills for quitting.

6. *Introduce and define the concept of "triggers for smoking."* As part of the learned-habit aspect of smoking, smokers should be informed of the relationship between triggers, urges to smoke, and smoking behavior. (See Figure 6.2 for a diagram that can be drawn on a wipe board or pad as concepts are presented.) A "trigger" is defined as a situation, event, or behavior (may include thoughts and feelings) that is commonly associated with smoking a cigarette, so that being in the situation brings on the urge to smoke. After several days of self-monitoring smoking using Wrap Sheets, smokers will be asked to identify trigger situations, as well as what they are thinking and feeling at the time of the urge, on the Triggers for Smoking form (see Figure 5.2).

TRIGGERS FOR SMOKING

Think about the different times or situations in which you usually smoke. These situations may trigger your smoking in different ways. For example, you may automatically light up a cigarette whenever you get in the car. The trigger here is "getting in the car." We call such situations "Triggers for Smoking."

You can begin to understand your own triggers for smoking by looking over the Wrap Sheets you keep this week. After keeping Wrap Sheets for 3 days, list below as many of your own triggers as possible. In addition to the event or what you were doing when smoking, also list how you are feeling (your mood) and what you might be thinking at the time.

Learning about your own triggers can help you quit and quit for keeps. Read the example below before beginning to list your own trigger situations.

	Event or What You're Doing	Feeling	Thinking
EX:	*Driving to work*	*Tense, frustrated*	*How will I ever get anything done today!*
1.	Coffee in the morning	Tired	
2.	Talking on the phone	Relaxed	
3.	Arguing with husband	Angry	He's so selfish-he'll never change
4.	Break at work	Frustrated	It's time for a smoke
5.	Watching TV	Bored	
6.	After dinner	Content	A cigarette would be great right now
7.			
8.			

FIGURE 5.2. Triggers for Smoking.

Facilitators should be advised that a subset of smokers will state that they smoke "constantly" as a matter of habit, not in response to specific triggers. Although internal physiological cues may be triggers to smoke, these smokers should still be encouraged to examine the circumstances that commonly accompany their smoking (e.g., with coffee, while on breaks at work, with alcohol, while socializing, when anxious) as a means of identifying their triggers for smoking.

7. *Provide a rationale and explanation for nicotine fading.* Note that although this protocol utilizes nicotine fading as an intervention to address the physiological dependence on nicotine, pharmacotherapy is also commonly used as part of an intensive smoking cessation treatment. Information regarding pharmacological treatment of nicotine dependence can be found in Chapter 7. The specific rationale for the choice of a pharmacological agent and its role in combating physical addiction to nicotine should be substituted in this section of the protocol if pharmacotherapy rather than nicotine fading is employed.

Nicotine fading is a nonaversive procedure that addresses both pharmacological and psychological factors. The nicotine-fading rationale is that cigarette smoking is physically addicting for many smokers and that gradually reducing their dependence on nicotine will reduce the intensity of their withdrawal symptoms at quit day, thus making quitting less difficult. Smokers work toward a target quit day by switching to cigarettes with progressively lower nicotine content over a period of several weeks (brand fading), while also reducing the number of cigarettes smoked daily (rate fading). Facilitators should point out that smokers are to smoke their regular brand the first week and to smoke "normally," as described previously. Smokers frequently report mild withdrawal symptoms throughout the brand-switching phase.

Facilitators should provide smokers with the following rationale for the use of nicotine fading. Smokers are told that nicotine is physically addicting and that people vary in the degree to which they are physically dependent. However, many smokers will experience withdrawal symptoms on quitting. The typical withdrawal symptoms that may be experienced are irritability, sad or depressed mood, change in sleeping habits, difficulty concentrating, change in appetite, drowsiness, and craving for a cigarette. Withdrawal symptoms are typically worse during the first week after quitting and generally do not last beyond 2 weeks. Smokers are informed that, although withdrawal symptoms may vary depending on the number of cigarettes and the nicotine content of the brand smoked, they are always worse when people quit cold turkey. By gradually reducing their dependence on nicotine through nicotine fading, smokers will reduce the intensity of their withdrawal symptoms at quit day, thus making quitting less difficult.

It is helpful at this point to elicit discussion from smokers about withdrawal symptoms experienced during past quit attempts. Smokers are generally quite able and willing to discuss past experiences with withdrawal symptoms. This discussion also serves to reinforce the premise that nicotine is physically addicting.

The nicotine fading procedure helps smokers reduce their physical dependence on nicotine prior to quit day. Smokers are told that there are two ways to accomplish nicotine fading:

a. *Brand fading* involves changing brands in 30%, 60%, and 90% decrements, on a weekly or biweekly basis, prior to quitting. Smokers should be provided with a list of the more common cigarette brands and their nicotine yields as a means of helping them decide which brands to use in their fading schedule. This information is published by the Federal Trade Commission (Federal Trade Commission, 1997).

b. *Rate fading* involves having smokers gradually reduce the number of cigarettes they smoke daily. Smokers may set a goal of reducing their daily smoking rate by a minimum of 10–15% per week prior to quitting. It is very important that smokers do not reduce their daily smoking rate below 10 cigarettes per day. Smoking less than 10 cigarettes per day may increase the reward value of those remaining cigarettes and could actually make it harder to quit.

Another important component of nicotine fading involves tracking changes in estimated nicotine intake through self-monitoring of estimated nicotine yields during the fading process. After recording their smoking rates, smokers can calculate and plot their estimated intake of nicotine each day. This self-monitoring of daily nicotine yield provides smokers with positive feedback regarding their efforts, because these levels invariably go down if they follow the basic brand-changing instructions. Compliance with this procedure has been observed to increase smokers' self-confidence in their ability to quit. More details of these procedures are available in Foxx and Brown (1979).

Important points to reiterate to smokers about nicotine fading include the following:

a. By quit day, the smoker's nicotine level will be at its lowest. Although this does not guarantee success, it should make it as easy as possible to quit by virtue of having reduced the physical dependence prior to quitting.

b. Withdrawal symptoms may occur during the fading process prior to quit day. These occurrences should be presented to smokers as evidence that the fading process is working and that withdrawal distress will be less intense at quit day. Better to experience the withdrawal symptoms while still smoking than all at once on quit day.

c. Facilitators should discuss with smokers that they may not like the taste of the cigarette brands they switch to during brand fading. Smokers can be told tactfully that this is probably for the best, as it will likely be easier for them to quit smoking if their last experiences with cigarettes are less enjoyable.

d. Smokers should be cautioned not to compensate when switching to a lower nicotine brand by smoking more cigarettes, inhaling more deeply, smoking more of the cigarette, or covering the entire filter with fingers or lips in order to bypass the filtering system of low tar and nicotine cigarettes.

Rate fading is closely associated with the use of self-management strategies that are described in Session 2. Rather than merely reducing the number of cigarettes smoked, rate fading should be accomplished by learning to avoid particular cigarettes in specific trigger situations. Thus, as smokers are applying newly learned coping skills to avoid smoking in trigger situations, they should begin to reduce their smoking rate by a minimum of 10–15% per week prior to quitting. Smokers who wish to make further reductions in their smoking should feel free to do so, but facilitators should caution smokers not to set unrealistically high goals. The ideal goal is one that can reasonably be accomplished, which will then serve to enhance smokers' self-efficacy for quitting smoking.

One drawback of brand fading is that it may not work for smokers who are already smoking brands with the lowest nicotine content. If their regular brand is already at the lowest possible nicotine yield (currently 0.05 mg nicotine), they may change to another brand of equal nicotine yield in order to disrupt the taste and "comfort" associated with smoking their regular brand. Furthermore, some prospective quitters may find smoking reduced-nicotine cigarettes aversive or may have a strong desire to quit right away without undergoing a fading process over several weeks. Finally, it should be noted that actual reductions in nicotine intake may be less than those suggested by the published nicotine yield of the cigarette brand, as smokers may compensate by smoking more cigarettes or changing their smoking behaviors, as mentioned previously. Smokers should be cautioned about this possibility and advised to keep such changes to a minimum. However, for this reason, nicotine fading is recommended primarily as a smoking cessation strategy rather than as both a cessation strategy and a possible harm reduction approach (with the goal of staying on a reduced nicotine brand) if cessation fails.

8. *Provide the homework assignments to be completed prior to Session 2.* Facilitators should confirm the date and time of the next session, review assignments to be completed before the next session, and answer any questions that smokers might have about the assignments.

Prior to Session 2

Do for the first time:

1. Complete Wrap Sheets daily for each cigarette smoked, while smoking normally.
2. After completing Wrap Sheets for several days, complete Triggers for Smoking Worksheet.

SESSION 2

Session 2 Objectives

1. To review the cognitive social learning theory rationale for smoking cessation treatment.
2. To review self-monitoring of smoking behavior (Wrap Sheet) assignment.
3. To review Triggers for Smoking Worksheet.
4. To introduce the self-management approach to managing trigger situations and the use of three self-control strategies.
5. To introduce and demonstrate the Benson (deep breathing) relaxation approach.
6. To review the rationale and explanation of nicotine fading and to assign (or explain to smokers how to choose) the 30% nicotine content reduction brand.
7. To preview the homework assignments to be completed prior to Session 3.

Session 2 Handouts and Worksheets

1. Managing Triggers for Smoking Worksheet
2. Deep breathing relaxation exercise
3. Wrap Sheets

Session 2 Content

1. *Review cognitive social learning rationale*. Facilitators should reiterate that smoking behavior continues for many reasons.
   a. Smoking is a *learned habit*—a behavior pattern that has been overlearned through years of repetition. Smokers must learn about their own unique behavior patterns and identify triggers and effective coping strategies for each trigger situation.
   b. Smoking is a *physical addiction*—the drug nicotine produces a physical dependence, characterized by both tolerance and withdrawal symptoms (the defining characteristics of a physical addiction). Withdrawal symptoms typically last from one to two weeks and are generally worse when one quits cold turkey.
   c. For many people, smoking also serves as a means to *manage negative moods*. Some smokers learn to rely on cigarettes to cope with upsetting situations and to combat negative feelings such as depression, anxiety, anger, and frustration.
   Effective treatment must address each aspect of smoking that is relevant to a given in-

dividual. Facilitators should inform smokers that the current treatment accomplishes this goal. Smokers are also reminded that the other critical ingredient in quitting smoking is their own effort.

2. *Review the self-monitoring of smoking behavior (Wrap Sheet) assignment.* The facilitators should begin by asking smokers what they have learned about their smoking patterns from having completed the Wrap Sheets. A general question to pose for consideration is whether people have noticed a pattern to their smoking. Generally if smokers have completed Wrap Sheets, they have no difficulty discussing their observations about their smoking patterns. Facilitators should focus the discussion on what smokers have noticed about the times of day when they smoke, the activities they engage in while smoking, and the moods that they associate with smoking. Often smokers notice things that they had not previously realized, although in other instances completing the Wrap Sheets merely confirms what they already knew about their smoking. The importance of completing the Wrap Sheets should be emphasized to smokers; frequently, they will learn new information about their smoking despite previously thinking that they knew their smoking patterns.

   After they have self-monitored their smoking behavior, some smokers will report having smoked fewer cigarettes as a result of completing the Wrap Sheets. This is not uncommon, as self-monitoring is a reactive procedure that often results in a self-recorded smoking rate at least several cigarettes per day less than the real baseline (Abrams & Wilson, 1979a). Smokers should be reassured that it is all right if completing the Wrap Sheets has resulted in their smoking fewer cigarettes, despite the fact that their instructions were to smoke normally during the baseline period. From this point on in the treatment, reductions in smoking will be welcomed.

3. *Review Triggers for Smoking assignment.* Facilitators should remind smokers that triggers for smoking are situations, behaviors, thoughts, or moods that are commonly associated with smoking a cigarette and that serve as a signal to smoke. Facilitators should ask what smokers have learned about their triggers for smoking after having completed the Wrap Sheets. As homework from Session 1, smokers will have previously completed the Triggers for Smoking Worksheet. They should be encouraged to refer to the form in responding to this question. Smokers may need to be reminded to include thought and feeling components in identifying particular trigger situations. Smokers should also be reminded that once they quit smoking, trigger situations that they have identified are likely to become high-risk situations for relapse.

4. *Introduce the self-management approach to managing trigger situations.* Facilitators can begin the discussion about managing trigger situations by asking the question, "How can you deal with trigger situations without smoking?" This will generate a discussion in which smokers offer their own ideas about how to avoid smoking in trigger situations. Facilitators should keep in mind that many good suggestions about quitting come from other smokers, and tell this to the group. Facilitators are only one source of information about quitting smoking, and other group participants represent an equally valuable source of knowledge.

   After a brief discussion about dealing with trigger situations, facilitators should introduce the idea of planning in advance to manage triggers. A systematic plan can be developed for changing certain behaviors and thoughts so that the individual can successfully not smoke in trigger situations. Facilitators should introduce the notion of "self-control" and contrast this with the idea of "willpower." Self-control should be presented as "the development of a systematic and strategic plan to manage trigger situations without smoking," whereas willpower involves "trying to exert sheer will over quitting, without any particular plan or strategy."

It may also be useful for the facilitator to mention that willpower is not a helpful concept, as it is generally used by smokers as an explanation for why they have been unable to change their behavior. For example, people are commonly heard to say, "I will never be able to quit smoking, I don't have enough willpower." The concept of self-control or self-management of behavior provides smokers with an alternative way of thinking that is more optimistic. The idea is that if smokers can learn a systematic approach and set up specific strategies for quitting, this will make it easier to be successful. We often use the example of willpower being akin to a weight lifter trying to lift a 250-pound barbell over his/her head without using any particular technique or proper body mechanics. That is, the weight lifter is trying to do this by using brute force. The person who uses self-control strategies utilizes technique and proper body mechanics and therefore should have an easier time accomplishing the task, while fully utilizing all of his/her abilities. The bottom line is that facilitators should try to disabuse smokers of the notion of willpower. Another strategy is to encourage smokers to think about other areas of their lives in which they have been successful in making important changes. Smokers can be encouraged to recognize that they can apply these same strengths and abilities to quitting smoking as well.

The following are the three core self-control strategies that form the basis of the self-management approach. These should be introduced to smokers at this point in Session 2:

a. *Avoid trigger situations*. The most effective strategy that anyone can use to manage a trigger situation is to avoid it completely. It is obvious that if an individual does not come in contact with a trigger situation, this situation cannot exert any influence over his/her behavior (i.e., the situation cannot serve as a signal for him/her to smoke). Examples of avoiding trigger situations include forgoing the morning routine of drinking coffee, avoiding social situations that involve alcohol (at least temporarily after quitting), avoiding former smoking "hangouts," and immediately leaving the dinner table after a meal instead of lingering over dessert and smoking.

b. *Alter trigger situations*. In instances in which the smoker cannot or is unwilling to avoid a trigger situation, significantly altering the trigger situation is a second useful strategy. In regard to triggering behaviors, the smoker might choose to drink orange juice in the morning instead of coffee, to go for a walk or jog instead of watching TV, or to sit in the nonsmoking section of a restaurant instead of the smoking section. Examples of changing or altering triggering thoughts would be a smoker telling him/herself that "a cigarette won't change this difficult situation" or "I don't need a cigarette," rather than saying "I need a cigarette to cope with this situation."

c. *Use an alternative or a substitute in place of the cigarette*. The use of an alternative behavior or thought in place of a cigarette is useful either alone or in conjunction with avoiding or altering the trigger situation. Examples of behavioral alternatives include using a relaxation technique rather than smoking a cigarette in a stressful situation; chewing sugarless gum or eating sugarless candy, fruit, or vegetables (e.g., carrot or celery sticks); calling a friend; or doing needlework to keep one's hands busy. Examples of using thought alternatives include thinking any of the following thoughts: "I'm doing great—I can do without this cigarette," "One cigarette *can* hurt," or "This feeling is a signal that I need to use a coping technique now."

Facilitators should ask smokers to plan for and begin using the self-control strategies to manage trigger situations in the second week. The Managing Triggers for Smoking Worksheet (Figure 5.3) is then introduced to record these efforts. Smokers should be encouraged to intervene in only two or three (no more) trigger situations this week. They should systematically decide on, use, and record the strategies on their worksheets. Smokers should come to group sessions prepared to discuss how effective these strategies were. Facilitators can entertain discussion about whether smokers should begin with the easiest trigger situations or the most difficult ones. The former is often a good idea for people who are lacking in confidence, and the latter might be recommended only for people who are enthusiastic and confident that they can tackle more difficult situations first. In general, smokers usually have a good sense of which trigger situations are useful to attack at the early stage of treatment. Facilitators should note that while smokers are addressing trigger situations, they will also be cutting down on the number of cigarettes (i.e., nicotine and rate fading), which is discussed in further detail later in the session.

5. *Introduce the Benson deep breathing relaxation approach.* One particular substitute or alternative behavior that can be useful in many situations is relaxation. Facilitators should

MANAGING TRIGGERS FOR SMOKING WORKSHEET

How did you manage your triggers for smoking this week?

Continue to keep a record of your triggers for smoking and the strategies you used to deal with them. This week, reduce the number of cigarettes you smoked last week by 10% and smoke only your newly assigned lower-nicotine brand.

Trigger	Strategy
Example: Driving to work	*Chew gum, listen to relaxing music, keep cigarettes in trunk*
Coffee in the morning	Drink orange juice instead, leave house earlier
Talking on the phone	Chew on toothpick—keep toothpicks by phone
Arguing with husband	Go for a walk, deep breathing relaxation
Break at work	Drink water, take break with nonsmokers
Watching tv	Eat carrots, read a book, go for a walk
After dinner	Don't linger at table, wash the dishes

FIGURE 5.3. Managing Triggers for Smoking Worksheet.

introduce the idea that relaxation is a skill that can be learned with practice and that it can be useful in the course of smoking cessation in at least two different ways. First, daily use of a relaxation procedure may help to reduce a smoker's overall level of stress, which may make quitting smoking somewhat easier. Second, once a smoker has acquired the relaxation skill or ability to relax, he/she can use it in a "portable" way just prior to or at the moment of an actual stressful trigger situation to cope with that situation and avoid the urge to smoke. There are many different types of relaxation procedures, but one that we have found most useful in working with smokers is a deep-breathing relaxation approach called the Benson Relaxation Procedure (Benson, 1975).

Facilitators should now refer smokers to the Deep Breathing Relaxation Exercise handout (Figure 5.4). In session, the facilitators should review the content of the handout with smokers and provide brief explanations for the various aspects of the procedure. They should also ask for and respond to any questions about the relaxation approach. It should be emphasized that this is a deep-breathing form of relaxation and that smokers should find 10 or 20 minutes during which they can practice by sitting in a comfortable chair in a

---

DEEP BREATHING RELAXATION EXERCISE

This is one of the simplest relaxation methods, based upon a meditative, deep-breathing technique. There are five things you need to do to prepare for this exercise.

Getting Ready:
1. Choose a quiet, comfortable environment where there are few distractions and where you won't be disturbed.
2. Choose a time of day when you are least likely to be disturbed by others and you won't be worried about having to get somewhere right after your practice session.
3. Choose a word or phrase to repeat, either silently or aloud, while practicing your relaxation. This will help you to keep your mind from wandering during the practice session. The words "one" or "calm" are often recommended, but any simple, pleasing word will do.
4. Develop a passive, "let it happen" attitude while practicing. Don't worry about how well you are performing or about distracting thoughts. Simply continue repeating your special word or phrase.
5. Select a comfortable position. This is important to prevent undue muscular tension. A comfortable sitting position in a soft chair is probably best, as lying down may result in your falling asleep.

Those are the preliminaries. The procedure itself is very simple. There are five steps.

Relaxing:
1. Sit quietly in a comfortable position.
2. Close your eyes.
3. Relax all your muscles as fully and deeply as possible.
4. Breathe easily and naturally through your nose. BECOME AWARE OF YOUR BREATHING. As you breathe out, say "one" or your special word or phrase either silently to yourself or aloud. For example, breathe in...then out, "one," in ...out, "one," etc.
5. Continue for 10–20 minutes. Open your eyes to check the time, if you wish, but do not use an alarm. When you finish, sit quietly for several minutes, at first with your eyes closed and later, with your eyes open. Do not stand up for a few minutes.

FIGURE 5.4. Deep Breathing Relaxation Exercise. From *The Relaxation Response*, by Herbert Benson, M.D., with Miriam Klipper. Copyright © 1975 by William Morrow & Company, Inc. Reprinted by permission of HarperCollins Publishers Inc.

quiet place where they will not be interrupted or disturbed. Smokers should be encouraged to take a passive "let it happen" attitude toward the relaxation technique and to focus on slow rhythmic deep breathing. We usually inform smokers that tension or stress is associated with rapid, shallow breathing, and therefore slow, deep breathing contributes to a state of relaxation. Facilitators can also inform smokers that once they have practiced this approach on a daily basis for 7 to 10 days, they can readily develop the ability to use this approach anywhere at any time. That is, in a stressful situation that they might encounter, they can merely focus on their breathing and relax themselves in a matter of 1 or 2 minutes by merely breathing slowly and deeply. Smokers should also be encouraged to choose a word such as "one" or "calm" to say silently to themselves between breaths.

We have found it useful to ask smokers to spend 2 or 3 minutes in the session practicing this technique. Ask everyone in the group to choose a word that they will say silently, to get in a comfortable position in the chair they are sitting in, and to close their eyes if they are comfortable doing so. At that point they can begin to breath slowly and rhythmically. The facilitator should allow this to continue for several minutes. Facilitators should also engage in the procedure with smokers in order to reduce their inhibitions. We find that after 2 to 3 minutes of this, smokers are generally able to achieve a very relaxed state and are sometimes quite surprised at how relaxed they become. This brief demonstration should serve to encourage their continued practice in order to acquire this skill on an ongoing basis. Smokers are encouraged to practice this skill daily for 10 to 20 minutes. Facilitators can also encourage smokers to begin to think of other healthy ways in which they can manage their stress.

It is also very useful to explain to smokers how they can combine relaxation with coping imagery. For example, they might form an image of urges as waves in the ocean that rise and fall or wax and wane. Waiting out an urge and riding on top of it, like a surfer, can help to cope with the urge until it fades and washes out against the shore. An alternate metaphor might be that of the rise and fall of a roller coaster. Smokers should be encouraged to develop their own images that may be more personally meaningful to them.

6. *Review nicotine fading and assign 30% reduction brand.* Facilitators should briefly review the rationale for using nicotine fading; namely, that nicotine is a physically addicting drug. Despite the fact that people vary in the degree to which they are physically dependent on nicotine, many smokers will experience physical withdrawal symptoms on quitting. Withdrawal symptoms are generally worse in the first week after quitting and typically do not last beyond 2 weeks.

At this point, facilitators should hand out a Nicotine Fading Schedule (Figure 5.5) for the following week if specific cigarette brands are to be assigned to smokers. However, it is recommended that smokers not be given schedules that show brands for weeks beyond the upcoming one. If smokers are to tailor their own nicotine fading schedules, a general nicotine fading handout indicating percent reduction of estimated nicotine intake for each brand and a list of cigarette brands and their nicotine contents can be provided. Nicotine fading is a flexible procedure that can be done in various ways. Facilitators typically discuss a 3-week fading schedule in which smokers will switch to brands with published nicotine yields that are 30%, 60%, and 90% lower than their regular baseline brand of cigarette with each progressive fading change. Facilitators should encourage smokers to buy

NICOTINE FADING SCHEDULE

Week	Cigarette brand	Nicotine yield
WEEK 1	Regular brand: Marlboro, king, nonmenthol, filter, hard pack	1.1 mg
WEEK 2	30% reduction: Benson & Hedges, 100s, lights, nonmenthol, filter, soft pack	0.8 mg
WEEK 3	60% reduction: Merit, ultralight, king, nonmenthol, filter, soft pack	0.4 mg
WEEK 4	90% reduction: Now, king, nonmenthol, filter, soft pack	0.1 mg

FIGURE 5.5. Nicotine Fading Schedule.

their new brand immediately after the end of the current session and to begin smoking them the following day.

Facilitators should explain the concept of daily nicotine yield to smokers, including the fact that it is based on published nicotine yields that may differ somewhat from the actual amount of nicotine that they are ingesting. Facilitators should also explain to smokers how to calculate their daily nicotine yield by multiplying the number of cigarettes smoked each day by the published nicotine yield of their regular baseline brand cigarette. Smokers should then calculate their average daily nicotine yield for their baseline week on the Nicotine Fading Worksheet (Figure 5.6).

NICOTINE FADING WORKSHEET

Week 1 – Regular brand: _Marlboro King_

Average number smoked per day:		Mg. nicotine per cigarette		Average nicotine per day
20	×	1.1	=	22

Week 2 – 30% Reduction of nicotine   Brand: _Benson & Hedges 100's_

Average number smoked per day:		Mg. nicotine per cigarette		Average nicotine per day
18	×	0.8	=	14.4

Week 3 – 60% Reduction of nicotine   Brand: _Merit Ultra-Lights_

Average number smoked per day:		Mg. nicotine per cigarette		Average nicotine per day
17	×	0.4	=	6.8

Week 4 – 90% Reduction of nicotine   Brand: _Now King_

Average number smoked per day:		Mg. nicotine per cigarette		Average nicotine per day
15	×	0.1	=	1.5

FIGURE 5.6. Nicotine Fading Worksheet.

Finally, smokers should be cautioned not to compensate for the lower nicotine yield of their new cigarette brand by inhaling more deeply, puffing more frequently, or smoking more of each cigarette. Facilitators should acknowledge that some smokers may have trouble reducing the daily number of cigarettes they smoke or may even smoke a few more cigarettes daily when they first switch to their new brand. However, generally within a few days, smokers are able to adjust and reduce their daily rate to one that is lower than (or at least equivalent to) their baseline daily smoking rate.

Facilitators should also discuss the use of rate fading in conjunction with brand fading. Reductions in rates should be closely associated with the use of self-management strategies described earlier in this session. Specifically, rate fading should be accomplished in the context of learning to avoid particular cigarettes in specific trigger situations. Facilitators should suggest to smokers that as they are applying newly learned coping skills to avoid smoking in trigger situations, they should begin to reduce their smoking rates by a minimum of 10–15% per week prior to quitting. Smokers who wish to make further reductions in their smoking should feel free to do so, but facilitators should caution smokers not to set unrealistically high goals. The ideal goal is one that can reasonably and readily be accomplished. Facilitators should be sensitive to the fact that many smokers will have low self-efficacy beliefs regarding quitting smoking. The quitting process should involve a series of success experiences that build self-efficacy. It is generally better to have smokers set smaller goals that they can reasonably accomplish rather than set more challenging goals that they may fail to achieve. Facilitators may want to reiterate that, in some instances, merely maintaining the same smoking rate, rather than reducing the rate, may be a reasonable accomplishment. However, even under these circumstances, smokers should still be working at self-management strategies to reduce smoking in specific trigger situations.

7. *Preview the homework assignments to be completed prior to Session 3.* Facilitators should confirm the date and time of the next session, review assignments to be completed before the next session, and answer any questions that smokers might have about the assignments.

Prior to Session 3

Do for the first time:

1. Complete the Managing Triggers for Smoking Worksheet, identifying which self-control strategies are applied in specific trigger situations and how effective they are.
2. Practice deep breathing relaxation daily.
3. Accomplish nicotine fading through brand (smoke 30% nicotine-reduction brand) and rate (10–15% rate reduction, if possible) fading strategies.

Continue to do:

4. Complete Wrap Sheets.

SESSION 3

Session 3 Objectives

1. To review the self-management approach and the use of three self-control strategies.
2. To review the homework assignment to practice managing triggers using self-management strategies.
3. To review the Benson (deep breathing) relaxation homework assignment.
4. To review self-monitoring of smoking behavior (Wrap Sheet) assignment.
5. To introduce the concept of making broader lifestyle changes that support quitting smoking.
6. To review the nicotine fading assignment and assign (or explain to smokers how to choose) the 60% nicotine-content reduction brand.
7. To preview the homework assignments to be completed prior to Session 4.

Session 3 Handouts and Worksheets

1. Nonsmoking Game Plan: Lifestyle Change Worksheet
2. Managing Triggers for Smoking Worksheet
3. Wrap Sheets

Session 3 Content

1. *Review self-management approach and self-control strategies.* Facilitators should remind smokers that the first step in managing triggers is to identify their own triggers for smoking. It is also important to focus on specific details about trigger situations, such as moods and thoughts experienced during those situations. The Wrap Sheets provide an important source of information about triggers for smoking.

   Facilitators should review the concept of self-control as the development of a systematic plan for changing certain behaviors and thoughts in order to successfully refrain from smoking in trigger situations. Self-control is different from willpower: the latter involves trying to exert sheer will without any plan or strategy. Facilitators should briefly review and provide examples of the three ways to practice and strengthen self-control skills.
   a. *Avoid* trigger situations.
   b. *Alter* trigger situations
   c. Use an *alternative* in place of a cigarette.
2. *Review assignment to practice managing triggers using self-management strategies.* Facilitators should engage smokers in discussing their experiences in using the three self-control strategies to manage trigger situations. How did smokers do at *avoiding* trigger situations? Smokers can be reminded that avoiding a trigger situation altogether is likely to be the most effective coping strategy, and therefore it should be used whenever possible. How did smokers do at *altering* trigger situations? In what ways did smokers alter trigger situations, and how helpful were these changes? Finally, how successful was the use of *al-*

ternatives or substitutes in place of a cigarette? What alternatives did smokers find helpful? Which were not helpful?

While discussing the use of these self-control strategies, smokers should be encouraged to share information with the group regarding which strategies and approaches they were and were not able to use successfully. Facilitators should acknowledge and reinforce examples of the successful use of particular strategies and suggest that others in the group may want to try out those strategies. The group can also be engaged in a problem-solving process about strategies that did not work successfully. Facilitators and other group members can offer suggestions to smokers about how to improve in these areas. If a particular strategy was not successful, the smoker may want either to try a different strategy in the future or to fine-tune and thus improve the same strategy that he/she used initially. Facilitators can reiterate that quitting smoking is a process of figuring out what techniques and approaches will and will not work for them. The analogy is of a buffet or smorgasbord of approaches to sample, many of which will be suggested by other group members. The successful quitter will have attempted various approaches and sorted through them to see what works and what doesn't until he/she finally arrives at a personalized set of approaches that are effective for him/her.

Smokers should be reminded of the link between self-management and rate fading and that their goal for the past week was to reduce their cigarette intake by approximately 10–15%. Facilitators should ask the group how they did in this regard. What were their strategies for achieving this rate reduction? Did they decide to systematically eliminate smoking in certain trigger situations or times of day? Facilitators should remember that nicotine fading sometimes results in a temporary increase in smoking of the lower nicotine brand, so that for some people, merely *not increasing* their smoking rate may be a reasonable accomplishment.

Smokers should be informed that their homework for this week will be to continue using the self-control strategies to successfully avoid smoking in trigger situations and to continue to accomplish the rate-fading goal of reducing the amount of cigarettes smoked by an additional 10–15%. Smokers should also be reminded that today's trigger situations are tomorrow's high-risk situations for relapse. Working on managing triggers now will increase their chances of successfully quitting smoking by enabling them to deal more successfully with high-risk situations.

3. *Review assignment to practice Benson (deep breathing) relaxation.* Smokers should be reminded that relaxation is a skill that can be learned with practice. Facilitators should briefly review the rationale for the deep-breathing relaxation. Facilitators should explain to smokers that this relaxation technique can be used not only for general relaxation on a daily basis but also in specific stressful situations on a moment's notice. Facilitators should remind smokers that the homework for this session was to practice the relaxation technique daily for 10 to 20 minutes.

Facilitators should inquire as to how smokers did with this assignment and engage them in a brief discussion of their experiences. Did smokers practice daily? Did they go beyond the daily practice and attempt to use the relaxation approach in an actual trigger situation? Did they have any difficulties in practicing or using the relaxation procedure? Facilitators should discuss difficulties encountered during the relaxation technique, including finding a time and place to practice. In our experience, we find that smokers typically do not practice this approach daily for the amount of time prescribed. However, they should be encouraged to do so and also to practice using the technique in a "portable" fashion in stressful situations.

Facilitators should also inquire as to whether smokers incorporated imagery into their use of the relaxation technique to help them cope with urges to smoke. If so, what images did they use? Was the use of imagery in combination with deep breathing helpful in fighting off urges? Were some images more helpful than others? In reviewing smokers' experiences, facilitators should promote the exchange of ideas among smokers and should explicitly encourage smokers to try out different approaches that other smokers have found helpful. Here again, smokers should be encouraged to use their successes and failures as learning experiences to guide them in deciding what strategies will work for them and which ones need to be revised.

4. *Review self-monitoring of smoking behavior (Wrap Sheet) assignment.* Smokers should be asked what they have learned about their smoking patterns from doing their Wrap Sheets during the past week. For example, during what times of day did they find they were smoking? What activities were they engaged in while smoking? What moods have they experienced in relation to smoking particular cigarettes? Facilitators should engage smokers in this discussion for 5 to 10 minutes and should remind smokers that their homework is to continue with the Wrap Sheets again this week. Facilitators should stress the importance of the Wrap Sheets for identifying and managing trigger situations, as well as for calculating daily nicotine yield during nicotine fading.

5. *Introduce the concept of lifestyle change to support quitting smoking.* Facilitators should introduce the notion that quitting smoking involves more than putting down cigarettes. There are very important lifestyle changes that smokers can make in order to help them remain abstinent. These types of changes have been detailed on the Nonsmoking Game Plan: Lifestyle Change Worksheet (Figure 5.7). Facilitators should have smokers look at the worksheet while previewing each component of the lifestyle change plan. Rather than engaging in a complete discussion of each topic, the task at this session is to introduce these topics to smokers to prepare them to complete the worksheet for homework. Completed worksheets will be discussed at the next session. Key issues related to the specific topics are as follows:
   a. *What will you do to make cigarettes unavailable to you?* The intent of this question is to engage smokers in thinking about their potential exposure to cigarettes on quit day and thereafter. We presume that exposure to cigarettes and other smoking cues will increase the likelihood of relapse. We generally encourage smokers to prepare for quit day by making sure that they have gotten rid of all cigarettes in their houses and cars, as well as looking in other places in which there may be a few remaining cigarettes (e.g., in coat pockets, desk drawers at work, etc.).
   b. *What will you do to increase time spent in nonsmoking places or time spent doing nonsmoking activities?* As with the previous question, the intent of this question is to prod smokers to reduce exposure to smoking cues in the environment. For many smokers, there are places they have spent time in which they tend not to smoke, even though they are still smokers. Some people do not smoke in their bedrooms, others do

NONSMOKING GAME PLAN: LIFESTYLE CHANGE WORKSHEET

As part of your Nonsmoking Game Plan, you can plan to make changes in your daily behaviors that can help you remain a nonsmoker. Below, list specific answers to some general lifestyle questions important to quitting smoking and remaining a nonsmoker.

1. What will you do to make cigarettes unavailable to you?
   a. _Temporarily avoid friends who smoke_
   b. _Make sure I've gotten rid of all cigarettes_
   c. _____

2. What will you do to increase time spent in nonsmoking places or time spent doing nonsmoking activities?
   a. _Go to the movies_
   b. _Sit in nonsmoking section at restaurants_
   c. _Visit nonsmoking friends_

3. How can you develop a "buddy system" or get support from others when quitting?
   a. _Jogging with Chris in the morning_
   b. _Call John when I feel like having a cigarette_
   c. _____

4. What will you do to manage stress successfully?
   a. _Deep breathing relaxation_
   b. _Exercise daily_
   c. _Work less overtime while quitting_

5. What will you do to keep from gaining weight?
   a. _Exercise daily_
   b. _Eat at home more – healthy meals_
   c. _Cut up carrots and celery for snacking_

6. What will you do to become more physically active?
   a. _Daily jogging_
   b. _Take stairs, not elevator, at work_
   c. _Do yardwork_

FIGURE 5.7. Nonsmoking Game Plan: Lifestyle Change Worksheet.

not smoke in their offices near their computers. Smokers can be encouraged to think of places in their homes or at work in which they typically do not smoke; these places are relatively "safer" places to spend time once they quit smoking. Similarly, there are places outside the home or workplace in which smoking does not take place that are good places for smokers to spend time in the early stages of quitting smoking. Examples here include the homes of nonsmoking friends, libraries, movie theaters, health clubs or gyms, and nonsmoking sections of restaurants. The same logic applies to nonsmoking *activities*. Smokers should be encouraged to think of activities they perform in which they tend not to smoke. Some smokers walk or do some other type of exercise, others do not smoke while spending time with nonsmoking friends.

c. *How can you develop a "buddy system" or get support from others when quitting?* This issue is addressed in more detail in Session 5; however, smokers should begin to think now about ways in which they can positively engage friends and family members in their effort to quit smoking. Some smokers find a "buddy" who will quit smoking with them on their quit day; others find someone who will begin an exercise program with them. In general, smokers should be encouraged to figure out what behaviors from others they do and do not find supportive and then to solicit supportive behaviors from others while assertively giving feedback about behaviors they do not find supportive.

d. *What will you do to manage stress successfully?* This is obviously a very broad issue but quite likely an important one. We have already introduced the Benson Relaxation Procedure as one means of managing stress. In the context of this Lifestyle Change worksheet, smokers should be encouraged to detail more specifically in what ways they will apply the relaxation skills they have learned and practiced. For example, if a smoker knows that he/she becomes anxious in social situations and typically uses smoking as a way to relax, he/she may decide to use relaxation for 5 minutes prior to entering into a social situation and to focus on deep breaths during the course of the social situation. Smokers may also wish to pursue information on other stress-reducing activities such as biofeedback, progressive muscle relaxation, guided imagery, or time management. Exercise is stress reducing and represents another viable option for smokers. Exercise is discussed as a separate category below.

e. *What will you do to keep from gaining weight?* This is a complex issue that facilitators can begin to address in the context of the lifestyle change plan discussion. We know that this is an important issue because many smokers relapse to smoking due to concerns about or actual weight gain following initial cessation. This issue has generally been associated with women smokers, although it cannot be assumed that all men are devoid of concerns about weight gain. Facilitators can conceptualize this issue in both behavioral and cognitive terms. That is, while encouraging smokers to make behavioral changes in an effort to avoid or minimize weight gain, facilitators must also be prepared to address smokers' attitudes and expectations about weight gain while they are quitting smoking.

f. *What will you do to become more physically active?* There seems to be an inverse relationship between cigarette smoking and exercise. People who smoke often do not have the desire, either physically or mentally, to exercise; people who exercise regularly generally do not have the desire to smoke. Smokers should be encouraged to adopt or increase physical activity during the process of quitting smoking. Commonly, smokers who do not wish to engage in vigorous exercise might adopt a walking program, ride a bicycle, or begin swimming at the local YMCA. Others embrace the idea of a more vigorous aerobic or anaerobic exercise program and may join a health club, begin jogging, lift weights or do circuit weight training, or take an aerobics class. Facilitators should caution smokers to obtain medical clearance from their physicians before beginning to engage in any type of vigorous exercise. Facilitators should remind smokers that, in addition to being a good smoking cessation activity in its own right, exercise helps to reduce stress and burns calories to help minimize weight gain.

6. *Review nicotine fading assignment and assign 60% reduction brand.* Facilitators can briefly review the idea that nicotine is physically addicting and that nicotine fading allows smokers to gradually withdraw from nicotine while continuing to smoke before quit day. Nicotine fading involves:

   a. Changing brands to those with progressively lower nicotine content.
   b. Reducing the number of cigarettes smoked.
   c. Calculating changes in daily nicotine yield of cigarettes smoked to provide feedback on how the procedure is working.

   Facilitators should engage smokers in a discussion of how they fared during nicotine fading. Did they pick one brand and stick to it, or did they smoke more than one brand this week? Smokers will invariably talk about whether they were able to smoke the new brand without increasing the number of cigarettes. They also have various reactions to the taste and experience of smoking a different brand.

   Facilitators should take a few minutes a session to have each person calculate this past week's daily nicotine yield on the Nicotine Fading Worksheet. In order to do this, they will have to know the nicotine yield of the brand they smoked during the past week. Facilitators should provide assistance when needed to smokers in calculating their nicotine yield. Facilitators should then reinforce the *reductions* in daily nicotine yield that smokers have experienced this past week. One of the nice features of nicotine fading is that smokers invariably experience lower nicotine yields. These changes should be attributed to smokers' own efforts in the service of increasing their self-efficacy. Once again, smokers should be cautioned not to compensate for the lower nicotine yield of their new cigarette brand by smoking more cigarettes, inhaling more deeply, puffing more frequently, or smoking more of each cigarette.

   Facilitators should now hand out the nicotine fading schedule for the next week or encourage smokers to pick out the brand they will smoke that represents a 60% reduction in nicotine yield from baseline. Once again, smokers should be encouraged to buy their new brand right after the session and to begin smoking it the next day.

7. *Preview the homework assignments to be completed prior to Session 4.* Facilitators should confirm the date and time of the next session, review assignments to be completed before the next session, and answer any questions that smokers might have about the assignments.

Prior to Session 4

Do for the first time:

1. Complete the Nonsmoking Game Plan: Lifestyle Change Worksheet, specifying lifestyle change goals for each category listed.

Continue to do:

2. Complete the Managing Triggers for Smoking Worksheet.
3. Practice deep breathing relaxation daily.

4. Complete Wrap Sheets.
5. Accomplish nicotine fading by fading both brand (smoke 60% nicotine-reduction brand) and rate (10–15% rate reduction, if possible).

SESSION 4

Session 4 Objectives

1. To provide process comments to smokers pertinent to their current experience in the smoking cessation treatment.
2. To review the homework assignment to practice managing triggers for smoking using self-control strategies.
3. To review the homework assignment to set goals regarding making broader lifestyle changes that support quitting smoking.
4. To review the homework assignment to practice the Benson (deep breathing) relaxation approach.
5. To review self-monitoring of smoking behavior (Wrap Sheet) assignment.
6. To introduce relapse-prevention concepts of identifying and coping with high-risk situations; to provide an opportunity for smokers to begin practice of these skills during the session.
7. To introduce the abstinence violation effect concept and how to cope with a possible slip.
8. To review nicotine fading assignment and assign (or explain to smokers how to choose) the 90% reduction brand.
9. To assist smokers in preparing for the upcoming quit day.
10. To preview the homework assignments to be completed prior to Session 5.

Session 4 Handouts and Worksheets

1. Coping with High Risk Situations Worksheet
2. Managing Triggers for Smoking Worksheet
3. Nonsmoking Game Plan: Lifestyle Change Worksheet
4. Wrap Sheets

Session 4 Content

1. *Provide process comments to smokers pertinent to their current experience in the smoking cessation treatment*
   a. *Learning ways to manage trigger situations now is critical for successful quitting.* Facilitators should remind smokers that this is an important phase of their treatment. Their efforts at finding effective ways to manage trigger situations for smoking are critical in determining how successful they will be in quitting smoking. Smokers should be reminded that developing effective strategies for managing triggers is a trial-and-error process. Even strategies that do not work can provide valuable information. Rather

than become discouraged, it is critical that smokers use this information to refine their approaches until they develop strategies that do work.

b. *Efforts to manage trigger situations now will help with high-risk situations for relapse.* It is also important to remind smokers that the trigger situations they are working on today represent potential high-risk situations for relapse once they initially quit smoking. Thus the efforts that they are now putting into devising effective ways of managing trigger situations will be rewarded once they quit smoking. Having effectively avoided smoking in key trigger situations will make it that much easier to remain abstinent when those same high-risk situations are encountered after quitting.

c. *Withdrawal symptoms mean that nicotine fading is working.* Facilitators might also want to comment on the process of nicotine fading. Smokers have made two brand changes and will make a third and final brand change during the coming week. They are likely experiencing some withdrawal symptoms during the fading process. Facilitators should frame this as evidence that the procedure is working. Facilitators should point out to smokers that, as a result of experiencing symptoms of withdrawal while still smoking, they can expect to experience lower levels of physical withdrawal on quitting. The overall result is that quitting should be easier than it would have been had they quit "cold turkey." Smokers should be congratulated on their successful efforts with nicotine fading, and facilitators should encourage internal attributions in this regard to enhance their self-efficacy about the prospects of successfully quitting smoking.

2. *Review the homework assignment to practice managing triggers for smoking using self-control strategies.* Facilitators should engage smokers in a discussion of their experiences using self-control strategies to manage trigger situations. The guidelines for this discussion are similar to those from Session 3. Given that smokers are now 1 week away from quit day, efforts should be intensified and should be meeting with reasonable success. Facilitators should achieve a healthy balance during this discussion between generating examples of how smokers are successfully managing triggers (and reinforcing those efforts) and reviewing situations in which smokers are reporting difficulties (and helping them solve any problems with their use of strategies in those situations). The novice facilitator will sometimes spend excessive amounts of session time with smokers who are having difficulties at the expense of those who are doing well. This can be a problem for at least three reasons: smokers who are doing well are not being reinforced by "airtime" in the session; smokers who are having difficulties are not being exposed to positive models (i.e., successful smokers) and to positive examples of the successful use of strategies; and a sense of pessimism may pervade the group.

As in Session 3, smokers should be reminded that today's trigger situations are tomorrow's high-risk situations for relapse. Working now on managing triggers will increase their chances of successfully quitting smoking by enabling them to deal more successfully with high-risk situations. Finally, the homework for the coming week is to continue using the self-control strategies to reduce the number of cigarettes smoked by an additional 10%.

3. *Review the homework assignment to set goals regarding making broader lifestyle changes that support quitting smoking.* Facilitators should reiterate the notion that in order to in-

crease their chances of success at remaining nonsmokers, smokers should make important lifestyle changes. These types of changes have been detailed on the Nonsmoking Game Plan: Lifestyle Change Worksheet. Each component of this lifestyle change plan was previewed by facilitators in Session 3, and smokers were to have completed this plan for homework. At this session, facilitators should spend a few minutes discussing each topic in detail, eliciting from smokers the changes that they plan to make.

a. *What will you do to make cigarettes unavailable to you?* Facilitators should ask smokers what ideas they have come up with to prevent unnecessary exposure to cigarettes and cigarette cues. Have they gotten rid of all cigarettes in their houses and cars, as well as looking in other places where cigarettes might remain (e.g., in coat pockets, desk drawers at work, etc.)? If smokers live with, or are frequently exposed to cigarette smokers, this is an important topic to discuss. For example, it may be more difficult for a smoker to rid his/her house of cigarettes if his/her spouse smokes. However, facilitators should help smokers in solving such problems. For instance, many smokers have successfully enlisted the support of spouses by having them agree not to smoke in the house or to bring cigarettes into the house.

b. *What will you do to increase time spent in nonsmoking places or time spent doing nonsmoking activities?* Facilitators should ask smokers what they plan to do to increase time spent in nonsmoking places or nonsmoking activities. The presumption is that the more time that smokers are able to spend in places or engaged in activities in which smoking is not permitted, the more protected they are from the risk of relapse. Most smokers are able to identify a range of "safe" places and activities. This concept has intuitive appeal for them, as they generally realize that the less they are exposed to cigarettes and related cues, the less likely they are to smoke. The smokers who are at greatest risk and who may require extra attention in this discussion are those who live with or work with smokers and those who discount the notion of trying to stay as far away from smoking cues as possible. As with other aspects of group cessation treatment, smokers usually can generate useful ideas with prompting from facilitators and with exposure to input and ideas from other group members.

c. *How can you develop a "buddy system" or get support from others when quitting?* Facilitators should ask smokers in what ways they can positively engage friends and family members in their effort to quit smoking. Facilitators should encourage smokers to be assertive with others in their lives by stating what behaviors of the other person they do and do not find helpful in their efforts to quit smoking. Interestingly, we find that different smokers react quite differently to the same type of behavior by a friend or family member. Some smokers feel supported and validated by having others frequently ask them about how they are doing in their quitting efforts, whereas others find it annoying and stressful. Therefore, smokers should be encouraged to figure out what behaviors from others they do and do not find supportive and to play an active role in encouraging supportive behaviors while discouraging nonsupportive behaviors.

d. *What will you do to manage stress successfully?* Facilitators should inquire what approaches smokers intend to use for managing stress. At this stage in treatment, smokers should be able to articulate specific applications of the Benson Relaxation Procedure that will help them cope with urges to smoke in trigger situations. Another helpful notion to introduce here is that of developing a positive addiction to replace smoking. This might involve setting aside 45–60 minutes daily to engage in some activity that can be done easily and does not take a lot of mental energy to accomplish. The activity should be noncompetitive, generally done alone, and one the smoker believes has some mental, physical, or spiritual value. The activity is generally one that the smoker feels can be improved upon with practice, but this is a subjective judgment. Finally, the smoker must be able to accomplish the activity without self-criticism and must be able to be completely accepting of him/herself while engaging in the activity. Some activities that might become positively addicting include brisk walking, meditation, bike riding, yoga, taking a hot bath or spending time in the sauna, reading, and listening to classical music. Exercise is a class of activity that can be stress reducing; it is discussed as a separate category later.

e. *What will you do to keep from gaining weight?* Facilitators should ask smokers what plan they have to minimize weight gain and to address concerns they might have about gaining weight. As stated in Session 3, facilitators should encourage smokers to make behavioral changes in an effort to avoid or minimize weight gain, while also focusing on their own attitudes and expectations about weight gain while quitting smoking.

Behavioral suggestions should focus largely on making wise and healthy food choices, particularly right after quitting smoking, as well as on the expenditure of calories via exercise. Indulging oneself by eating foods rich in sugars and carbohydrates is likely to be counterproductive. Snacking as much as possible on fruits, vegetables, and other low-calorie foods, as well as maintaining a generally balanced diet, is the best means of avoiding weight gain after quitting. Physical activity will help to burn calories and increase metabolism, which will also help to prevent weight gain. However, facilitators must also be alert to cognitive issues surrounding weight gain. Many smokers attempt to quit smoking but tell themselves that if they gain even 4 or 5 pounds, they will resume smoking. In effect, they are saying that they would rather smoke than be overweight, however they define it. These attitudes are most likely rooted in the perceptions of thinness that are prevalent in our society and perpetuated by the media. The goal for the facilitator is to encourage the smoker to make a reasoned judgment about the relative merits of quitting smoking versus a modest and (hopefully) temporary weight gain. Smokers can be encouraged to do as much as possible to avoid gaining weight but also to be prepared to tolerate a modest weight gain should they in fact gain weight. In the event that they successfully quit smoking but do gain weight, they can then devote their efforts to losing whatever weight they may have gained during the quitting process.

f. *What will you do to become more physically active?* Facilitators should inquire about smokers' plans for physical activity. Smokers can be reminded that cigarette smoking seems to be inversely related to exercise. While there may be exceptions to this "rule," smokers generally see the wisdom of this and are often enthusiastic about beginning an exercise program in conjunction with quitting smoking. Other smokers may view exercise much more negatively and may need help reconceptualizing physical activity in ways that may not involve vigorous exercise. In either event, smokers should be encouraged to increase their physical activity during the process of quitting smoking. Facilitators should suggest that smokers set modest goals for exercise at first and increase gradually, because being overly ambitious at first often leads beginners to discontinue an exercise program. Once again, facilitators should remind smokers that exercise also helps to reduce stress and burns calories to help minimize weight gain, which are important during the process of quitting smoking.

4. *Review assignment to practice Benson (deep breathing) relaxation.* The homework for Session 4 was to practice the relaxation technique daily for 10 to 20 minutes. Facilitators should inquire as to how smokers did with this assignment and briefly discuss their experiences. Facilitators should continue to help solve problems encountered during the relaxation technique. Smokers should once again be reminded that relaxation is a skill that can be learned with practice. Finally, facilitators should reinforce the idea that this relaxation technique can be used for both general relaxation on a daily basis and in a more "portable" manner to deal with specific stressful situations that occur during the course of the day.

5. *Review self-monitoring of smoking behavior (Wrap Sheet) assignment.* Smokers should be asked what they have learned about their smoking patterns from doing their Wrap Sheets during the past week. The guidelines for this discussion are essentially similar to those from Session 3. Facilitators should remind smokers that their homework is to continue with the Wrap Sheets this week. Facilitators should reiterate the importance of the Wrap Sheets with regard to managing trigger situations and calculating daily nicotine yield during nicotine fading.

6. *Introduce-relapse prevention concepts: Identifying and coping with high-risk situations.* A high-risk situation for relapse is defined as a situation that could lead to resumption of smoking. To help smokers identify high-risk situations, facilitators should ask them the following question: "If you were to slip and smoke a cigarette after quit day, in what situation would it be?" Facilitators should also provide smokers with information from the smoking research literature suggesting that the most common high-risk situations for relapse are those involving: (a) negative mood; (b) positive mood, especially in social situations involving alcohol; and (c) social interactions with other smokers (Lichtenstein, Antonnuccio, & Rainwater, 1977; Shiffman, 1982). Smokers should be asked to identify as many high-risk situations as possible, in preparation for developing specific coping strategies in each of these high-risk situations.

For each high-risk situation identified, smokers are encouraged to develop a full set of coping strategies to deal with the situation without smoking. They are reminded that these high-risk situations are functionally similar (if not identical) to the trigger situations they have previously addressed and that the same self-management strategies (i.e., avoid, alter, or use an alternative/substitute) can be applied to cope with these situations. Facilitators should emphasize the importance of planning for potential surprise high-risk situations. Smokers should think about upcoming events in their lives, such as a wedding they are invited to or a holiday gathering with family members. Maintaining an awareness of possible high-risk situations and being prepared with specific coping strategies is the most effective way for smokers to be successful at maintaining abstinence from smoking. The hardest thing to do is to cope with a high-risk situation that was not anticipated or to cope with one that was anticipated but not planned for.

Facilitators should introduce the Coping with High-Risk Situations Worksheet (Figure 5.8) and ask smokers to work on one high-risk situation in the session. That is, smokers should write down one high-risk situation that they anticipate and indicate what specific coping strategies they would use to avoid smoking in that situation. Smokers should be encouraged to be as specific as possible in listing the high-risk situation and in indicating the type of coping strategy or strategies they would use to avoid smoking. Facilitators should give smokers several minutes to work on this in the session, and they should review one smoker's responses as a means of providing an example for others prior to their completing the assignment this week on their own.

7. *Introduce abstinence violation effect concept and how to cope with a possible slip.* The typical response to a "slip" or episode of continued smoking following quit day is one of self-defeating attributions and negative emotional reactions. This response has been termed the abstinence violation effect, or AVE, and has been postulated to result in a resumption of full-blown smoking following an initial slip (Marlatt & Gordon, 1985). Smokers are informed of the following: (a) a slip (an instance or several instances of smoking) is different from a relapse (a return to baseline level of smoking); (b) if one does slip, he/she is likely to feel bad, guilty, even somewhat depressed; (c) this negative emotional reaction is likely to involve negative attributions of oneself as "weak" or as a "failure" due to being "unable to quit smoking"; and (d) he/she is likely to think that "one slip makes me a smoker again," which serves as a rationalization for a return to smoking at one's baseline rate.

The main task following a slip is to prevent the slip from becoming a relapse. Smokers are instructed that the AVE is a natural reaction to having a slip and that it is crucial to

---

NONSMOKING GAME PLAN: COPING WITH HIGH-RISK SITUATIONS WORKSHEET

High-Risk Situations Week of <u>May 12th</u>

For each specific high-risk situation, describe the event, persons you might be with, what you might be doing, thinking, or feeling at the time. List the specific coping strategies you will use to avoid smoking in each case. Remember: Avoid, Alter, use Alternatives.

High-Risk Situations	Specific Coping Strategies
1. Happy hour on Fridays with coworkers	Don't go for one month, then go briefly with nonsmoking friend
2. Stress at work—project deadline	Enlist coworkers' help, deep breathing, take breaks
3. Seeing someone smoking	Remember my reasons for quitting, think about how well I'm doing
4. Lunch with Sally	Sit in nonsmoking section, ask Sally not to smoke in the car
5. Anniversary of my husband's death	Be with family, keep busy, remind myself that smoking won't help
6.	
7.	
8.	
9.	
10.	

FIGURE 5.8. Nonsmoking Game Plan: Coping with High-Risk Situations Worksheet.

fight off this negative emotional reaction by doing the following: (a) think of the slip as a mistake rather than as evidence that you are weak or are a failure; (b) respond to it as you would to other mistakes (i.e., use it as a learning experience, figure out what you did wrong and how to correct it or avoid doing it next time); (c) realize that one cigarette does not mean that you are a smoker unless you allow it to; (d) redouble your coping efforts and remind yourself of all the successful, hard work you have put in so far; and (e) do not smoke the next cigarette, and remember that the depressed, guilty, angry feelings will decrease with each passing hour and day.

Finally, smokers should be cautioned not to hear this as "permission" to slip or as a message that it is "okay" to slip. Remind smokers that the surest way to quit smoking is not to have any slips. However, should they have a slip, they can recover and still successfully quit smoking.

8. *Review nicotine fading assignment and assign 90% reduction brand.* Facilitators should engage smokers in a discussion of how they fared in smoking their 60% reduction brand. The guidelines for this discussion are essentially similar to those from Session 3. Facilitators should take a few minutes a session to have each person calculate the past week's daily nicotine yield on the Nicotine Fading Worksheet. In order to do this, they will have to know the nicotine yield of the brand they smoked during the past week. Facilitators should provide assistance when needed to smokers in calculating their nicotine yield. Facilitators should then point out and reinforce the *reductions* in daily nicotine yield that smokers have experienced in the past week. Again, reductions in nicotine yield of cigarettes smoked the past week should be attributed to smokers' own efforts, in the service of increasing their self-efficacy. Finally, the caution should be repeated that smokers should not compensate for the lower nicotine yield of their new cigarette brand by smoking more cigarettes, inhaling more deeply, puffing more frequently, or smoking more of each cigarette.

Facilitators should now hand out the nicotine fading schedule for the next week or encourage smokers to pick out the brand they will smoke that represents a 90% reduction in nicotine yield from baseline. Once again, smokers should be encouraged to buy the brands right after the session and to begin smoking their new brand the next day.

9. *Assist smokers in preparing for the upcoming quit day.* Facilitators should remind smokers that their quit day is on the morning of their next session. Smokers are to quit smoking upon awakening that day. They will then receive the support of the group session after (hopefully) not having smoked a cigarette for less than 12 hours. This is a manageable goal that smokers can focus on; smokers very much want to come to the session reporting that they have been successful. Facilitators should remind smokers that in order to quit on the morning of quit day, they must prepare themselves the night before, both mentally and physically. Among other things, they should make sure that they have permanently gotten rid of any remaining cigarettes before going to bed. It is also helpful to have a specific, perhaps hour-by-hour, plan for not smoking for the first day or even the first several days after quitting.

It helps to suggest to smokers that they review their reasons for quitting smoking throughout the upcoming week. It is important for smokers to remain in touch with the reasons that led them to attempt to quit smoking in the first place. Smokers should also be encouraged to follow through on all the assignments for the coming week, as they are particularly important in prepare for quitting. Specifically, facilitators should urge smokers to be thorough in identifying high-risk situations and developing coping strategies. It is also important that smokers follow through with the lifestyle changes they have indicated on their Nonsmoking Game Plan: Lifestyle Change Worksheet. Finally, smokers should be actively engaged in the nicotine-fading process, smoking the assigned 90% reduction brand, and continuing with rate fading by applying the self-control strategies for dealing with trigger situations.

10. *Preview the homework assignments to be completed prior to Session 5.* Facilitators should confirm the date and time of the next session, review assignments to be completed before the next session, and answer any questions that smokers might have about the assignments.

Prior to Session 5

Do for the first time:

1. Complete the Coping with High-Risk Situations Worksheet, identifying high-risk situations and specific coping strategies to avoid smoking.

Continue to do:

2. Continue to work on applying self-control strategies for trigger situations and complete the Managing Triggers for Smoking Worksheet.
3. Continue to work on accomplishing lifestyle change goals, as specified on the Nonsmoking Game Plan: Lifestyle Change Worksheet.
4. Practice deep breathing relaxation daily.
5. Complete Wrap Sheets.
6. Accomplish nicotine fading by fading both brand (smoke 90% nicotine reduction brand) and rate (10–15% rate reduction, if possible).

SESSION 5

Session 5 Objectives

1. To discuss with smokers their quit day experiences (smokers were to quit smoking as of the morning of today's session).
2. To review the homework assignment to identify and develop coping strategies for dealing with high-risk situations for relapse.
3. To review the concept of the abstinence violation effect and how to cope with a possible slip, should it occur (as well as applying it to any slips that may have already occurred).
4. To review smokers' progress regarding making broader lifestyle changes that support quitting smoking.

5. To introduce the concept of social support for nonsmoking and to assist smokers in maximizing their social support for quitting smoking.
6. To review smokers' final experiences with nicotine fading prior to quitting.
7. To assist smokers in making specific plans for maintaining abstinence over the next several days (prior to the next session).
8. To preview the homework assignments to be completed prior to Session 6.

Session 5 Handouts and Worksheets

1. Social Support for Nonsmoking Worksheet
2. Coping with High-Risk Situations Worksheet
3. Nonsmoking Game Plan: Lifestyle Change Worksheet

Session 5 Content

1. *Discuss with smokers their quit day experiences.* Facilitators should be aware that, beginning with this session, smokers' experiences in attempting to quit smoking will be different and that group members need to be reminded to take a nonjudgmental and supportive approach to fellow group members. We recommend beginning this session with a statement such as the following:

> "We expect that people in the group may be at different places at this point. Everyone reacts to quitting somewhat differently. Some people have had many withdrawal symptoms . . . some fewer. Some people react emotionally to quitting smoking . . . some don't. Some people may have smoked . . . some have not. But whatever your own experience has been, we ask that you please remember that 'we're all in this together' and we're here to support each other."

Beginning with a statement such as this should also help to normalize the experience of the smoker. Thus if a smoker is reacting with strong emotions to quitting or has smoked a cigarette during the day, he/she should feel more comfortable sharing the experience with the group following an acknowledgment such as this by the facilitator.

Facilitators should now ask group members how their quit day experiences have gone so far. Everyone in the group should get several minutes to share their quit day experience. Facilitators should, of course, reinforce the successes of those who have not smoked, but special care needs to be taken to encourage those who have. A good general strategy is to help those who are not faring as well to find the success in what they have done. For example, if someone smoked one cigarette during the day, it can be pointed out to them that there must have been many other instances during the day when they resisted the urge to smoke. Facilitators can acknowledge smokers' negative reactions to having had a slip but can also mention that this will be discussed later in the session.

In conjunction with asking smokers how they have fared so far, facilitators can also ask about possible withdrawal symptoms. Smokers will likely report a range of withdrawal reactions, from very mild to very severe. Facilitators should remind smokers that withdrawal symptoms are worse in the first week after quitting and generally run their course within the first 2 or 3 weeks and that they should be considerably lessened by having gone through the nicotine-fading procedure prior to quitting.

Facilitators should remind anyone who has smoked of the distinction between a slip and a relapse and of the discussion of what they must do to keep a slip from becoming a relapse (i.e., abstinence violation effect). This topic is covered more fully in this session when reviewing the abstinence violation effect.

Facilitators should now engage smokers in a more guided discussion of their quit day experiences. Facilitators should ask smokers to discuss the types of plans they made for dealing with quit day. What specific types of strategies have they planned? What are their expectations for the next several days? How do they plan to be successful at staying abstinent during this time? Other topics are also worthy of discussion here. Smokers should briefly discuss coping with urges to smoke. Many smokers think (irrationally) that urges will not cease unless they succumb and smoke a cigarette. Smokers should be reminded that urges are time limited. Urges begin, increase until they reach their peak, and then subside. This entire process generally takes only several minutes. Smokers should remind themselves of this when they have an urge. Smokers who are quitting often tend to notice only the times of the day when urges are at their peak and erroneously come to think of the day as consisting of one continuous and intense urge. This type of misperception is, in fact, more likely to result in a return to smoking than is a more accurate view of the process. Facilitators can also point out that smokers sometimes experience a type of panic reaction when they think in terms of quitting "forever" or "for the rest of my life." Just as in Alcoholics Anonymous, it is helpful for smokers to think about quitting "one day at a time" or even one hour or one urge at a time during more difficult periods. It is much less overwhelming and much easier to manage one day or one hour than it is to conceive of doing anything for the rest of one's life. The use of coping imagery in combination with relaxation skills to combat urges has already been discussed and can be reiterated here.

Although it has been only a matter of hours, smokers should be encouraged to think about the benefits that they are experiencing from quitting smoking. Have they noticed any benefits of quitting? At this point, perhaps they are aware of being proud of themselves for quitting thus far, or they may even notice having a few extra dollars in their pocket from not purchasing cigarettes today. Smokers should be encouraged to reward themselves for increasing periods of time not smoking. Facilitators should encourage smokers to contract with themselves for rewards based on the length of time they do not smoke. What reward will they provide themselves after not smoking for a full day? After 1 week? One month? Six months? One year? Rewards should become more sizable for longer periods of abstinence. Smokers may or may not want to link rewards to the amount of money they have saved from not smoking, but in either event they should be encouraged to calculate the amount of money saved after various periods of time not smoking. It is not uncommon for smokers to plan a special vacation as a reward for a year of not smoking. One former heavy smoker quit smoking, along with her husband, who was also a heavy smoker. They decided to purchase a new automobile with the money they were saving, as the amount they had previously spent on cigarettes was equal to the monthly car payment.

These intrinsic and extrinsic rewards serve as the type of self-reinforcement that will help smokers to maintain abstinence from smoking.

2. *Review assignment to identify and cope with high-risk situations.* Facilitators should review the definition of a high-risk situation for relapse (a situation that could lead to resumption of smoking). Facilitators should remind smokers that the most common high-risk situations for relapse are those involving: (a) negative mood; (b) positive mood, especially in social situations involving alcohol; and (c) social interactions with other smokers. Facilitators should reiterate to smokers that maintaining an awareness of possible high-risk situations and being prepared with specific coping strategies is the most effective way for smokers to be successful at maintaining abstinence from smoking. For homework, smokers were to use the Coping with High-Risk Situations Worksheet (Figure 5.8) to identify as many high-risk situations as possible. For each high-risk situation identified, they were to develop a full set of coping strategies to deal with the high-risk situation without smoking by using self-management strategies (i.e., avoid, alter, or use an alternative or substitute).

Using this worksheet, facilitators should elicit examples of high-risk situations and specific coping strategies from group members. Facilitators should reinforce smokers' examples that provide specificity regarding situations and corresponding coping strategies and review problem situations in which smokers may have had difficulty identifying situations and/or useful coping strategies. As before, time should be balanced between showcasing adaptive and useful examples for the group to hear and providing assistance to those smokers who are having difficulty with the assignment. Facilitators should inform smokers that their assignment is to complete a new Coping with High-Risk Situations Worksheet for the next session.

3. *Review abstinence violation effect concept: How to cope with a possible slip.* Facilitators should lead the group in a discussion of the typical cognitive and emotional reactions to a slip and how to prevent a slip from becoming a relapse. Facilitators can reiterate the following: (a) a slip (an instance or several instances of smoking) is different from a relapse (a return to baseline level of smoking); (b) if one does slip, he/she is likely to feel frustrated, guilty, even somewhat depressed; (c) this negative emotional reaction is likely to involve negative attributions of oneself as "weak" or as a "failure" due to being "unable to quit smoking"; and (d) a person is likely to think that "one slip makes me a smoker again," which serves as a rationalization for a return to smoking at one's baseline rate.

As discussed previously, the main task that one faces if a slip does occur is to prevent the slip from becoming a relapse. Smokers are instructed that their negative emotional reaction to a slip is fairly natural and that it is crucial to fight off this reaction by doing the following:

a. Think of the slip as a "mistake" rather than as evidence that you are weak or are a failure.

b. Respond to it as you would to other mistakes (i.e., use it as a learning experience, figure out what you did wrong and how to correct it or avoid doing it next time).

c. Realize that one cigarette does not mean that you are a smoker unless you allow it to.

d. Redouble your coping efforts, reminding yourself of all the successful, hard work you have put in so far.

e. Do not smoke the next cigarette and realize that the depressed, guilty, angry feelings will decrease with each passing hour and day of abstinence.

Although special attention should be paid to those individuals who have already slipped, discussion of the abstinence violation effect is relevant to all group members. Finally, facilitators should remind smokers not to misinterpret this message as "permission" to slip.

4. *Review smokers' progress regarding lifestyle changes that support quitting smoking.* To increase their chances of success at remaining abstinent, smokers should make important lifestyle changes. These changes are detailed on the Nonsmoking Game Plan: Lifestyle Change Worksheet (Figure 5.7). Each component of this lifestyle change plan was discussed at length in Session 4, and smokers were to have completed this plan and begun implementing the lifestyle changes. At this session, facilitators should spend a few minutes discussing each topic, eliciting from smokers the changes that they have been engaged in according to their plans. Facilitators should positively reinforce those who have followed through with specific plans. Brief problem solving should be initiated with those smokers who have been unable to make lifestyle changes. This effort should focus on helping them to remove real or perceived barriers that appear to be preventing their follow-through. Smokers should be encouraged to continue to engage in these lifestyle changes, as they are consistent with helping them remain abstinent. Facilitators should not spend time trying to convince or persuade smokers who seem unwilling or otherwise reluctant to make lifestyle changes.

5. *Introduce concept of and assist smokers in planning to maximize social support for nonsmoking.* Social support can be a source of motivation for quitting and of positive reinforcement for successfully maintaining abstinence. Social support may also provide a buffer against the stress of quitting or other stressful events that might precipitate a relapse. Facilitators should inform smokers that social support can be a positive factor in their success in quitting smoking and should contrast this with the negative social influences that they might also encounter that can interfere with successful quitting. Examples of negative social influence include a family member, friend, or acquaintance who doubts the smoker's ability to quit smoking in light of past failures or who otherwise tries to undermine the importance of the smoker's determination to quit smoking. Facilitators should instruct smokers to identify sources of positive social support in their environment and to acknowledge and express appreciation for the support they are receiving related to quitting smoking. In line with this, facilitators should also encourage them to identify potential sources of support or specific supportive behaviors that they would like someone close to them to engage in and to ask for this support from that individual. Finally, facilitators should encourage smokers to identify sources of negative social influence and to express their concerns to those individuals and ask them to discontinue the behavior(s) in question. Facilitators should now introduce the Social Support for Nonsmoking Worksheet (Figure 5.9) and ask smokers to complete the form prior to the next session. The forms require smokers to comment on the four specific areas just alluded to: (a) What kinds of behaviors from others have people found supportive regarding quitting smoking? (b) What kinds of behaviors from others have people found *not supportive* regarding quitting smoking? (c) What can people do to ask for positive social support (behaviors) from others? and (d) What can people do to ask that others reduce or eliminate *negative* and *nonsupportive* behaviors that interfere with their quitting efforts?

SOCIAL SUPPORT FOR NONSMOKING WORKSHEET

Getting support and encouragement from others while you quit and work at being a nonsmoker can be very helpful. Complete this handout to help you determine what other people do that is helpful or not helpful to you and what you can do to ask them to be more helpful.

<u>Supportive Behaviors for Nonsmoking:</u>
List behaviors from others that you consider to be helpful or supportive to your nonsmoking efforts:
1. _Wife is quitting smoking with me_
2. _Greg asks how I'm doing_
3. _Sara doesn't smoke in front of me_
4. _____

<u>Nonsupportive Behaviors for Nonsmoking:</u>
List behaviors from others that you consider to be <u>not helpful</u> or that <u>interfere</u> with your efforts to quit smoking:
1. _Son left cigarettes on kitchen table_
2. _Joan offered me a cigarette_
3. _____
4. _____

<u>Requesting Behavior Changes from Others:</u>
What can you ask or request of others to have them engage in more actions or behaviors that you find supportive of nonsmoking?
1. _Express appreciation to wife for quitting_
2. _Tell Greg that he's being helpful to me_
3. _Thank Sara for being so considerate_
4. _____

What can you ask or request of others to have them engage in fewer (or eliminate completely) behaviors that you find not helpful or interfere with your efforts to quit smoking?
1. _Ask son to keep cigarettes in his room_
2. _Tell Joan I'm quitting—please don't offer cigarettes_
3. _____
4. _____

FIGURE 5.9. Social Support for Nonsmoking Worksheet.

6. *Review smokers' final experiences with nicotine fading.* Facilitators should briefly discuss with smokers how they fared in smoking their 90% reduction brand. Although smokers have already quit, it is still useful for facilitators to take a few minutes to have each person calculate their past week's daily nicotine yield on the Nicotine Fading Worksheet. As before, facilitators should provide assistance when needed to smokers in calculating their nicotine yield. Facilitators should reinforce the cumulative *reductions* in daily nicotine yield, attributing this success to smokers' own efforts to increase their self-efficacy. Smokers should again be reminded that to the extent that they accomplished the fading procedure and experienced physical withdrawal symptoms during the process, their physical withdrawal should be lessened considerably on quitting. The end result is that they should have a somewhat easier time quitting than they would have had they chosen to quit cold turkey.

7. *Assist smokers in making plans for maintaining abstinence over the next several days*. Today is quit day, and this marks the beginning of the acute relapse-prevention phase of treatment. Facilitators should remind smokers that their next session is scheduled in 3 days (give exact date) to provide them with a manageable time frame during which to remain abstinent. Smokers should again be encouraged to follow through on all the assignments for this coming week, as they are particularly important during these first several days of cessation. Specifically, facilitators should urge smokers to continue to be diligent at identifying high-risk situations and developing coping strategies. Smokers should make an active effort to involve themselves in making the lifestyle changes they have indicated on their change plans. Finally, smokers should pay special attention to issues related to social support for nonsmoking over the next several days and try to maximize their positive social support and minimize negative social influences. It is particularly important during this early relapse prevention phase that smokers make every effort to minimize stressful events and situations in their lives and that they avoid highly tempting, high-risk situations.

8. *Preview the homework assignments to be completed prior to Session 6*. Facilitators should confirm the date and time of the next session, review assignments to be completed before the next session, and answer any questions that smokers might have about the assignments.

Prior to Session 6

Do for the first time:

1. Complete the Social Support for Nonsmoking Worksheet, identifying ways of maximizing positive and minimizing negative social influences regarding quitting smoking.

Continue to do:

2. Continue to work on identifying high-risk situations and specific coping strategies to avoid smoking and complete the Coping with High-Risk Situations Worksheet.
3. Continue to work on accomplishing lifestyle change goals as specified on the Nonsmoking Game Plan: Lifestyle Change Worksheet.
4. Practice deep breathing relaxation daily.

SESSION 6

Session 6 Objectives

1. To discuss with smokers their quitting experiences.
2. To review the concept of the abstinence violation effect and how to cope with a possible slip should it occur (as well as applying it to any slips that may have already occurred).
3. To introduce new strategies for coping with urges to smoke.

4. To review the homework assignment to identify and develop coping strategies for situations high in risk for relapse.
5. To review smokers' experiences in attempting to maximize social support for quitting smoking.
6. To review smokers' progress regarding making broader lifestyle changes that support quitting smoking.
7. To assist smokers in making specific plans for maintaining abstinence over the next several days (prior to the next session).
8. To preview the homework assignments to be completed prior to Session 7.

Session 6 Handouts and Worksheets

1. Coping with High-Risk Situations Worksheet
2. Social Support for Nonsmoking Worksheet
3. Nonsmoking Game Plan: Lifestyle Change Worksheet

Session 6 Content

1. *Discuss quitting experiences of the past several days.* Facilitators should remind smokers that today is the 4th day of abstinence and should inquire about how smokers are doing. Facilitators should engage smokers in a discussion of how the time since the last session has gone and should once again provide several minutes for each group member to share his/her experiences. It is important to reinforce the successes of those who have not smoked but also to be attentive to the needs of those who have. As in the previous session, facilitators should encourage those who have smoked to recognize the successes that they have had relative to their baseline level of smoking. Facilitators can again acknowledge smokers' negative emotional reactions to having had a slip, but this will be covered more fully later in the session.

   Facilitators should ask about possible withdrawal symptoms that smokers may be experiencing. Facilitators can remind smokers that withdrawal symptoms are typically worse in the 1st week after quitting and should begin to improve no later than the 2nd or 3rd week after quitting. Facilitators can also remind smokers that the withdrawal symptoms they are experiencing should be less severe than they would have been had they quit smoking their regular brand cold turkey, given the nicotine-fading procedure in which they participated.

   For those who have smoked, facilitators should distinguish between a slip and a relapse and briefly review the things they can do to prevent a slip from becoming a relapse.

   As in the previous session, facilitators should now engage smokers in a more guided discussion of their quit day experiences. Facilitators should ask smokers what types of coping strategies they have been using and what success they have been having with these strategies. Facilitators should continue to help smokers to solve problems in improving the use of coping strategies or developing new ones in instances in which the strategies have been ineffective. Facilitators should also engage smokers in a discussion of what they expect over the next several days and how they will plan to cope with some of the high-risk situations or difficulties that they might encounter.

Facilitators should ask smokers if they have begun to notice any short-term benefits of quitting. At this time in the quitting process, smokers are often able to recognize that they are breathing more easily, beginning to smell and taste more than in the past, saving money, feeling less inconvenienced by nonsmoking areas and policies, and developing a strong sense of accomplishment if they have remained abstinent. Smokers should be encouraged to share any positive experiences or perceived benefits that they have noticed about quitting smoking with the rest of the group. Facilitators should encourage participation by all members in this exercise.

Smokers should also be encouraged to reward themselves for quitting smoking for increasing periods of time. Facilitators should reiterate the suggestion made previously that smokers might want to contract with themselves to provide self-rewards based on increasing periods of time not having smoked. Smokers should also be encouraged to calculate the amount of money saved from not smoking, and it may be suggested that at a minimum, the money saved from not smoking should equal the value of the reward that is to be delivered after a given period of time not smoking. For instance, a smoker may determine that, after 6 months of not smoking, he/she will have saved a total of $500.00. This amount of money is then available to reward him/herself for not smoking during this period of time.

2. *Review abstinence violation effect concept: How to cope with a possible slip.* Facilitators should reengage the group in a discussion of the types of cognitive and emotional reactions to a slip and how to prevent a slip from becoming a relapse. At this point smokers have heard this previously, so facilitators may begin to phase out some of the specific details. However, facilitators should make the point that a slip is different from a relapse, that a negative emotional reaction is likely to occur if they do slip, and that a slip, in conjunction with this emotional reaction, frequently leads to a resumption of smoking. Furthermore, smokers should be encouraged to fight off this emotional reaction by viewing their slip as a mistake rather than as evidence that they are failures, to use the slip as a learning experience, to redouble their coping efforts, and to reaffirm that they will not smoke the next cigarette. Gradually, these negative feelings will pass with increasing amounts of time spent not smoking. Facilitators should address comments to the entire group but should pay special attention to the experiences and reactions of smokers who have had slips since quit day. From this session to the end of treatment, slips are increasingly likely to occur, and helping smokers to "process" their slips within the context of the abstinence violation effect is an important intervention. Facilitators should realize that other group members can be extremely helpful in this regard and should make every effort to encourage appropriately supportive comments from others in the group.

3. *Introduce strategies for coping with urges to smoke.* An important set of relapse prevention strategies involves being able to effectively cope with urges to smoke. In this session, facilitators can suggest to smokers a range of different strategies for their consideration, some of which have already been discussed in other contexts throughout the treatment. Almost all smokers will have urges, and facilitators should make smokers aware that having urges is an expected part of quitting smoking. It is important to normalize urges, as some smokers will consider that they are doing poorly or failing merely because they are experiencing urges. Instead, facilitators should recognize their accomplishment of successfully cop-

ing with these urges. In this way, facilitators can model the type of self-reinforcement that we want smokers to adopt.

Another psychoeducational component involves explaining the nature of urges. Under the duress of quitting and experiencing withdrawal symptoms, many smokers adopt the irrational belief that urges will not cease unless they succumb and smoke a cigarette. Smokers should be reminded that urges are time limited. Rather than believing that urges will not cease until they finally smoke a cigarette, smokers should work hard to remind themselves that urges have a beginning, a middle, and an end and that the entire process generally takes only several minutes. Many smokers who are quitting notice only the times of the day at which urges are at their peak and erroneously believe that the day consisted of one continuous and intense urge. This type of misperception is, in fact, more likely to result in a return to smoking than is a more accurate view of the process. Facilitators should also point out to smokers that they will likely experience an anxious or panicky reaction if they think in terms of quitting "forever" or "for the rest of my life." Facilitators should point out that it is more helpful for smokers to think about quitting one day at a time or even one hour or one urge at a time during difficult periods. It is much less overwhelming and much easier to manage one day or one hour than it is to conceive of quitting smoking (or doing anything, for that matter) for the rest of one's life.

Strategies for using coping imagery in combination with relaxation skills to combat urges have already been discussed and can be reiterated here. Smokers might imagine an urge as waves in the ocean that rise and fall or wax and wane. Waiting out an urge and riding on top of it, like a surfer, is an image that may help to cope with the urge until it fades and washes out against the shore. Another metaphor is that of the smoker as a sword-wielding samurai warrior, aggressively taking on urges as they occur and slicing through the urges with the sword. Finally, smokers should be encouraged to develop their own images that may be more personally meaningful to them. Smokers should be encouraged to incorporate imagery into their use of the relaxation to help them cope with urges to smoke.

Facilitators should make the point that, when confronted with an urge, smokers should *do something*; that is, they should take some active step(s) to cope with the urge rather than passively wait for the urge to pass. One strategy that is sometimes overlooked involves paying attention to the thoughts or beliefs that may accompany urges. For example, it is quite common that in a stressful situation a smoker will tell him/herself, "I need a cigarette to get through this situation." This thought has been repeated countless times in the past and becomes automatic, often without the smoker even realizing that he/she is saying this to him/herself. The problematic word in the sentence is "need." The point can be made that there are few things in life that are actually "needed" for survival (e.g., food, water, shelter, etc.) and that cigarettes are not one of those things. Smokers can be encouraged to substitute the phrase, "I really *want* a cigarette, but I don't *need* one—I will be okay without it."

Finally, in terms of doing something to cope with urges, behavioral strategies can also be effective. The basic self-management strategies learned for dealing with triggers and high-risk situations are applicable for coping with urges. Smokers should attempt to recognize the situations and circumstances that lead to urges or thoughts of smoking. They can be better prepared by avoiding these triggers altogether, by altering something about the nature of the trigger, or by substituting something else instead of the cigarette in those situations that cannot be avoided or altered. Smokers using nicotine gum are undoubtedly aware, but nevertheless should be reminded, that using a piece of gum in response to an urge to smoke is an excellent strategy. For smokers not using nicotine gum, other behavioral substitutes (e.g., regular chewing gum, carrots, cinnamon sticks, cut-up straws, and toothpicks) can serve the same purpose.

4. *Review assignment to identify and cope with high-risk situations.* Facilitators should remind smokers of the importance of being vigilant to high-risk situations and reiterate that the most common high-risk situations are characterized by negative mood, positive mood coupled with social situations that involve alcohol, and social interactions with other smokers. The most effective way for smokers to remain abstinent is to maintain an awareness of potential high-risk situations and be prepared with specific coping strategies for dealing with these situations. Following Session 5, smokers were to continue using the Coping with High-Risk Situations Worksheet to identify as many high-risk situations as possible and to fully develop coping strategies for dealing with each high-risk situation.

   Facilitators should engage smokers in a discussion about this assignment, specifically about how they are doing in anticipating high-risk situations and coping effectively with them. The discussions should be a mix of examples that provide instances of high-risk situations and coping strategies that the smokers were able to use in those situations, as well as examples of difficulties smokers may be having in either identifying situations or using coping strategies. If there are situations in which a smoker had a slip, discussion should center around whether he/she was able to anticipate the high-risk situation or, alternatively, whether it was a situation that he/she anticipated but was unable to cope with effectively. Facilitators should maintain a healthy balance in the discussion between bringing out adaptive and effective examples of coping with high-risk situations and talking about slips and other situations that people were unable to cope with effectively. Facilitators should again inform smokers that their assignment for the next session is to complete a new Coping with High-Risk Situations Worksheet (Figure 5.8) prior to Session 7. Facilitators should point out that, as smokers go through the process of quitting, last week's high-risk situations may become irrelevant, and new high-risk situations may begin to emerge, thus necessitating ongoing work on this assignment. Smokers should specifically try to anticipate situations or circumstances in the next week that might put them at risk for smoking, such as a party or a date for lunch with an "old smoking buddy."

5. *Review experiences in attempting to maximize social support for nonsmoking.* Facilitators should review the concept that positive social support can be a source of motivation for quitting and remaining abstinent, as well as a buffer against stressors, including the stress of quitting smoking. Positive social support can be an important factor in smokers' success at quitting smoking, whereas negative types of social influence can interfere with successful quitting. Facilitators should engage smokers in a discussion of their homework for this session. The assignment was to identify examples of both positive social support and negative social influence from others, and to ask for more of the positive social support and less

of the negative social influence from friends and family members. Smokers should be asked to refer to the Social Support for Nonsmoking Worksheet (Figure 5.9) and to share their responses with the rest of the group. Facilitators should guide this discussion one topic at a time and encourage participation from everyone.

Facilitators should ask smokers whether they have made any attempts to increase positive social support or to decrease negative social influence and ask them to discuss their experiences in trying to do so. Once again, facilitators should be aware that different smokers might respond in quite different ways to the same type of behavior by someone in their lives. A behavior that is interpreted as supportive by one person may be interpreted as being a negative influence by another. Facilitators should stress to smokers that it is their own unique personal reaction that is important and that the overall goal is to increase positive social influence and decrease negative social influence.

The issue of assertiveness, the ability to express one's thoughts and feelings directly, can be relevant to this discussion. For a smoker who has a spouse or other family member who smokes, the most effective type of social support intervention may be for the smoker to ask this family member not to smoke in the house, not to bring cigarettes in the house, and/or not to smoke in front of him/her. Some smokers may be lacking in assertiveness and may find this type of request very difficult to accomplish. Treatment strategies to enhance assertiveness skills are discussed in Chapter 6.

6. *Review smokers' progress regarding lifestyle changes that support quitting smoking.* Facilitators should once again review the importance of lifestyle changes in smokers' efforts to quit smoking and should engage smokers in a discussion of which lifestyle changes they have begun. Although of the six lifestyle changes from the Nonsmoking Game Plan: Lifestyle Change Worksheet are open for discussion, the facilitator should particularly focus on issues relating to managing stress, avoiding weight gain, and increasing physical activity and exercise. To what extent are smokers following through with their plans in this regard? What are some of the barriers that are preventing them from doing so?

7. *Assist smokers in making plans for maintaining abstinence over the next several days.* Facilitators should remind smokers of the date of the next session. Once again, this interval provides smokers with a manageable goal during which to remain abstinent over the next several days. However, as they may have to remain abstinent over a weekend, smokers should be encouraged to think about the challenges that this schedule will provide for them. Up until now (depending on the schedule of sessions), they may have remained abstinent during weekdays, when their routines are likely to be different from weekend routines. They should be particularly cautioned to think about high-risk situations they may encounter, including having free time, socializing over the weekend, or both. Smokers should again be encouraged to follow through on all assignments, including identifying high-risk situations and developing coping strategies, engaging in lifestyle change activities, and attempting to maximize positive social support and minimize negative social influence.

8. *Preview the homework assignments to be completed prior to Session 7.* Facilitators should confirm the date and time of the next session, review assignments to be completed before the next session, and answer any questions that smokers might have about the assignments.

Prior to Session 7

Do for the first time:

1. Work actively to utilize strategies for coping with urges to smoke.

Continue to do:

2. Continue to work on identifying high-risk situations and specific coping strategies to avoid smoking and complete the Coping with High-Risk Situations Worksheet.
3. Continue to implement ways of maximizing positive and minimizing negative social influences per the Social Support for Nonsmoking Worksheet.
4. Continue to work on accomplishing lifestyle change goals as specified on the Nonsmoking Game Plan: Lifestyle Change Worksheet.

SESSION 7

Session 7 Objectives

1. To discuss with smokers their quitting experiences
2. To review the concept of the AVE and how to cope with a possible slip should it occur (as well as applying it to any slips that may have already occurred).
3. To introduce new strategies for managing thoughts that can encourage relapse.
4. To review the use of strategies for coping with urges to smoke.
5. To review the homework assignment to identify and develop coping strategies for dealing with high-risk situations for relapse.
6. To review smokers' experiences in attempting to maximize social support for quitting smoking.
7. To assist smokers in making specific plans for maintaining abstinence over the next week (prior to the next session).
8. To preview the homework assignments to be completed prior to Session 8.

Session 7 Handouts and Worksheets

1. Strategies for Identifying and Counteracting Resumption Thoughts handout
2. Coping with High Risk Situations Worksheet
3. Social Support for Nonsmoking Worksheet
4. Nonsmoking Game Plan: Lifestyle Change Worksheet

Session 7 Content

1. *Discuss quitting experiences of past several days.* Facilitators should remind smokers that today is the eighth day of abstinence and should inquire about how they are doing. Facilitators should again engage smokers in a discussion of how they have been doing since the last session and should once again provide several minutes for each group member to

share his/her experiences. Facilitators should continue to reinforce the successes of those who have not smoked, while being attentive to the needs of those who have. For those who have smoked, facilitators should again distinguish between a slip and a relapse and briefly review the types of things that they can do to prevent a slip from becoming a relapse. Facilitators can discuss smokers' negative reactions to a slip, but this will be covered more fully later in the session.

Facilitators should ask about possible withdrawal symptoms that smokers may be experiencing. Facilitators can remind smokers that withdrawal symptoms are typically worse in the 1st week after quitting and should begin to improve no later than the 2nd or 3rd week after quitting. Facilitators can also remind smokers that the withdrawal symptoms they are experiencing should be less severe than they would have been had they quit smoking their regular brand cold turkey, given the nicotine-fading procedure in which they participated.

Facilitators should ask smokers what types of coping strategies they have been using and what success they have been having with these strategies. Facilitators should continue to help smokers to improve the use of coping strategies or to develop new ones in instances in which the strategies have been less than effective. Facilitators should also engage smokers in a discussion of what they expect over the next week and how they will plan to cope with some of the high-risk situations or difficulties that they might encounter.

2. *Review abstinence violation effect concept: How to cope with a possible slip.* Facilitators should review common cognitive and emotional reactions to a slip and how to prevent a slip from becoming a relapse. If they have had a slip, smokers should be encouraged to fight off this emotional reaction by viewing their slip as a mistake rather than as evidence that they are failures, to use the slip as a learning experience, to redouble their coping efforts, and to reaffirm that they will not smoke the next cigarette. Gradually these negative feelings will pass with increasing amounts of time spent not smoking. Facilitators should address comments to the entire group but should pay special attention to the experiences and reactions of smokers who have had slips since quit day. From this session to the end of treatment, slips are increasingly likely to occur, and helping smokers to "process" their slips within the context of the AVE is an important intervention. Facilitators should realize that other group members can be extremely helpful in this regard and should encourage appropriately supportive comments from others in the group.

3. *Introduce strategies for managing thoughts that can encourage relapse.* Another important set of relapse prevention strategies involves being able to identify and manage thoughts that might be conducive to smoking and thus lead to relapse. This section outlines a number of cognitive strategies smokers can use to help resist lingering smoking urges and strengthen their resolve to remain ex-smokers. Facilitators can offer the observation that, in many ways, the notion of willpower has to do with having effective skills in managing one's thinking in problem situations. Because practicing new ways of thinking is something smokers can do on their own without anyone's knowledge, they can use these skills in almost every situation in which they experience urges or temptations to smoke. Facilitators can provide smokers with the Strategies for Identifying and Counteracting Resumption Thoughts handout (Figure 5.10) for a summary of the concepts presented.

a. *Identifying smoking resumption thoughts.* Rationalizations to resume smoking are the most dangerous kind of thoughts because they often develop without smokers really

STRATEGIES FOR IDENTIFYING AND COUNTERACTING RESUMPTION THOUGHTS

Types of Smoking Resumption Thoughts:
1. Nostalgia–longing for the times when one could smoke; "It sure was fun to smoke while sitting around the campfire drinking a beer."
2. Testing control–due to overconfidence or curiosity, testing out one's control by smoking one or more cigarettes; "I bet I could smoke just one cigarette and then put them down."
3. Crisis–telling oneself that it is okay to smoke under "exceptional" circumstances, such as in a crisis; "Ordinarily I wouldn't smoke, but I'm under so much pressure right now, I need a cigarette."
4. Unwanted changes–worrying that changes (such as weight gain, irritability, inability to concentrate, withdrawal symptoms) one feels may be associated with nonsmoking; "I'm not willing to regain the weight I lost this summer, even if I have to start smoking again."
5. Self-doubts–self-doubts can undermine efforts to remain abstinent; "This is so hard for me—maybe I'm just meant to be a smoker."

Strategies to Counteract the Effects of These Thoughts:
1. Challenging–the most straightforward way to counteract thoughts about smoking is to directly confront or challenge them; "I cannot have one cigarette without smoking more."
2. Benefits of nonsmoking–another useful strategy is to think about the personal benefits of not smoking; "The best feeling in the world will be breathing freely again and not being congested once I've quit smoking."
3. Remembering unpleasant smoking experiences–another strategy is to recall specific unpleasant aspects of smoking; "I won't have to worry about my wife feeling like she's kissing an ashtray when she kisses me."
4. Distractions–another effective means of coping is for smokers to simply divert their attention from any aspect of smoking; "I'm going to ignore this urge and imagine, in vivid detail, that I'm skiing down my favorite slope in Colorado."
5. Self-rewarding thoughts–another strategy involves thinking about one's successes and strengths; "Good job! It wasn't easy but I didn't smoke in that tempting situation."

FIGURE 5.10. Strategies for Identifying and Counteracting Resumption Thoughts.

being aware of them, and they directly undermine the goal of abstinence. Dealing with rationalizations involves recognizing rationalizations and learning to cope with them by means of effective strategies. Following are categories of rationalizations or smoking resumption thoughts that facilitators should share with smokers, followed by some specific strategies to help cope with these thoughts.

   i. *Nostalgia.* Some temporary ex-smokers begin to long for the times when they could smoke as if reminiscing about some long-lost friend. Nostalgic thoughts may go like this: "I remember when I could smoke while watching the football game in the cold," or "It sure was fun to light up a smoke while sitting around the campfire in late summer." The main feature of these mismanaged thoughts is that they imply that the ex-smoker has given up something important.

  ii. *Testing control.* Sometimes after a period of abstinence, temporary ex-smokers become pleased with their success at stopping and act overconfident. Too often, though, this kind of thinking leads to self-statements such as "I'll bet I could smoke just one and then put it down!" or "I'm stronger than most people, because I can pick up cigarettes and then lay them down without any problems." Curiosity also can be a problem: "I wonder what it would be like to smoke one cigarette." Unfortunately, these tests often result in a resumption of smoking. Smokers are better off admitting the challenge of remaining an ex-smoker and granting their adversary, the urge to smoke, a lot of power and influence.

   iii. *Crisis*. At times of crisis, many temporary ex-smokers say to themselves something like, "I'll handle this situation better if I have a cigarette," or "This was so difficult, I deserve a cigarette." However, it is possible for these thoughts to be anticipated and counteracted. The rationalization for starting to smoke in a crisis is the same used by the overweight person who justifies excessive eating by saying, "It was a special occasion." Crises and special occasions have a way of becoming regular events.

   iv. *Unwanted changes*. Many temporary ex-smokers worry that changes they experience may be associated with their nonsmoking. For example, upon quitting, many individuals have concerns such as weight gain, irritability, inability to concentrate and to work effectively, and withdrawal symptoms. All of these concerns take the form of *worrying* along the following lines:

> "I think I'm beginning to gain lots of extra weight—I'd rather look slim than be an ex-smoker."
>
> "I'm being very short and irritable around my family—maybe it's more important for me to be a good parent and spouse than it is for me to be an ex-smoker now."
>
> "I'm really not getting any work done these days since I've stopped smoking."
>
> "These withdrawal symptoms are unbearable—I'm not sure they're ever going to stop."

Although some of these changes may occur, specific strategies should enable smokers to cope with the changes and even prevent them from happening. Controlling these thoughts is critical, as is taking active steps to manage one's weight, relax around others, and continue working effectively at home or in the office.

   v. *Self-doubts*. Self-doubts can undermine smokers' efforts to remain abstinent. The topic can be almost anything from nicotine addiction and lack of self-control to previous unsuccessful attempts to quit. The self-statements can take the following forms: "I'm one of those people who doesn't have any self-control," "I'm really addicted to smoking; I can't control myself," or "I tried to quit many times in the past, and none of these efforts really worked out; why should I expect this one to last!" Facilitators should suggest that smokers imagine how angry they would be if a neighbor or an acquaintance said these things to them, yet they accept them when they come in the form of self-statements.

b. *Challenging smoking resumption thoughts*. Facilitators should suggest the following strategies to help smokers attack their negative thoughts about smoking:

   i. *Challenging*. Smokers can use other thoughts to directly confront or challenge their thoughts about smoking. Smokers should also consider the logic of their thought processes. Here is a case in point:

> George was well on his way to being a successful ex-smoker when he began to think back on how enjoyable it had been to smoke while relaxing after work. With this thought running through his mind (nostalgia), he began to seriously consider having just one cigarette a day to relax (testing and overconfidence). He remem-

bered the good times when he was a smoker (nostalgia). Fortunately, George recognized that this pattern of thinking was directly undermining his motivation to remain an ex-smoker. He wrote down a number of his challenges on an index card and read them every time he found himself thinking about resuming smoking. These were George's *challenges*:

"I cannot have just one cigarette without smoking more."

"I can use the relaxation exercises to unwind from work instead of smoking."

"I can still have good times without smoking."

"I won't let these thoughts continue to run through my mind because they are undermining my motivation."

This example shows how mismanaged thoughts can be identified, challenged, and effectively controlled.

ii. *Benefits of nonsmoking.* It is useful at this point for smokers to think about personal benefits of not smoking. Thoughts about these benefits can be powerful antidotes to rationalizations to resume smoking. Smokers can consider:

Physical improvements—more stamina, greater activity, improved breathing, less coughing

Economic benefits—more money available for casual spending

Interpersonal improvements—increased attractiveness to others, congratulatory comments from friends

Reduced health risk—decreased risk of heart and lung disease

Feelings of accomplishment—increased sense of self-mastery, self-control

To return to the example of George, he began to pay more attention to the fact that he felt more strength when playing tennis, that his girlfriend had remarked how proud she was of his progress, and that he no longer awoke coughing in the middle of the night. Thinking about the emerging benefits of nonsmoking helps smokers to see the results of their efforts in a positive light.

iii. *Remembering unpleasant smoking experiences.* Another strategy is specific recollection of the unpleasant aspects of smoking. Smokers may already have experienced some of the physiological effects of chronic smoking, as these often compel people to quit the habit in the first place (smoker's cough, upset stomach, headaches, shortness of breath, etc.). Smokers should think back to how they felt the morning after they smoked heavily: How did their throats feel and their mouths taste? Clear memories of these experiences can help smokers overcome some of the lingering smoking urges and combat the mismanaged thinking that pulls them toward resumption.

iv. *Distractions.* Another effective means of coping is for smokers to simply divert their attention from any aspect of smoking. Smokers may want to concentrate on pleasant, enjoyable subjects (e.g., vacation spot, relaxation, personal accomplishments, etc.) that help them take their minds off smoking.

Barbara, for instance, loved to go to the mountains for her annual vacation. She was able to remember every turn in her favorite hiking trail. For distracting thoughts, Barbara recalled walking along that trail, seeing the special reminders of past good times. She was able to pick up anywhere she left off in imagining brief episodes of this distraction during the busy working day.

v. *Self-rewarding thoughts.* The final strategy to recommend to smokers involves reminding themselves of the successes and strengths they have already shown. In our culture, statements about one's accomplishments, if made out loud, are looked down on as being vain, egocentric, boastful, and conceited, but these positive self-statements can be made silently and can act as powerful incentives and guides to maintain motivation. For example, if a smoker avoids smoking in a situation he/she anticipated would be difficult, he/she can think to him/herself: "Good job! It wasn't easy, but I didn't smoke in that situation. I'm proud of myself."

Facilitators can suggest several ways in which smokers can utilize this information and practice changing mismanaged thoughts. Quite simply, it is important to write down smoking resumption thoughts, as well as adaptive, coping thoughts that can be used to challenge them. This can be done by taking a piece of paper, drawing a line vertically down the middle, and writing resumption thoughts in the left-hand column and the corresponding challenging thought across from it on the right. Alternatively, smokers can carry 3" × 5" index cards with the smoking resumption thought on one side and the challenge to that thought on the other side. In either case, it is important that smokers take out their lists or index cards and read them frequently, adding to them as new thoughts occur to them.

4. *Review the use of strategies for coping with urges to smoke.* Facilitators can remind smokers that urges are to be expected and are not a sign of failure. Smokers should be reminded that urges are time limited. Rather than believing that urges will not cease until they finally smoke a cigarette, smokers should work hard to remind themselves that urges have a beginning, a middle, and an end and that the entire process generally takes only several minutes.

Facilitators can review smokers' use of strategies for using coping imagery in combination with relaxation skills to combat urges. Overall, smokers should be encouraged to take an active role in coping with urges to smoke. Smokers should pay attention to the thoughts or beliefs that may accompany urges and to actively challenge those thoughts.

Finally, smokers should attempt to recognize the situations and circumstances that lead to urges or thoughts of smoking. They can be better prepared by avoiding these triggers altogether, by altering something about the nature of the trigger, or by substituting something else instead of the cigarette in those situations that cannot be avoided or altered.

5. *Review assignment to identify and cope with high-risk situations.* Facilitators should remind smokers that as they go through the process of quitting, previous high-risk situations may become irrelevant, and new high-risk situations are likely to emerge. Thus they need to keep a continual focus on what situations are currently high risk . For homework, smokers were to complete the Coping with High-Risk Situations Worksheet (Figure 5.8) to identify as many high-risk situations as possible and to fully develop coping strategies for dealing with each situation.

As before, facilitators should engage smokers in a discussion of this assignment, specifically with regard to how they are doing anticipating high-risk situations and coping effectively with them. As before, the discussion should be a mix of successes and difficulties. If there are situations in which a smoker had a slip, discussion should center around whether he/she was able to anticipate the high-risk situation or, alternatively, whether it was a situation that he/she anticipated but was unable to cope with effectively.

Facilitators should inform smokers that their assignment for next session is to complete a new Coping with High-Risk Situations Worksheet (Figure 5.8). Smokers should specifically try to anticipate situations or circumstances in the next week that might put them at risk for smoking.

6. *Review experiences in attempting to maximize social support for nonsmoking.* As before, facilitators should ask smokers to discuss attempts they have made to increase positive social support or to decrease negative social influence regarding quitting smoking. As with other aspects of treatment, facilitators should reinforce smokers for accomplishments that reflect adaptive coping and should help smokers to come up with solutions to situations that pose problems.

Facilitators should be particularly attentive to situations involving other smokers and how the group members are dealing with this challenge. As discussed at the previous session, assertiveness is a relevant skill in these situations. Smokers should be encouraged to act assertively if another's smoking is acting as a strong cue for them to smoke. Treatment strategies to enhance assertiveness skills are discussed in Chapter 6. Another, related issue is how smokers view the prospect of speaking with someone else about changing that person's behavior. Here again, assertiveness training is relevant, as smokers may have to first understand that they have the right to ask someone else to make a behavior change that would affect them positively.

7. *Assist smokers in making plans for maintaining abstinence over the next week.* Facilitators should remind smokers that the next session (Session 8) is the last. Smokers can be encouraged to focus on the goal of remaining abstinent for the next week and also to anticipate what plans they will make to assure that they remain abstinent after the group ends. Smokers should be encouraged to follow through on all assignments, including managing thoughts, identifying high-risk situations, developing coping strategies, coping with urges to smoke, attempting to maximize positive and minimize negative social influences, and engaging in lifestyle change activities.

8. *Preview the homework assignments to be completed prior to Session 8.* Facilitators should confirm the date and time of the next session, review assignments to be completed before the next session, and answer any questions that smokers might have about the assignments.

Prior to Session 8

Do for the first time:

1. Work actively to utilize strategies for identifying and challenging smoking resumption thoughts, using the Strategies for Identifying and Counteracting Resumption Thoughts handout (Figure 5.10) as a reference.

Continue to do:

2. Continue to work actively to utilize strategies for coping with urges to smoke.
3. Continue to work on identifying high-risk situations and specific coping strategies to avoid smoking, and complete the Coping with High-Risk Situations Worksheet (Figure 5.8).
4. Continue to implement ways of maximizing positive and minimizing negative social influences regarding quitting smoking per the Social Support for Nonsmoking Worksheet (Figure 5.9).
5. Continue to work on accomplishing lifestyle change goals as specified on the Nonsmoking Game Plan: Lifestyle Change Worksheet (Figure 5.7).

SESSION 8

Session 8 Objectives

1. To discuss with smokers their quitting experiences.
2. To review the concept of the abstinence violation effect and how to cope with a possible slip should it occur (as well as applying it to any slips that may have already occurred).
3. To review the use of strategies for managing thoughts that can encourage relapse.
4. To review the homework assignment to identify and develop coping strategies for dealing with high-risk situations for relapse.
5. To review smokers' progress regarding making broader lifestyle changes that support quitting smoking.
6. To offer some final remarks and observations about planning for the future.

Session 8 Content

1. *Discuss quitting experiences of the past week.* Facilitators should inform smokers that today is the 15th day of abstinence and should inquire about how they are doing. Facilitators should again engage smokers in a discussion of how they have been doing since the last session and should once again provide several minutes for each group member to share his/her experiences. Facilitators should continue to reinforce the successes of those who have not smoked, while being attentive to the needs of those who have. For those who have smoked, facilitators should remind them of the distinction between a slip and a relapse and briefly review the types of things that they can do to help prevent a slip from becoming a relapse.

2. *Review abstinence violation effect concept: How to cope with a possible slip.* In the context of reviewing the abstinence violation effect, facilitators should pay special attention to the experiences and reactions of smokers who have had recent slips. Helping smokers to "process" their slips within this context is an important intervention. Facilitators should realize that other group members can be extremely helpful in this regard and should encourage appropriately supportive comments from others in the group.

3. *Review the use of strategies for managing thoughts that can encourage relapse*. Facilitators should review the important set of relapse prevention strategies that involve identifying and managing thoughts that might be conducive to smoking and thus lead to relapse. The first step in the process is for smokers to identify thoughts that directly undermine their goal to remain ex-smokers. Facilitators should review the categories of rationalizations or smoking resumption thoughts that were discussed at the last session. The second step in the process is for smokers to counteract the effects of these thoughts using the strategies discussed in the last session. Facilitators should review these strategies for counteracting smoking resumption thoughts.

4. *Review assignment to identify and cope with high-risk situations*. Facilitators should remind smokers that, as they go through the process of quitting, previous high-risk situations may become irrelevant and new high-risk situations are likely to emerge. Thus they need keep a continual focus on what situations are currently high risk. Smokers were to continue using the Coping with High-Risk Situations Worksheet (Figure 5.8) to identify as many high-risk situations as possible and to fully develop coping strategies for dealing with each high-risk situation.

    As before, facilitators should discuss with smokers the completion of this assignment, specifically how they are doing regarding anticipating high-risk situations and coping effectively with them. As before, the discussion should be a mix of examples both of coping well with high-risk situations and of any difficulties they may be having. Any situation in which a smoker had a slip is fair game for discussion as to whether he/she was able to anticipate the high-risk situation or, alternatively, whether it was a situation that he/she anticipated but was unable to cope with effectively.

5. *Review smokers' progress regarding lifestyle changes that support quitting smoking*. One final time, facilitators should review the importance of lifestyle changes in smokers' efforts to quit smoking and should engage smokers in a discussion of which lifestyle changes they have initiated. Although all of the six lifestyle changes from the Nonsmoking Game Plan: Lifestyle Change Worksheet (Figure 5.7) are open for discussion, the facilitator should particularly focus on issues relating to managing stress, avoiding weight gain, and increasing physical activity and exercise. To what extent have smokers followed through with their plans? If they have not, what are some of the barriers that are preventing them from doing so?

6. *Offer final remarks and observations about planning for the future*. Facilitators should spend the last portion of Session 8 discussing with smokers what they should expect and what they will do now that the treatment program is ending. Those smokers who have either partially or fully relapsed should be congratulated for the positive efforts they did make and should be implored not to be discouraged. Smokers can be reminded that quitting smoking is essentially a trial-and-error process that takes many people a period of years and that they learn valuable information about what will and will not work for them in each successive cessation attempt. These smokers should be encouraged to reexamine their reasons for quitting. They should also be encouraged to maintain the positive lifestyle changes (e.g., exercise, stress management) they have made in the program, as well as any modifications to their smoking behavior pattern that might promote future cessation (e.g., no longer smoking in one's house or car). Finally, these smokers should be en-

couraged to select a new quit day and to utilize the same strategies they learned in treatment to prepare themselves to be successful in quitting.

Those smokers who have thus far quit smoking successfully should be congratulated for their efforts. Facilitators should shift the discussion toward possible barriers that may exist to their becoming lifelong nonsmokers. Facilitators should inform smokers that one particular barrier to be cognizant of at this point is becoming overconfident. This is one of the greatest risks for relapse for those who have not smoked. Paradoxically, many smokers have a tendency to react to abstinence by interpreting it to mean that they are now invulnerable to relapse and can have an occasional cigarette. To the extent that they smoke one and do not immediately relapse, this sense of invulnerability is reinforced and is likely to lead eventually to one or more subsequent cigarettes. This process invariably leads to relapse, as rarely are regular, addicted smokers able to become infrequent, occasional smokers. The other, more obvious type of risk to these abstinent smokers is that of succumbing to future high-risk situations. Smokers should be encouraged to continue to be vigilant to high-risk situations and to be prepared with a plan for how to cope in those situations. Facilitators should also urge smokers to be prepared for a generic type of upsetting situation that they might not now be able to anticipate. In our experience, the other long-term risk of relapse occurs when smokers have some type of unanticipated crisis, become stressed or upset, and reach for a cigarette in response to the situation. Finally, these smokers should also be encouraged to continue to use all the coping strategies and maintain all the lifestyle changes that have thus far supported their efforts at abstinence.

At this point, all smokers should be acknowledged for their efforts and should be encouraged to celebrate their efforts and their successes. Smokers should be reminded to reward themselves for success at quitting smoking (if applicable) and for all the hard work they have devoted to their effort to quit smoking. Facilitators would, of course, at this point wish all smokers good luck, perhaps share some personal feelings of having enjoyed working with people in the group, and bid farewell to participants as a group and individually.

6

Comorbidity Treatment
SKILLS TRAINING FOR COPING WITH DEPRESSION AND NEGATIVE MOODS

Richard A. Brown

Some smokers may need coping skills training and support in addition to the standard eight-session treatment program described in Chapter 5. We recently found that cognitive-behavioral coping skills training to deal with depression and other negative moods (CBT-D) combined with standard smoking cessation treatment yielded significantly better outcomes than standard smoking cessation treatment alone (ST) at 12-month follow-up for two particular subgroups of smokers with past major depressive disorder (MDD; Brown et al., 2001). Smokers with a recurrent depression history showed 28.0% abstinence with CBT-D versus 16.7% abstinence with ST; similarly, heavy smokers (> 25 cigarettes per day) with past MDD achieved 30.4% abstinence with CBT-D versus 15.2% abstinence with ST. Smokers who have experienced an exacerbation of depressed mood or depressive symptoms during past quit attempts might also be expected to benefit from the addition of depression coping skills training. Likewise, these skills may be useful for smokers in recovery from alcohol or drug problems, particularly if they have experienced MDD in the past. More generally, the modules in this chapter may be useful for smokers who have failed to quit smoking in the past with less intensive treatment programs, who show signs of increased severity of nicotine dependence, and/or who need more intensive support for relapse prevention than is provided in the standard behavioral treatment described in Chapter 5.

PROGRAM STRUCTURE

The treatment content in this chapter is designed to be integrated into the content of the behavioral treatment described in Chapter 5. As with intensive behavior treatment, the rationale for this comorbidity treatment is that smoking is a learned habit, a physical addiction, and a means of managing negative moods. Coping skills for dealing with the learned habit and physical addiction components of smoking are taught in the intensive behavioral treatment; however, management of negative moods is only briefly covered, primarily in the context of handling triggers. This chapter presents a full set of coping skills to deal with the stress and negative-mood components of smoking. Thus this comorbidity treatment consists of the integration of the coping skills provided in intensive behavioral treatment (Chapter 5) with the negative-mood coping skills content from this chapter. A comprehensive list of objectives begins each session, with content relevant to managing negative mood presented in **boldface** in the lists of objectives and handouts and worksheets for each session. The mood management components in this chapter are organized to match the program structure detailed in Chapter 5 such that there are eight sessions over a 7-week time period (Table 6.1). Session numbers in this chapter correspond to those in Chapter 5 (e.g., Session 1 content from this chapter is intended to be added to Session 1 content from Chapter 5).

The 90-minute sessions suggested for the intensive behavioral treatment allow considerable time during sessions not only for working with the behavioral treatment content but also for group discussion and for sharing of smokers' cessation-related experiences. The comorbidity treatment content can be readily integrated with the 8-week intensive behavioral treatment, either within a 90-minute or a 120-minute session. If a 90-minute format is chosen, facilitators should recognize that they will need to be very time efficient and that sessions will be "all business," somewhat to the exclusion of extended group discussion and sharing of experiences. Facilitators may need to occasionally remind smokers of the need to limit discussion due to the large amount of session content; however, most smokers will readily adapt to this situation. On the other hand, 120-minute sessions will probably allow sufficient time for thorough coverage of treatment content while also allowing time for group discussion. The drawback, of course, is that 2-hour group sessions may be more difficult to schedule and may present a less attractive option for smokers when they are deciding whether or not to make a commitment to participate in treatment.

A third option is to keep the 90-minute session length but to extend the total number of treatment sessions, resulting in a 10- to 14-session program. Although some of the comorbidity treatment content can be integrated with the relapse-prevention coping skills following quit day, care must still be taken to incorporate the basic mood coping skills content in sessions prior to quit day, so that smokers will be armed with some ability to cope with possible negative-mood or depressive reactions that may occur upon initial quitting.

COMORBIDITY MODULE SESSION 1

Integrated Session 1 Objectives

1. To introduce the group facilitators, the structural details of the treatment program, and ground rules for the conduct of the group sessions.
2. To conduct a warm-up exercise to help smokers get acquainted with other group members in a way that sets the tone for a supportive and positive group experience.
3. To present a positive focus and framework for quitting smoking, emphasizing the learning

TABLE 6.1. Treatment Schedule and Session Content for Mood Management Component

Phase of treatment	Preparation/cessation				Quit day		Maintenance	
Timeline (Days)	−28	−21	−14	−7	0	+3	+7	+14
Week No.	One	Two	Three	Four	Five	Five	Six	Seven
Session No.	1	2	3	4	5	6	7	8
Focus content of session	Cognitive social learning rationale Social learning model of depression Daily mood monitoring Introduction to thought-changing methods	Introduction to ABC method Introduction to positive and negative thoughts method	Intervention strategies—ABC method Intervention strategies—positive and negative thoughts method Introduction to increasing pleasant activities	Intervention strategies—increasing pleasant activities	Introduction to social skills and assertiveness	Intervention strategies—social skills and assertiveness	Continued intervention—social skills and assertiveness	Planning for the future Review specific coping strategies How to use specific strategies in the future
Review		Social learning model of depression Daily mood monitoring Homework	Daily mood monitoring Review ABC Method Worksheet Review inventory of thoughts Homework	Daily mood monitoring Review top 20 pleasant events Review ABC(D) Worksheet Review Positive/Negative Thoughts Worksheet Homework	Daily mood monitoring Review Contract and Weekly Plan for Pleasant Activities Review ABC(D)/Positive/Negative Thoughts Worksheet Apply changing thoughts to quitting Homework	Daily mood monitoring Review Contract and Weekly Plan for Pleasant Activities Review ABC(D)/Positive/Negative Thoughts Worksheet Apply changing thoughts to quitting Homework	Daily mood monitoring Review A Plan for Assertiveness Worksheet Review Contract and Weekly Plan for Pleasant Activities Review ABC(D)/Positive/Negative Thoughts Worksheet Homework	Review A Plan for Assertiveness Worksheet

gained in past quit attempts, the advantages of learning specific coping skills to aid in quitting, and the benefits of participating in a group program with the support of other group members.

4. To present the cognitive social learning theory rationale for smoking cessation treatment.
   a. **To present the social learning model of depression and its application to smoking cessation.**
   b. **To introduce daily mood monitoring and to give out the Daily Mood Rating Form for completion between first and second sessions.**
   c. **To provide a rationale and an explanation for the use of skills to identify and change negative ways of thinking.**

5. To introduce self-monitoring of smoking behavior and to give out Wrap Sheets for completion between first and second sessions.
6. To introduce and define the concept of triggers for smoking.
7. To provide a rationale and an explanation of the use of nicotine fading.
8. To preview the homework assignments to be completed prior to Session 2.
   a. **Includes homework for managing negative mood.**

Integrated Session 1 Handouts and Worksheets

1. Written Program Schedule
2. Wrap Sheets
3. Triggers for Smoking Worksheet
4. **Daily Mood Rating Form (Table 6.2)**
5. **ABC Overview (Table 6.3)**
6. **Positive and Negative Thoughts Overview (Table 6.4)**

Session 1 Comorbidity Treatment Content

1. *Present the social learning model of depression and its application to smoking cessation.* Facilitators should explain to smokers that smoking consists of the following three components: *learned habit, physical addiction,* and *means of managing negative mood* (all covered in detail in Chapter 5). To the extent that the smoker feels that his/her smoking serves as a means of coping with negative moods or has certain characteristics that might predispose him/her to have cessation-related mood issues, treatment must focus on learning to manage or cope with negative moods. Treatment must also focus on initial quitting, as well as on helping to maintain abstinence and prevent relapse. Smokers should be told that this treatment will help them learn skills to cope with negative mood situations more effectively.

   The cognitive social learning model of depression can be applied to the experience of negative moods. The model proposes that our experiences are made up of thoughts, feelings, and behaviors. Furthermore, reciprocal and bidirectional relationships exist among thoughts, feelings, and behaviors such that each one affects the others. Figure 6.1 illustrates the reciprocal relationships among the three.

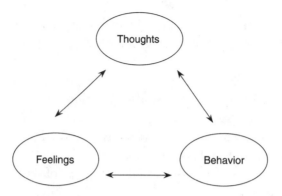

FIGURE 6.1. Social learning model of depression.

Facilitators should define each of these terms:

a. *Behaviors* are things that we do, our actions. Others can observe the actions and can agree either that they happened or that they didn't happen.

b. *Thoughts* are what we say to ourselves. They are constant and ongoing. Facilitators can suggest to smokers that it is best to conceive of thoughts in complete sentences. For example, a smoker may indicate that he/she is thinking about "family problems." However, this does not covey much specific information as to *what* he/she is thinking about the family problems. In contrast, the complete sentence, "I have family problems but I believe they can be resolved" conveys much more specific information about what the smoker is thinking.

c. *Feelings* describe an emotional state at a particular time. Feelings are best described in a single word, such as "sad," "happy," "angry," "anxious," and so forth. The term "mood" will also be used at times and is, for our purposes, synonymous with "feelings."

Facilitators should ask smokers in the group to give depressive and nondepressive examples of behaviors and thoughts. Examples of depressive behaviors might include crying, sleeping too much, or sitting around the house with the curtains closed, whereas nondepressive behaviors might include laughing, talking with good friends, or watching a favorite TV show. Examples of depressive thoughts would be, "Nobody cares about me," or "I'll never quit smoking"; examples of nondepressive thoughts would be, "Today's going to be a good day," or "I will successfully quit smoking." In relation to feelings, facilitators should ask smokers to give examples of negative moods and positive moods more generally, rather than specifically depressive and nondepressive examples. Negative mood examples might include feeling sad, angry, irritable, anxious, bored, enraged, or frustrated; positive mood examples might include being happy, calm, joyous, thankful, excited, relaxed, or content.

Once smokers have distinguished between depressive and nondepressive behaviors and thoughts and between positive and negative feelings, group facilitators should pose the following question: "Of these three—thoughts, feelings, and behavior—which is hardest to change *directly*?" The answer is that it is hardest to change feelings directly. It is nearly impossible to go from feeling sad or angry to feeling happy without first changing some aspect of one's behavior or one's thoughts. We cannot change our feelings or mood directly; however, we can learn to change aspects of our behavior and our thoughts, which will, in turn, have a direct impact on improving feelings. In fact, often feelings can't help but change when one engages in nondepressive behaviors and thoughts.

Facilitators might pose an example to the group to illustrate this point. They might ask group members what each of them would do to change their feelings or mood if they were feeling particularly "down" or depressed. More specifically, they might challenge group members to indicate how they would change their moods directly. Typically, a group member might say, "I would call a friend," to which the facilitator would reply by pointing out that this would be an example of changing behavior, which would in turn improve mood. Another group member might offer that, "I would think of all the things for which I am thankful," to which the facilitator would reply that this represents an example of changing thoughts to improve mood. Again, the basic point is that one cannot change mood or feelings directly but that changing aspects of thoughts and/or behavior can powerfully influence mood.

Facilitators should then explain that the goal of this aspect of the treatment program is to teach smokers skills to change their thoughts and behavior to help them cope more effectively with negative moods and negative mood situations. Learning and applying these coping skills will help to replace the role of cigarettes in coping with negative mood.

Facilitators should explain to smokers that the social learning model of depression fits nicely within the learned-habit component of smoking outlined earlier. Many times smoking is related to negative moods. Once the negative mood occurs, for whatever reason, the vicious cycle of negative thoughts, behaviors, and feelings may become activated and may lead to smoking a cigarette (see Figure 6.2).

The integration of the social learning model of depression with the previously developed model of smoking behavior is important for quitting smoking for several reasons. First, many people smoke as a way to manage their moods. Therefore, it is important to learn alternative ways of coping with negative mood states without smoking. Second, it is important to actively maintain a positive mood while quitting smoking in order to combat possible feelings of sadness, anger, or depression that may occur during the quitting pro-

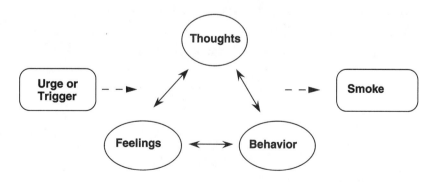

FIGURE 6.2. Integration of social learning model of depression and learned habit model of smoking.

cess. Finally, because many slips or relapses to smoking occur in negative mood situations, learning how to manage these situations more effectively may help to forestall slips or prevent slips from becoming relapses.

2. *Introduce daily mood monitoring*. The rationale for daily mood monitoring is that, in order to gain control over mood (i.e., by learning coping skills), it is necessary to learn how to identify negative mood and to distinguish different mood states. It is also important to gain an awareness of the factors that may affect mood.

   Using the Daily Mood Rating Form (Table 6.2), smokers should rate their moods at the end of each day on three dimensions: (a) depressed versus happy, (b) angry/irritable versus calm, and (c) anxious versus relaxed. These three dimensions represent the primary mood states that affect smoking and smoking cessation. Smokers should rate their moods on a 1–9 scale, with a high score ("9" being the highest) representing a positive mood and a low score ("1" being the lowest) representing a negative mood. Ideally, smokers should rate their moods about an hour before going to bed so that they can look back on the entire day. Each mood rating should represent an average of their mood experience for the day. Smokers should attend to events or situations that were associated with either positive moods or negative moods. Once smokers have had practice rating their moods for a day or two, they should begin to record events or situations that were associated with both positive moods and negative moods.

3. *Provide a rationale and explanation for changing thoughts*. Facilitators should explain to smokers that they will learn two different skills for identifying and changing negative ways of thinking. Smokers will choose one of the skills to focus on during treatment but will have the opportunity to learn about both. The two skills for changing thoughts follow:

   a. *The ABC method* is a useful skill for people who tend to overreact to situations or events by becoming extremely upset.

   b. *Increasing positive/decreasing negative thoughts* is a useful set of skills for people who tend to be chronic negative thinkers.

   For homework, smokers should read the descriptions of these techniques in the ABC Overview (Table 6.3) and the Positive and Negative Thoughts Overview (Table 6.4). These techniques are discussed in Session 2, and smokers are given a more detailed description of them for homework. During Session 3, smokers are asked to choose which of these techniques they prefer to focus on during treatment. Facilitators can explain that it is better to master one skill and do it well than to work only halfway on both skills.

4. *Review mood component homework assignments for next session*. Facilitators should confirm the date and time of the next session, review assignments to be completed before the next session, and answer any questions that smokers might have about the assignments.

Prior to Session 2

Do for the first time:

   a. Complete Daily Mood Rating Form at the end of each day.
   b. Read ABC Overview.
   c. Read Positive and Negative Thoughts Overview.

TABLE 6.2. Daily Mood Rating Form

INSTRUCTIONS: At the end of each day, about an hour before going to bed, rate your mood on three dimensions for that day. If your mood was *negative* (depressed, angry/irritable, or anxious), mark a *lower* number on the chart for that day for each mood. If your mood was *positive* (happy, calm, or relaxed), mark a *higher* number for each mood. Write down events or situations that might have contributed to your mood, either positively or negatively over the past week.

EXAMPLE
Date: Monday, 5/14

Happy	9	8	7	**6**	5	4	3	2	1	Depressed
Calm	9	8	7	6	5	**4**	3	2	1	Angry/irritable
Relaxed	9	8	7	6	**5**	4	3	2	1	Anxious

Date: _____

Happy	9	8	7	6	5	4	3	2	1	Depressed
Calm	9	8	7	6	5	4	3	2	1	Angry/irritable
Relaxed	9	8	7	6	5	4	3	2	1	Anxious

Date: _____

Happy	9	8	7	6	5	4	3	2	1	Depressed
Calm	9	8	7	6	5	4	3	2	1	Angry/irritable
Relaxed	9	8	7	6	5	4	3	2	1	Anxious

Date: _____

Happy	9	8	7	6	5	4	3	2	1	Depressed
Calm	9	8	7	6	5	4	3	2	1	Angry/irritable
Relaxed	9	8	7	6	5	4	3	2	1	Anxious

Date: _____

Happy	9	8	7	6	5	4	3	2	1	Depressed
Calm	9	8	7	6	5	4	3	2	1	Angry/irritable
Relaxed	9	8	7	6	5	4	3	2	1	Anxious

Date: _____

Happy	9	8	7	6	5	4	3	2	1	Depressed
Calm	9	8	7	6	5	4	3	2	1	Angry/irritable
Relaxed	9	8	7	6	5	4	3	2	1	Anxious

Date: _____

Happy	9	8	7	6	5	4	3	2	1	Depressed
Calm	9	8	7	6	5	4	3	2	1	Angry/irritable
Relaxed	9	8	7	6	5	4	3	2	1	Anxious

Events or situations that resulted in *positive* moods:
Going for a walk, dinner with friends, coworker complimented me, watched favorite TV show

Events or situations that resulted in *negative* moods:
Son lied to me, long wait at doctor's office, dishwasher broke, late for dinner

185

TABLE 6.3. ABC Overview

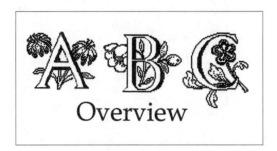

In managing negative mood, it is helpful to take a look at your thinking patterns. A method developed by a well-known psychologist, Dr. Albert Ellis, can help you understand the connection between what you think and how you feel. This method is called the ABC technique.

The <u>A</u> stands for <u>A</u>ctivating event, the event you feel upset about.

The <u>B</u> stands for <u>B</u>eliefs about the activating event, or what you tell yourself about the event.

The <u>C</u> stands for the emotional <u>C</u>onsequences, or reaction to the event.

The ABC technique is not intended to help you avoid <u>reasonable</u> emotional reactions to events but rather to avoid <u>emotional overreactions</u>. To best describe the ABC technique, look at the following example:

> Jack reports that he is angry and sad (emotional consequence: <u>C</u>) because he did not get a raise in pay at work (activating event: <u>A</u>). He is so upset that he does not go to work for the next two days.

In this example, Jack might conclude that <u>A</u> (the activating event) caused <u>C</u> (the emotional consequence). This is not surprising, because people commonly believe that events cause their emotional reactions:

<u>A</u>   →?→   <u>C</u>
<u>A</u>ctivating Event   <u>C</u>onsequence

However, this is not accurate. When Jack felt angry and sad, it was not <u>A</u> (the activating event) that <u>caused</u> his emotional reaction; rather it was <u>B</u> (his beliefs or what he said to himself) that resulted in <u>C</u> (his emotional reaction).

<u>A</u> → <u>B</u> → <u>C</u>
<u>A</u>ctivating Event <u>B</u>eliefs <u>C</u>onsequence

In the example, Jack's beliefs or self-talk included statements such as:
"I should have gotten a raise."
"Since I didn't, I must be a total failure."
"I didn't get it because the boss hates me."

The ABC technique correctly identifies Jack's beliefs or self-talk statements as leading to his emotional overreaction. Jack's beliefs or self-talk about why he didn't get a raise are directly related to his feelings of anger and sadness.

<u>A</u> → <u>B</u> → <u>C</u>
<u>A</u>ctivating Event <u>B</u>eliefs <u>C</u>onsequence
Not getting a raise *"I must be a total failure."* *Angry and sad*

> Many times it is not what happens that makes us upset; rather, it is what we tell ourselves about the situation. If, at times, your thinking patterns cause you to overreact, as in this example, the ABC technique can help you.

In future sessions, we will discuss how you can change your emotional overreactions (<u>C</u>) by learning to evaluate and change what you say or believe (<u>B</u>) about upsetting events (<u>A</u>).

TABLE 6.4. Positive and Negative Thoughts Overview

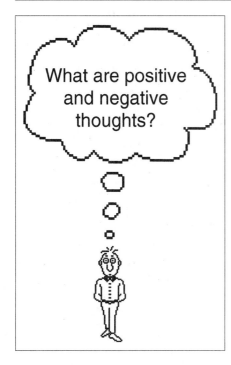

POSITIVE THOUGHTS are thoughts that have a good effect on your mood and reflect the positive point of view. For example, they may be thoughts about:
- *your good qualities:* "I am smart," "I am a good worker," "I am fun at parties."
- *good parts of your life:* "My family is great," "I really enjoy my job," "My friends are the best."
- *good thoughts about the future:* "Things will work out," "I have a lot to look forward to."

NEGATIVE THOUGHTS are thoughts that have a negative effect on your mood, usually because they focus either on:
- *bad points:* "I am stupid," "The only luck I ever have is *bad* luck," "My spouse is always complaining," "My kids are never satisfied", or . . .
- *negative feelings about the world or the future:* "No one cares about me," "What's the use, nothing's going to improve."

Managing Thoughts

When your mood becomes depressed, you have a larger number of negative thoughts. These thoughts, which may have been originally caused by feelings of depression, in turn produce more depressed feelings. Thus a destructive downward spiral begins. By breaking up this process, you can reduce feelings of depression and maintain a more pleasant state of mind.

Reducing the number of negative thoughts you have will not automatically increase the number of positive thoughts you have. So, you *also* need to learn techniques for increasing positive thinking.

Three techniques for reducing negative thoughts and five techniques for increasing positive thoughts are included in the next session. In future sessions, we will teach specific techniques that will help you reduce negative thoughts and increase positive thoughts.

Note. The section on positive and negative thoughts was adapted from: *Control Your Depression,* (pp. 140–154), by P. M. Lewinsohn, R. F. Munoz, M. A. Youngren, and A. M. Zeiss, 1986, New York: Prentice Hall.

COMORBIDITY MODULE SESSION 2

Integrated Session 2 Objectives

1. To review the cognitive social learning theory rationale for smoking cessation treatment.
   a. To review the social learning model of depression and its application to smoking cessation.
   b. To review self-monitoring of daily mood (Daily Mood Rating Form) assignment.
2. To review self-monitoring of smoking behavior (Wrap Sheet) assignment.
3. To review Triggers for Smoking Worksheet.
   a. To discuss the use of the ABC method for changing negative ways of thinking.
   b. To discuss the positive and negative thoughts method for changing negative ways of thinking.

    c. **To instruct smokers to choose either the ABC method or the positive and negative thoughts method and do the corresponding homework assignment.**

4. To introduce the self-management approach to managing trigger situations and the use of three self-control strategies.

5. To introduce and demonstrate the Benson (deep breathing) relaxation approach.

6. To review the rationale and explanation of nicotine fading and to assign (or explain to smokers how to choose) the 30% nicotine content reduction brand.

7. To preview the homework assignments to be completed prior to Session 3.

    a. **Includes homework for managing negative mood.**

Session 2 Handouts and Worksheets

1. Managing Triggers for Smoking Worksheet
2. Deep breathing relaxation exercise
3. Wrap Sheets
4. **ABC Method: Changing Faulty Thinking (Table 6.5)**
5. **ABC Method Worksheet: Identifying Faulty Thinking (Table 6.6)**
6. **Strategies for Increasing Positive and Decreasing Negative Thoughts (Table 6.7)**
7. **Inventory of Thoughts (Table 6.8)**
8. **Daily Mood Rating Form (Table 6.2)**

Session 2 Comorbidity Treatment Content

1. *Review the social learning model of depression and its application to smoking cessation.* Facilitators should remind smokers of the reciprocal relationships between thoughts, feelings, and behaviors. One cannot change feelings or mood *directly*, but rather indirectly through changing thoughts and behavior. This aspect of the treatment will teach them coping skills to change aspects of their thoughts and of their behavior, which will in turn have a positive impact on their mood.

    Learning skills to manage negative moods is important for quitting smoking. Many smokers use cigarettes to manage negative moods: They smoke when they are stressed, upset, angry, or bored. Developing alternative ways of coping with negative moods may be necessary to help these individuals quit smoking successfully. In a similar vein, maintaining a positive mood while quitting smoking may be necessary to ward off feelings of sadness, anger, or depression that may occur when quitting. Finally, many slips or relapses occur in negative mood situations; therefore, learning to manage these situations more effectively may help to avoid slips or prevent slips from becoming relapses.

2. *Review daily mood monitoring assignment.* Facilitators should inquire about smokers' experiences in rating their moods since the last session. As many group members as time permits should be provided the opportunity to share their experience in rating their moods. In the early stages of learning mood coping skills, people often have trouble identifying specific moods and rating the degree to which they experience a particular mood. Facilitators may ask group members specific questions to assist them. Did they find it dif-

ficult to identify and assign a numerical rating to one or more of their moods? Did identifying and rating moods get easier with practice or not? Were they able to identify factors that influenced their moods? For example, they may have noticed that on evenings when they were home by themselves, they were more depressed and anxious than on evenings when they were out with friends, when they felt happy and relaxed.

Facilitators can point out that being able to identify and rate the degree to which they experience particular moods can be a first step in gaining control over mood. Smokers begin to recognize that moods do not materialize out of thin air but rather are related to what one thinks and does. Positive ways of thinking and behaving breed positive moods. Finally, smokers should be asked to continue rating their moods on the Daily Mood Rating Form between now and the next session.

3. *Discuss ABC method for changing thoughts.* Facilitators should remind smokers that they will have a choice to work on one of two different skills: (1) changing faulty thinking or (2) increasing positive and decreasing negative thoughts. Group members should have read introductory handouts on each skill that were distributed in Session 1. What follows is the basis for presentation and discussion of the ABC method during this treatment session (see also Table 6.5).

The ABC method promotes the idea that "It's not what happens to us that makes us upset, but rather what we tell ourselves about what happens." Facilitators should present the following overview to smokers, using a handout or writing this material on a board or flip chart. In the ABC method, the A stands for the <u>A</u>ctivating event, the event you feel upset about. The <u>B</u> stands for the <u>Beliefs</u> about the activating event, or what you tell yourself about the event. The <u>C</u> stands for the Emotional <u>Consequence</u> or overreaction.

Smokers should be informed that the ABC technique is not intended to help them to avoid *reasonable* emotional reactions to events but rather to avoid *emotional overreactions*. Emotional overreactions are potential trigger situations for smoking. They are better dealt with by changing one's way of thinking rather than by smoking. Following quit day, situations involving an emotional overreaction represent high risks for relapse.

The following example can be used to illustrate the ABC technique: Jack reports that he is angry and sad (emotional consequence: <u>C</u>) because he did not get a raise in pay at work (activating event: <u>A</u>). He is so upset that he does not go to work for the next 2 days. In this example, Jack might conclude that <u>A</u> (not getting a raise) caused <u>C</u> (feeling angry and upset). This is not surprising, because people commonly believe that events directly cause their emotional reactions. However, this is not accurate. It was <u>B</u> (Jack's beliefs or what he said to himself) that resulted in <u>C</u> (his emotional reaction).

In the example, Jack's *beliefs* or self-talk included: "I should have gotten a raise." "Since I didn't, I must be a total failure." "I didn't get it because the boss hates me." These *beliefs* about why he didn't get a raise led to Jack's feelings of anger and sadness. *Many times it is not what happens that makes us upset; rather, it is what we tell ourselves about the situation.*

Facilitators should indicate to smokers that the ABC technique may be quite helpful to them if they believe their thinking patterns at times cause them to overreact, as in this example. In future sessions, they will learn how they can change their emotional

TABLE 6.5. ABC Method: Changing Faulty Thinking

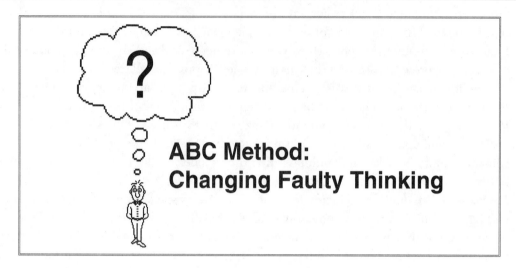

In previous exercises using the ABC technique, you learned to identify beliefs and self-talk statements that can result in emotional overreactions. The next step is to change these beliefs or self-talk in order to reduce or avoid emotional overreactions.

To change your emotional <u>C</u>onsequences (<u>C</u>), you need to <u>D</u>ispute (<u>D</u>) your <u>B</u>eliefs (<u>B</u>) about <u>A</u>ctivating events (<u>A</u>). If any beliefs are irrational or not constructive, then you can dispute and change them.

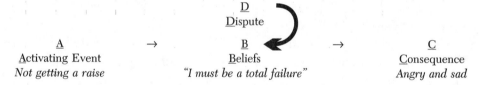

<u>A</u>		<u>B</u>		<u>C</u>
Activating Event	→	Beliefs	→	Consequence
Not getting a raise		*"I must be a total failure"*		*Angry and sad*

You can <u>D</u>ispute or challenge beliefs that are not constructive by *arguing against the beliefs*. Ask yourself the following questions to help you <u>D</u>ispute irrational or nonconstructive beliefs or self-talk:

1. What is the evidence for my belief?
2. What are the alternative views?
3. What's the worst that could happen now? What could I do if it did happen?
4. Is it helpful in some way for me to believe what I do?
5. What would I say to a friend in the same situation (or who had experienced the same <u>A</u>ctivating event)?

Challenging your irrational or nonconstructive beliefs in this way can lead to new, more constructive beliefs (counterthoughts) that will better fit the situation. By changing your beliefs, emotional overreactions will be replaced by new, more positive feelings.

overreactions (C) by learning to evaluate and change what they say or believe (B) about upsetting events (A). For now, smokers can begin to learn to identify beliefs and attitudes that cause them to overreact.

There are three kinds of unhelpful beliefs or thoughts that smokers can try to recognize: (a) highly evaluative words such as "should" and "must"; (b) "catastrophizing" words such as "awful" and "terrible"; and (c) overgeneralizing words such as "I'll never" and "nobody ever."

Smokers who choose to work on the ABC method should begin to evaluate their beliefs and self-talk during one upsetting situation that occurs this week. They should record this information on the ABC Method Worksheet: Identifying Faulty Thinking (Table 6.6). If time allows, facilitators can solicit examples from the group of the types of situations they might encounter in which the ABC method would apply. Smokers can be reminded to list the A, B, and C as accurately as possible, but to particularly focus their attention on trying to identify the unhelpful beliefs (B) that might produce the emotional overreaction (C). They should ask themselves: Have I identified all of the nonconstructive thoughts that led to my emotional overreaction? Are there others that I may need to identify? In summary, the ABC method is useful for decreasing *overreactions* to problems and difficulties. The goal is for smokers to change the way they think about problems and difficulties in order to gain control of their negative feelings and moods.

4. *Discuss the positive and negative thoughts method for changing thinking.* The positive and negative thoughts method is based on the notion that mood is related to the balance between positive and negative thoughts. When one experiences more positive thoughts than negative thoughts, mood is likely to be positive, that is, happy, content, relaxed, or some other positive mood state. However, when the number of negative thoughts outweighs the number of positive thoughts, the result is undoubtedly a negative mood state; the mood itself may be sadness, anger, anxiety, or something else, depending on the nature of the negative thoughts experienced.

The first step in using this approach is for smokers to identify negative and positive thoughts through self-monitoring. Then they can then learn techniques to increase positive and decrease negative thoughts. An important point for facilitators to highlight is that they will need to both increase positive thoughts and decrease negative thoughts in order to effectively change their moods. Merely increasing positive thoughts without decreasing negative thoughts (or decreasing negative thoughts without increasing positive thoughts) will not be nearly as effective. This approach is a useful strategy for smokers who tend to be chronic negative thinkers.

For smokers who choose to work with the positive and negative thoughts method, the first step in the process is to self-monitor thoughts to create an inventory of both positive and negative thoughts that they frequently experience. They can do this by carrying a 3" × 5" file card or a piece of paper around with them. One side is labeled "+" (for positive thoughts) and the other side "–" (for negative thoughts). Each time throughout the day that they become aware of a positive or negative thought, they should write down the thought, verbatim, on the appropriate side of the card or paper. At the end of each day, they should transcribe positive and negative thoughts identified that day onto a master list

TABLE 6.6. ABC Method Worksheet: Identifying Faulty Thinking

The ABC technique can help you identify faulty thinking patterns. To understand C (your feelings or emotional overreactions), you can first learn how to evaluate B (your beliefs, or self-talk) about A (activating events).

INSTRUCTIONS: *Step 1: Complete Box C; Step 2: Complete Box A; Step 3: Complete Box B*

Step 2, Box A

A = Activating Event

Describe Event:

I did not get a raise in my pay at work even

though other people did.

_____

_____

_____

_____

_____

_____

Step 3, Box B

B = Beliefs or Self-Talk

List each of the things you said to yourself about A that resulted in C:

1. I should have gotten a raise.

2. Since I didn't, I must be a total failure.

3. I didn't get it because my boss hates me.

_____

_____

_____

_____

Step 1, Box C

C = Emotional Consequence

Describe how you felt when A happened:

I felt:

Angry

Sad

Hurt

_____

_____

_____

Step 4: Place a check mark beside each statement in Box B that is nonconstructive or "irrational."

or inventory of thoughts that consists of a positive-thoughts column and a negative-thoughts column. Smokers should again be reminded to write down thoughts as complete sentences rather than as mere phrases.

Once smokers develop a sizable master list of both positive and negative thoughts, they should have an accompanying sense of the approximate ratio of positive to negative thoughts they typically experience. Should they so desire, the more quantitatively oriented smokers in the group can actually count the number of positive and negative thoughts they have over a period of days to determine a more exact ratio. In addition, by writing down their thoughts, smokers should also be developing a good idea of the specific thoughts (both positive and negative) that they tend to experience.

Once smokers have gained experience in self-monitoring, they can begin to practice using *specific strategies* to increase positive thoughts and reduce negative thoughts. They will read about these strategies for homework in the handout Strategies for Increasing Positive and Decreasing Negative Thoughts (Table 6.7); however, facilitators should also preview them in session.

The following techniques can be useful to *increase positive thoughts*:

a. *Priming* is a technique that reminds smokers of their positive thoughts so they can keep them in mind. The first step in priming is to make a list of common positive thoughts. If done diligently, the list of positive thoughts from the aforementioned master list or inventory of thoughts will serve as a good source of positive thoughts. Positive thoughts about oneself that are self-generated or offered by trusted friends or family members can be particularly helpful.

   Once smokers have generated a list of positive thoughts, they can list each one on a 3" × 5" index card so they end up with a "deck" of positive-thought cards. Facilitators should instruct smokers to carry these cards with them and to pull out different cards throughout the day. Each time they pull out a card, they should read it and think about it. They can also keep a few blank cards in the deck in order to add to their positive thoughts each day as new ones occur to them.

b. *Using cues* is closely related to the technique of priming. Oftentimes, people may have a sizable deck of thought cards but forget to use them during the day. Smokers should be encouraged to use cues in their daily routine to help them remember to think one or more positive thoughts. For example, they can think a positive thought each time that they eat a meal, talk on the telephone, brush their teeth, or comb their hair. Any daily activity can be used as a cue to think a positive thought.

c. *Giving yourself credit* is another positive-thought approach that builds on the notion of remembering to think positively. People often do not remember to give themselves credit for things that they accomplish. We have a tendency to focus on things we have done wrong or mistakes we have made. We also tend to focus on the things we did not accomplish rather than paying attention to those that we did accomplish. This approach involves having smokers remind themselves of the things they do accomplish each day by carrying an index card, writing down each task that is completed, and giving themselves credit. These accomplishments do not have to be large; even recognition of the smallest accomplishment can bring satisfaction. Examples of daily accomplishments that can be written down include dealing with a difficult customer at work,

TABLE 6.7. Strategies for Increasing Positive and Decreasing Negative Thoughts

INCREASING POSITIVE THOUGHTS

1. *Priming*. Priming is a technique that reminds you of your positive thoughts so you can increasingly have them in your mind. To prime yourself for positive thinking, first make a list of common positive thoughts. You can do this by carrying an index card with you for several days and writing down your positive thoughts as you have them. Positive thoughts about *yourself* are particularly helpful. You can even get some positive thoughts from people you trust who can tell you what your good points are.

   Once you have a list of positive thoughts, take them one by one and list each on its *own* index card so you have a "deck" *of positive cards.* Carry the cards with you and pull out different cards throughout the day. Each time you pull out a card, *read it and think about it.* Keep a few blank cards in the deck so you can add to your positive thoughts each day as new ones occur to you.

2. *Using Cues*. Use cues in your daily routine to remind yourself to think a positive thought. For example, think a positive thought each time you get in your car, enter your workplace, set your alarm clock, comb your hair, and so forth.

3. *Giving Yourself Credit*. People often don't give themselves credit for the things they accomplish. Instead, they focus on things they do wrong or imperfectly, or they blame themselves when things don't turn out right. To remind yourself of the things you accomplish each day, carry an index card and write down each task you complete during the day and give yourself credit. At the end of each day, look over your list and think about how much you really did accomplish. Accomplishments can be big or small. Some examples include:

   - Got to work only 5 minutes late in spite of terrible traffic.
   - Helped a coworker with a problem.
   - Wrote a memo.
   - Returned five phone calls.
   - Completed all of the work I had planned for today with just one exception.
   - Sent my sister a birthday card.
   - Cooked a tasty dinner.

4. *Time Projection*. Use this technique to get through stressful times. These stressful periods may be short (being stuck in traffic) or long (job loss, mourning). To use this technique, mentally travel forward in time to the point that, as best you can estimate, this stressful time will be over. For example, when stuck in traffic, think ahead a couple of hours to a time when you will be thoroughly involved in work and the traffic jam will be a remote memory. With stressful times of longer duration, think about how things will improve and you will recover over time. Look forward to a time in your life when you can put this stressful period behind you and the strong feelings that you have today will have faded. Remind yourself of other stressful periods in your past life and how you recovered from them. Remember that you *can* endure the pain and survive.

5. *Positive Self-Rewarding Thoughts*. Use this technique to reward yourself whenever you do something positive or think a positive thought. For example, you might be considering getting together with friends for an outing.

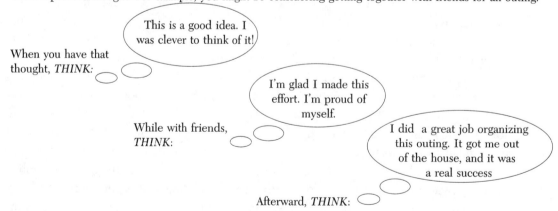

(continued)

TABLE 6.7. *(continued)*

DECREASING NEGATIVE THOUGHTS

1. *Thought Interruption.* As soon as you notice that you are thinking a negative thought, interrupt the thought by saying to yourself:

   "I'm going to stop thinking that now."

   Or state firmly and forcefully in your mind:

   "STOP!"

   Then, without getting upset, let your attention flow back to other ideas. If you do this consistently, you will begin to catch negative thoughts almost as soon as they begin. As you continue to practice this technique, you should have fewer and fewer negative thoughts.

2. *Worrying Time.* One of the many sources of depression is an inability to keep certain negative thoughts away. These thoughts may be bothersome ideas that move in on your train of thought again and again, draining your energy and getting in the way of whatever you're trying to do. If you feel like you need to spend some time mulling these thoughts over, reserve some "worrying time" to do so. Plan about one half-hour per day in your daily schedule for worrying time:

   My worrying time begins at _____:_____ a.m./p.m. and ends at _____:_____.

   During the rest of the day, quickly identify troubling thoughts when they occur and jot down a word or two to remind yourself of the thought later. Then put the thought out of your mind until worrying time. During your worrying time, refrain from doing *anything* except thinking—don't eat, drink, or talk. Give each troubling thought the attention you think it deserves without exceeding the time you have set aside.

3. *The Blow-Up Technique.* This approach is intended to make a disturbing negative thought less upsetting by blowing it completely out of proportion so that it seems so ridiculous that it ceases to be frightening. Here's an example of how it can work:

   > Wendy was scheduled for an interview for a new position at work. Although she had the experience necessary for the job, she began to worry that she might not be entirely qualified for the position. She began to think that she might embarrass herself at the interview, not being able to respond correctly to the questions asked. As the interview day drew near, she became more and more fearful and considered canceling the interview altogether. But, when she thought about it, she realized that she *was* qualified for the job. Just the same, she was afraid of looking stupid in the interview and ultimately being rejected for the job.
   >   To help herself feel less fearful, Wendy used the blow-up technique. She imagined the interview to be like a police investigation—with the interviewer in uniform, pacing around her. Wendy is dressed in a striped suit, sitting in a dark room under a bright lightbulb dangling from a long wire. Behind a two-way mirror, high government officials are watching and challenging her every statement. They only stop their challenges to confer by hotline with the president, who is in constant communication. The interviewer asks her questions like, "What is the square root of 37?" "What is the origin of the universe?" and "Who won the '42 World Series?" Wendy struggles, and finally admits that she doesn't know the answers to these questions. At this point, he interviewer whirls around, faces Wendy nose to nose, and screams, "Fool! We had no intention of giving you this job! Ha! Ha! Ha! Ha!!!" A door opens and a TV anchorman walks through with a cameraman and microphone: "We are here, live, with Wendy who didn't get the job. Wendy, what went wrong, and what does this mean . . . for America?"

   Using this technique, you can imagine a totally ridiculous scene. If the scene seems funny, it can reduce your fear and make the situation feel less threatening.

Note. This section on positive and negative and negative thoughts was adapted from: *Control Your Depression* (pp. 140–154) by P. M. Lewinsohn, R. F. Munoz, M. A. Youngren, and A. M. Zeiss, 1986, New York: Prentice Hall.

completing a planned exercise activity for the day, helping the children with homework, beginning work on an important project, helping a coworker with a problem, and
so forth. Looking over this list of tasks accomplished at the end of the day can be an effective way of giving oneself credit and improving one's mood.

d. *Time projection* can be a useful technique to help smokers get through stressful times.
These stressful periods may be short (being stuck in traffic) or long (job loss, mourning). To use this technique, smokers can mentally travel forward in time to the point
that, as best they can estimate, this stressful time will be over. For example, when stuck
in traffic, they can think ahead a couple of hours to a time when they will be thoroughly
involved in work and the traffic jam will be a remote memory. With stressful times of
longer duration, smokers can think about how things will improve and they will recover over time. They can look forward to a time in their lives when they can put this
stressful period behind them and the strong feelings of today will have faded. Facilitators can remind smokers to think about other stressful periods in their lives and how
they recovered from them.

The following techniques can be useful to *reduce negative thoughts*:

a. *Thought interruption* involves interrupting a negative thought in one of several ways.
Smokers can be instructed to practice stopping the negative thought by interrupting it
with another thought. Typically, smokers are taught to yell the word "stop!" after becoming aware that they are thinking one or more negative thoughts. They can then proceed to gradually fade the overt word "stop" until they are silently saying "stop" to
themselves rather than aloud. Another variation is for smokers to say to themselves,
"I'm not going to think that now," and gradually to fade this into saying it silently.

After interrupting one or more negative thoughts using this technique, smokers
should be instructed to switch to a positive thought or to a predetermined positive image (e.g., walking on the beach, being in the mountains, by a lake, etc.). Another effective strategy is to follow the use of thought interruption by occupying oneself in something active (e.g., washing the dishes, calling a friend, working on a crafts project, etc.).

b. *Worrying time* is another approach for reducing negative thoughts that is based on the
notion that worrying (i.e., having unwanted and intrusive negative thoughts) drains
people's energy and interferes with daily activities. If smokers feel that they need to
spend some time mulling these thoughts over, they can reserve some "worrying time"
to do so. Facilitators should suggest to smokers that they plan about one half-hour in
their daily schedule for worrying time. During the rest of the day, smokers can quickly
identify troubling thoughts when they occur and jot down a word or two to remind
themselves of the thought later. They can then put the thought out of their minds until
worrying time. During the worrying time, smokers should refrain from doing anything
except thinking (i.e., they should not eat, drink, or talk). Worrying time is a time to give
each troubling thought the attention that the individual thinks it deserves without exceeding the time they have set aside.

c. *The blow-up strategy* is an approach that is intended to make a disturbing negative
thought less upsetting by blowing it completely out of proportion. There are at least
two different variations of this approach. In one variation, one can exaggerate an upset-

ting thought until it seems completely ridiculous. If the scene seems funny, it can reduce one's fear and make the situation feel less threatening. For example, assume a smoker is upset about a situation because of the possible embarrassment of having made a mistake that others will find out about. In this instance, he/she can blow up the situation by imagining that news about the mistake is being broadcast nationwide via radio, TV, and newspaper and that every acquaintance, friend, and family member is contacting him/her to tell him/her how inept he/she is because of the mistake he/she has made.

The alternative to blowing up a disturbing situation to the point of ridiculousness is to think about the worst outcome that can possibly happen in a situation. Once this worst possible outcome is conceived, smokers can then go about doing their best to try to assure that this worst outcome does not take place, while also preparing themselves mentally for the possibility that it might occur. This two-pronged attack on a worrisome situation tends to provide smokers with a sense of control and tends to reduce unfocused negative thinking and worrying.

Smokers who choose to work on the positive and negative thoughts method should begin to keep track of their positive and negative thoughts on index cards and compile a master list of positive and negative thoughts on the Inventory of Positive and Negative Thoughts form (Table 6.8). They should take special care to write down those positive and negative thoughts that are most powerful or those that tend to occur over and over again.

TABLE 6.8. Inventory of Thoughts

INVENTORY OF POSITIVE AND NEGATIVE THOUGHTS

INSTRUCTIONS: For the next week, keep track of your positive and negative thoughts. Write down the positive and negative thoughts that are the most powerful or that tend to occur over and over again. You don't need to write down every thought you have, just the ones important to this exercise—those thoughts that send you clear positive or negative messages.

Positive Thoughts	Negative Thoughts
I can do this.	I'll never get everything done.
The weekend will be great.	I'll miss my cigarettes.
I like my job.	I can't trust my son.
I'm pretty successful.	I'm getting old.
I love the spring.	This is too stressful.
I have a great family.	My boss is an idiot.
I'm going to be a nonsmoker.	I'm lazy.
I'll save a lot of money.	
I did a good job on this.	

Regardless of whether smokers choose to work on the ABC method or the positive and negative thoughts method, facilitators can offer the following comments. Learning and applying techniques to change ways of thinking take practice; smokers should not expect results overnight. Furthermore, no one is content or happy all of the time; smokers should maintain reasonable expectations about what they can accomplish by practicing and applying the thought-changing techniques. The overall goal is to keep negative feelings at a more reasonable level so that one can deal with life's difficulties more constructively. This will, in turn, reduce the tendency to use cigarettes as a coping strategy in negative-mood situations.

4. *Review mood component homework assignments for next session.* Facilitators should confirm the date and time of the next session, review assignments to be completed before the next session, and answer any questions that smokers might have about the assignments.

Prior to Session 3

1. Read ABC Method: Changing Faulty Thinking (Table 6.5)
2. Read Strategies for Increasing Positive and Decreasing Negative Thoughts (Table 6.7)
3. After reading about each of these methods for changing thoughts, choose one.

Do for the first time:

4. Based on the method for changing thoughts selected, complete the corresponding assignment. If ABC method is selected, do ABC Method Worksheet: Identifying Faulty Thinking (Table 6.6) for an upsetting situation this week. If positive and negative thoughts method is selected, do Inventory of Positive and Negative Thoughts this week.

Continue to do:

5. Complete Daily Mood Rating Form at the end of each day

COMORBIDITY MODULE SESSION 3

Integrated Session 3 Objectives

1. To review the self-management approach and the use of three self-control strategies.
2. To review the homework assignment on practicing managing triggers using self-management strategies.
   a. **To review self-monitoring of daily mood (Daily Mood Rating Form) assignment.**
   b. **To review ABC method for changing negative ways of thinking, including the homework assignment (ABC Method Worksheet: Changing Faulty Thinking).**
   c. **To discuss the next step in the ABC method: disputing (D) unhelpful beliefs.**
   d. **To review the positive and negative thoughts method for changing negative ways of**

thinking, including the homework assignment (Inventory of Positive and Negative Thoughts).

    e. **To discuss the active use of strategies for increasing positive and decreasing negative thoughts.**

    f. **To preview increasing pleasant activity as an active coping strategy for maintaining a positive mood while in the process of quitting smoking.**

3. To review the Benson (deep breathing) relaxation homework assignment.

4. To review self-monitoring of smoking behavior (Wrap Sheet) assignment.

5. To introduce the concept of making broader lifestyle changes that support quitting smoking.

6. To review the nicotine fading assignment and assign (or explain to smokers how to choose) the 60% nicotine-content reduction brand.

7. To preview the homework assignments to be completed prior to Session 4.

    a. **Includes homework for managing negative mood.**

Session 3 Handouts and Worksheets

1. Nonsmoking Game Plan: Lifestyle Change Worksheet
2. Managing Triggers for Smoking Worksheet
3. Wrap Sheets
4. **Positive and Negative Thoughts Worksheet (Table 6.10)**
5. **Top 20 Pleasant Events form (Table 6.11)**
6. **A List of Pleasant Events (Table 6.12)**
7. **ABC Worksheet: Identifying Faulty Thinking (Table 6.6)**
8. **Daily Mood Rating Form (Table 6.2)**

Session 3 Comorbidity Treatment Content

1. *Review daily mood monitoring.* Facilitators should once again ask smokers about their experiences rating their moods since the previous session. Are identifying and rating their moods getting easier with practice? Were smokers able to identify factors that influenced their moods? Are they beginning to notice any relationship between their cigarette smoking and their moods? This information should be discussed in session, and as many smokers as possible should be provided with the opportunity to contribute.

    Facilitators can remind smokers that being able to identify and rate moods can be a first step in gaining control over them. Smokers should be asked to continue their mood ratings on the Daily Mood Rating Form between now and the next session. They should be reminded to rate their moods on all three dimensions each day.

2. *Review of ABC method for changing thoughts.* Prior to today's session, smokers were asked to choose one of the two skills to work on and to do the homework assignment relevant to that particular skill. At today's session, facilitators will review their work with these skills. The first of the two skills for changing thoughts is the ABC method. Facilitators should remind smokers that the ABC philosophy is that "it's not what happens to us that makes us upset, but rather what we tell ourselves about situations or circumstances." Homework for

today was to read the ABC Method: Changing Faulty Thinking. Facilitators should ask about smokers' reactions to these ideas and answer questions.

The written homework for today was to complete the ABC Method Worksheet for one upsetting situation this past week. Facilitators should ask smokers who worked on this skill how they did in using the ABC method for the upsetting situation. Several group members should offer examples from their homework assignments to review in session. At this point facilitators should only be looking for smokers to identify <u>A</u> (the activating event), <u>B</u> (the negative beliefs or self-talk about the event or situation), and <u>C</u> (the emotional consequences of what their feelings were about the situation). Facilitators should also ask smokers whether they have noticed that activating events and emotional reactions often trigger their smoking. In our experience, it is the rare cigarette smoker who does *not* instinctively reach for a cigarette in an emotionally upsetting situation. Thus this skill can be invaluable at protecting smokers from potential relapse in negative mood situations. Facilitators should emphasize the importance of identifying nonconstructive beliefs as a key building block for breaking the connection between beliefs and smoking behavior.

3. *ABC Method: Disputing ("D") Unhelpful Beliefs.* The next step is to discuss how to change non-constructive beliefs or thoughts in order to reduce or avoid emotional overreactions. The handout ABC Method: Changing Faulty Thinking (Table 6.5) was assigned as homework and is now reviewed in session. To change their emotional <u>C</u>onsequences (<u>C</u>), smokers need to <u>D</u>ispute (<u>D</u>) their <u>B</u>eliefs (<u>B</u>) about <u>A</u>ctivating events (<u>A</u>). If beliefs are irrational or not constructive, then smokers can dispute and change them. Facilitators can indicate to smokers that Disputing, or challenging, nonconstructive beliefs is a matter of arguing effectively against them. Smokers can ask themselves the following questions to help them Dispute irrational or nonconstructive beliefs:

a. What is the evidence for my belief?
b. What are the alternative views?
c. What is the worst that could happen now? What could I do if it did happen?
d. Is it helpful in some way for me to believe what I do?
e. What would I say to a friend in the same situation (or who had experienced the same Activating event)?

Several other tips for disputing nonconstructive beliefs include:

f. Arguing against "should" and "ought" thoughts with "why should I?"
g. Questioning self-talk that includes words such as "terrible" and "awful" with "I would have liked" or "Was it really awful?"
h. Challenging overgeneralizations with "just because it happened this time . . . does it really mean it will *always* happen?"

Challenging irrational or nonconstructive beliefs in this way can lead to new, more constructive beliefs (i.e., counterthoughts) that will better fit the situation. By changing their beliefs, smokers' emotional overreactions will be replaced by new, more positive feelings, which will, in turn, reduce the risk of relapse to smoking in upsetting situations.

Facilitators can now use the ABC examples previously solicited to work on disputing irrational beliefs and developing counterthoughts. It is important to solicit suggestions and ideas from the entire group during this process. As homework, smokers should complete the ABC(D) Worksheet: Changing Faulty Thinking (Table 6.9) for at least one upsetting

TABLE 6.9. ABC(D) Worksheet: Changing Faulty Thinking

The ABC technique can help you change faulty thinking patterns by Disputing your Beliefs about an Activating event.

Instructions

1. Complete box C.
2. Complete box A.
3. Complete box B.
4. Place an X by each statement in box B that is irrational or not constructive.
5. Complete box D. Use questions from ABC(D) overview to help you Dispute beliefs.
6. Complete "New Feelings" box.

Step 2, Box A

Activating Event
(Describe Event)

My boss noticed a mistake in my
monthly report.
_____
_____
_____

Step 3, Box B

Beliefs or Self Talk
(List each of the things you said to yourself about A that resulted in C.)

1. She thinks I'm stupid.
2. She won't trust me in the future.
3. I always make careless mistakes.
4. Maybe I'm not cut out for this work.

Step 1, Box C

Emotional Consequence
(Describe how you felt when A happened)

I felt:
ashamed
sad
depressed
anxious
_____
_____

Step 5, Box D

D Counterthoughts
(After disputing statements in Box B, list your counterthoughts.)

1. No evidence—she didn't seem too concerned.
2. She's always thought well of me—won't change.
3. Mistakes are rare—I'm usually careful.
4. I'm overreacting. I do a good job.

Step 6

New Feelings
(After reading your statement in Box D, describe how you feel about A.)

I feel:
slightly embarrassed
optimistic
more calm
_____
_____

situation this week. They should now be actively disputing the nonconstructive beliefs in addition to identifying the ABC of the situation. Smokers should be cautioned that acquiring skill at this approach takes time, and at this stage they may only be able to clearly work through an ABC(D) circumstance after time has passed and they are less upset by the activating event. However, with practice, they will eventually be able to change thoughts and feel less upset more immediately after the upsetting situation, if not during the situation itself.

4. *Review the Positive and Negative Thoughts Method.* The second of the two skills for changing thoughts is the Positive/Negative Thoughts Method. This method is based on the notion that mood is related to the balance between positive and negative thoughts. When negative thoughts far outweigh positive thoughts, the result is a depressive, anxious, angry, or otherwise negative mood in which smoking becomes a reliable and familiar coping strategy. For homework, smokers who chose this method were to have read the Positive and Negative Thoughts Worksheet and completed the Inventory of Positive and Negative Thoughts. Facilitators should inquire about smokers' experiences and reactions to this assignment. What are some specific examples of positive and negative thoughts smokers had? Did they have difficulty identifying and writing down specific positive and negative thoughts? Did they find themselves identifying more negative thoughts than positive?

Facilitators should remind smokers that it is extremely important to actually *write down* thoughts rather than just thinking about them. Also, it is very important to write down the thoughts as complete sentences, rather than as phrases or partial thoughts. Smokers can be told that writing down thoughts can be difficult and that it takes practice. The most difficult thing about learning to identify specific thoughts is that they are so automatic that one is often not aware of the content of any particular thought.

5. *Review strategies for increasing positive and decreasing negative thoughts.* Once smokers have gained experience in writing down positive and negative thoughts, they can begin to use *specific strategies* to increase positive thoughts and decrease negative thoughts. These techniques were discussed in Session 2 and are reviewed in this session.

Prior to the next session, smokers who chose this method should continue to monitor their positive and negative thoughts and practice using one technique for increasing positive thoughts and one technique for decreasing negative thoughts. Once they feel that they have mastered these first two techniques, they can go on to work with other techniques for either increasing positive thoughts or decreasing negative thoughts. Smokers can use the Positive and Negative Thoughts Worksheet (Table 6.10) to monitor their positive and negative thoughts and to indicate which techniques they have used, how effective they were, and what they might do differently next time to make them more useful.

Finally, it can be reiterated to smokers that these techniques will take practice to learn. No one is content or happy all of the time; the idea is to keep negative feelings at a more reasonable level to manage life's difficulties more constructively. Increasing their ability to do so will undoubtedly have a positive impact on smokers' ability to quit smoking and remain abstinent.

TABLE 6.10. Positive and Negative Thoughts Worksheet

INSTRUCTIONS: For the next week, continue to keep track of your positive and negative thoughts. Remember, you don't need to write down every thought, just the ones that send you clear positive or negative messages.

Positive Thoughts	Negative Thoughts
Quitting will feel good.	It's going to be a bad day.
I had a good day at work.	I have bad luck.
I'm a kind person.	My mother's a pain.
My new car is great.	Jim doesn't understand me.
I have lots of friends.	Withdrawal is terrible.
I'm going to quit—I can do it!	
Write down one technique that you used to increase positive thoughts:	Write down one technique that you used to decrease negative thoughts:
Priming	Thought interruption
How effective was it for you?	How effective was it for you?
1 2 ③ 4 5 Not Effective Very Effective	1 2 3 4 ⑤ Not Effective Very Effective

6. *Introduce Increasing Pleasant Activities.* Facilitators should provide a rationale for and a brief preview of the upcoming unit on increasing pleasant activities. The rationale for this approach has several facets. People often feel deprived when they quit smoking. It is important to add positive activities and experiences while quitting because smoking is often an important source of positive reinforcement for many people. Pleasant activities should help smokers feel more satisfied and less deprived and provide a source of rewards for quitting smoking. From the depression literature, it is well known that there is a direct relationship between pleasant activities and mood; specifically, the more enjoyable things one does in a day or a week, the better he/she is likely to feel. Because feelings of sadness and depression often accompany quitting smoking for people with past histories of depression or elevated depressive symptoms, maintaining a positive mood by increasing pleasant activities will not only help remediate depressed mood but also make it easier to quit smoking.

   For homework prior to the next session, smokers are asked to construct their own personalized list of pleasant events, using the Top 20 Pleasant Events form (Table 6.11), drawing ideas and items from the List of Pleasant Events (Table 6.12) that consists of 292 activities that many people find pleasurable.

7. *Review mood component homework assignments for next session.* Facilitators should confirm the date and time of the next session, review assignments to be completed before the next session, and answer any questions that smokers might have about the assignments.

TABLE 6.11. Top 20 Pleasant Events

INSTRUCTIONS: List 20 events that you enjoy and find pleasant. Choose events that you can do frequently, that you have control over, and that are affordable. If you have trouble thinking of pleasant events, refer to the list provided in Table 6.12 to give you ideas.

Examples:
    Have coffee, tea, Coke with a friend.
    Watch favorite TV show.
    Take a ride in the country.
    Help another person.

1. Washing the car
2. Playing tennis
3. Gardening
4. Driving in the country
5. Going to the theater
6. Playing cards
7. Breathing fresh air
8. Reading the newspaper
9. Watching my son play baseball
10. Calling my sister
11. Eating in a restaurant
12. Going dancing
13. Getting a haircut
14. Sailing
15. Reading a magazine
16. Working on my car
17. Listening to music
18. Eating ice cream
19. Shopping
20. Looking at the stars

TABLE 6.12. A List of Pleasant Events

1. Being in the country
2. Wearing expensive or formal clothes
3. Making contributions to religious, charitable, or other groups
4. Talking about sports
5. Meeting someone new of the same sex
6. Taking tests when well prepared
7. Going to a rock concert
8. Playing baseball or softball
9. Planning trips or vacations
10. Buying things for myself
11. Being at the beach
12. Doing art work (painting, sculpture, drawing, moviemaking, etc.)
13. Rock climbing or mountaineering
14. Reading the Scriptures or other sacred works
15. Playing golf
16. Taking part in military activities
17. Rearranging or redecorating my room or the house
18. Going to a sports event
19. Reading a "How to Do It" book or article
20. Going to races (horse, car, boat, etc.)
21. Reading stories, novels, nonfiction, poems, or plays
22. Hearing a speech on an interesting topic
23. Driving skillfully
24. Breathing clean air
25. Riding in an airplane
26. Exploring (hiking away from known routes, spelunking, etc.)
27. Having a frank and open discussion
28. Singing in a group
29. Thinking about myself or my problems
30. Working at my job
31. Going to a party
32. Going to church functions (socials, classes, bazaars, etc.)
33. Speaking a foreign language
34. Going to service, civic, or social club meetings
35. Going to a business meeting or a convention
36. Being in a sporty or expensive car
37. Playing a musical instrument
38. Making snacks
39. Snow skiing, sledding, playing in the snow
40. Being helped
41. Wearing informal clothes
42. Combing or brushing my hair
43. Acting
44. Taking a nap
45. Being with friends
46. Canning, freezing, making preserves, etc.
47. Solving personal problems
48. Just sitting and thinking
49. Seeing good things happen to my family or friends
50. Going to a fair, carnival, circus, zoo, or amusement park
51. Talking about philosophy or religion
52. Planning or organizing something
53. Listening to the sounds of nature
54. Dating, courting, etc.
55. Having a lively talk
56. Listening to the radio
57. Having friends come to visit
58. Competing in a sports event
59. Introducing people who I think would like each other
60. Giving gifts
61. Going to school or government meetings (court sessions, etc.)
62. Getting massages or backrubs
63. Getting letters, cards, or notes
64. Watching the sky, clouds, or a storm
65. Going on outings (to the park, a picnic, a barbecue, etc.)
66. Playing basketball
67. Buying something for my family
68. Photography
69. Giving a speech or a presentation
70. Reading maps
71. Gathering natural objects (wild foods or fruit, rocks, driftwood, etc).
72. Fishing
73. Loaning something
74. Being noticed as sexually attractive
75. Pleasing employers, teachers, etc.
76. Counseling someone
77. Going to a health club, sauna, hot tub, etc.
78. Learning to do something new
79. Going to a drive-in (Dairy Queen, McDonald's, etc.)
80. Complimenting or praising someone
81. Thinking about people I like
82. Being at a fraternity or sorority
83. Being with my parents
84. Horseback riding
85. Protesting social, political, or environmental conditions.
86. Talking on the telephone
87. Having daydreams
88. Kicking leaves, sand, pebbles, etc.
89. Playing lawn sports (badminton, croquet, shuffleboard, horseshoes, etc.)
90. Going to school reunions, alumni
91. Seeing famous people
92. Going to the movies
93. Kissing
94. Being alone

(continued)

TABLE 6.12. *(continued)*

95. Budgeting my time
96. Cooking meals
97. Being praised by people I admire
98. Doing favors for people
99. Being relaxed
100. Being asked for my help or advice
101. Thinking about other people
102. Playing board games (Monopoly, Scrabble, etc.)
103. Sleeping soundly at night
104. Doing heavy outdoor work (cutting or chopping wood, clearing land, farm work, etc.)
105. Reading the newspaper
106. Snowmobiling or dune-buggy riding
107. Being in a body-awareness, sensitivity, encounter, therapy, or "rap" group
108. Dreaming at night
109. Playing ping-pong
110. Brushing my teeth
111. Swimming
112. Running, jogging, or doing gymnastics,
113. Walking barefoot
114. Playing frisbee or catch
115. Doing housework or laundry; cleaning things
116. Being with my roommate
117. Listening to music
118. Knitting, crocheting, embroidery, or fancy needlework
119. Petting, necking
120. Amusing people
121. Talking about sex
122. Talking about politics or public affairs
123. Asking for help or advice
124. Going to banquets, luncheons, potlucks, etc.
125. Talking about my hobby or special interest
126. Watching attractive women or men
127. Smiling at people
128. Playing in the sand, a stream, the grass, etc.
129. Being with my husband or wife
130. Having people show interest in what I have said
131. Going on field trips, nature walks, etc.
132. Expressing my love to someone
133. Caring for houseplants
134. Having coffee, tea, a Coke, etc., with friends
135. Taking a walk
136. Collecting things
137. Playing handball, paddleball, etc.
138. Sewing
139. Suffering for a good cause
140. Remembering a departed friend or loved one, visiting a cemetery
141. Doing things with children
142. Beachcombing
143. Being complimented or told I have done well
144. Going to office parties or departmental get-togethers
145. Attending a concert, opera, or ballet
146. Playing with pets
147. Thinking up or arranging songs or music
148. Saying something clearly
149. Boating (canoeing, kayaking, motor-boating, sailing, etc.)
150. Pleasing my parents
151. Restoring antiques, refinishing furniture, etc.
152. Watching television
153. Talking to myself
154. Camping
155. Working in politics
156. Working on machines (cars, bikes, motorcycles, tractors, etc.)
157. Thinking about something good in the future
158. Playing cards
159. Completing a difficult task
160. Laughing
161. Solving a problem, puzzle, crossword, etc.
162. Being at weddings, baptisms, confirmations, etc.
163. Shaving
164. Having lunch with friends or associates
165. Playing tennis
166. Taking a shower
167. Driving long distances
168. Woodworking, carpentry
169. Writing stories, novels, plays, or poetry
170. Being with animals
171. Being in a city
172. Taking a bath
173. Singing to myself
174. Making food or crafts to sell or give away
175. Playing pool or billiards
176. Being with my grandchildren
177. Playing chess or checkers
178. Doing craft work (pottery, jewelry, leather, beads, weaving, etc.)
179. Scratching myself
180. Putting on makeup, fixing my hair, etc.
181. Designing or drafting
182. Visiting people who are sick, shut in, or in trouble
183. Cheering, rooting
184. Bowling
185. Being popular at a gathering
186. Watching wild animals
187. Having an original idea
188. Gardening, landscaping, or doing yard work
189. Reading essays or other academic literature
190. Wearing new clothes
191. Dancing
192. Sitting in the sun
193. Riding a motorcycle

(continued)

TABLE 6.12. *(continued)*

194. Working on my finances
195. Wearing clean clothes
196. Making a major purchase (car, bicycle, stereo, etc.)
197. Helping someone
198. Being in the mountains
199. Getting a job advancement (a promotion, a raise, a better job, getting accepted at a better school, etc.)
200. Hearing jokes
201. Winning a bet
202. Talking about my children or grandchildren
203. Meeting someone new of the opposite sex
204. Going to a revival or crusade
205. Talking about my health
206. Seeing beautiful scenery
207. Eating a good meal
208. Improving my health (having my teeth fixed, changing my diet, etc.)
209. Being downtown
210. Wrestling, boxing, or karate
211. Hunting or shooting
212. Playing in a musical group
213. Hiking
214. Going to a museum or exhibit
215. Writing papers, essays, reports, etc.
216. Doing a job well
217. Having spare time
218. Feeling the presence of the Lord in my life.
219. Doing a project in my own way
220. Doing "odd jobs" around the house
221. Being told I am needed
222. Being at a family reunion or get-together
223. Giving a party or get-together
224. Washing my hair
225. Coaching someone
226. Going to a restaurant
227. Seeing or smelling a flower or plant
228. Being invited out
229. Receiving honors (civic, military, etc)
230. Using cologne, perfume, or aftershave
231. Having someone agree with me
232. Reminiscing, talking about old times
233. Getting up early in the morning
234. Having peace and quiet
235. Doing experiments or other scientific work
236. Visiting friends
237. Writing in a diary
238. Playing football
239. Being counseled
240. Saying prayers
241. Giving massages or backrubs
242. Meditating or doing yoga
243. Seeing a boxing match
244. Going to a barber or beautician
245. Being with someone I love
246. Reading magazines
247. Sleeping late
248. Starting a new project
249. Being stubborn
250. Having sexual relations with partner
251. Going to the library
252. Playing soccer, rugby, hockey, lacrosse, etc.
253. Preparing a new or special food
254. Birdwatching
255. Shopping
256. Watching people
257. Building or watching a fire
258. Winning an argument
259. Selling or trading something
260. Finishing a project or task
261. Confessing or apologizing
262. Repairing things
263. Working with others as a team
264. Bicycling
265. Being with happy people
266. Playing party games
267. Writing letters, cards, or notes
268. Being told I am loved
269. Eating snacks
270. Staying up late
271. Having family members or friends do something that makes me proud
272. Being with my children
273. Going to auctions, garage sales, etc.
274. Thinking about an interesting question
275. Doing volunteer work; working on community service programs
276. Waterskiing, surfing, scuba diving
277. Receiving money
278. Defending or protecting someone; stopping fraud or abuse
279. Hearing a good sermon
280. Winning a competition
281. Making a new friend
282. Talking about my job or school
283. Reading cartoons, comic strips, or comic books
284. Borrowing something
285. Traveling with a group
286. Seeing old friends
287. Teaching someone
288. Using my strength
289. Traveling
290. Going to a play
291. Looking at the stars or moon
292. Being coached

Note. Adapted from "The Pleasant Events Schedule: Studies on Reliability, Validity, and Scale Intercorrelation" by D. J. MacPhillamy and P. M. Lewinsohn, 1982, *Journal of Consulting and Clinical Psychology, 50*(3), 363–380. Copyright © 1982 by the American Psychological Association. Adapted with permission.

Prior to Session 4

Do for the first time:

1. Complete Top 20 Pleasant Events using A List of Pleasant Events if necessary.

Continue to do:

2. Based on whichever method for changing thoughts smokers have chosen, they are to complete the corresponding assignment. If the ABC method was chosen, complete ABC(D) Worksheet for an upsetting situation this week. If the positive and negative thoughts method was chosen, complete the Positive and Negative Thoughts Worksheet for an upsetting situation this week.
3. Complete the Daily Mood Rating Form at the end of each day.

COMORBIDITY MODULE SESSION 4

Integrated Session 4 Objectives

1. To provide process comments to smokers pertinent to their current experience in the smoking cessation treatment.
2. To review the homework assignment to practice managing triggers for smoking using self-control strategies.
3. To review the homework assignment to set goals regarding making broader lifestyle changes that support quitting smoking.
4. To review the homework assignment to practice the Benson (deep breathing) relaxation approach.
5. To review self-monitoring of smoking behavior (Wrap Sheet) assignment.
6. To introduce relapse-prevention concepts of identifying and coping with high-risk situations; to provide an opportunity for smokers to begin practice of these skills during the session.
   a. To review self-monitoring of daily mood (Daily Mood Rating Form) assignment.
   b. To review the rationale for increasing pleasant activities, the development of Top 20 Pleasant Events lists.
   c. To preview the methods for making active plans to increase pleasant activities.
   d. To review ABC method for changing negative ways of thinking, including the homework assignment—the ABC(D) Worksheet—and to discuss the use of disputing (D) nonconstructive beliefs.
   e. To review the positive and negative thoughts method for changing negative ways of thinking, including the homework assignment (Positive and Negative Thoughts Worksheet).
   f. To discuss the active use of strategies for increasing positive and decreasing negative thoughts.
7. To introduce the abstinence violation effect concept and how to cope with a possible slip.
8. To review nicotine fading assignment and assign (or explain to smokers how to choose) the 90% reduction brand.

9. To assist smokers in preparing for the upcoming quit day.
10. To preview the homework assignments to be completed prior to Session 5.
    a. **Includes homework for managing negative mood.**

Session 4 Handouts and Worksheets

1. Coping with High Risk Situations Worksheet
2. Managing Triggers for Smoking Worksheet
3. Nonsmoking Game Plan: Lifestyle Change Worksheet
4. Wrap Sheets
5. **Daily Mood Rating Form (Table 6.2)**
6. **Contract for Increasing Pleasant Activities (Table 6.13)**
7. **Positive and Negative Thoughts Worksheet (Table 6.10)**

Session 4 Comorbidity Treatment Content

1. *Review daily mood monitoring.* Facilitators should inquire about smokers' experiences rating their moods since the previous session. At this point, smokers should be increasingly aware of factors that influence their moods and of the relationship between cigarette smoking and their moods. This information should be discussed in session, and as many smokers as possible should be provided with the opportunity to contribute to the discussion. It is possible that smokers are noticing increased negative moods despite beginning to learn coping skills to ameliorate negative moods. This may be due, in part, to the effects of nicotine fading, by which smokers are changing brands, smoking fewer cigarettes, and possibly experiencing withdrawal effects (some of which manifest as depressed, anxious, irritable moods). Increased negative mood may also reflect anticipatory anxiety as quit day draws near. Smokers should be asked to continue to rate their moods between now and the next session on the Daily Mood Rating Form and to use all three mood dimensions each day.

2. *Review increasing pleasant activities and Top 20 Pleasant Events form.* Facilitators should reiterate the rationale for increasing pleasant activities: Because people often feel deprived when they quit smoking, it is important to add positive activities and experiences at a time when they are taking away an important source of positive reinforcement. For homework, smokers were to list their own enjoyable activities on the Top 20 Pleasant Events form. Facilitators should ask smokers how they did in constructing their Top 20 lists. Smokers should be encouraged to share the contents of their lists with the rest of the group members and to add to their lists any new activities that they would find enjoyable.

3. *Preview methods for increasing pleasant activities.* The overall goal of the pleasant activities approach is to increase the number of daily or weekly pleasant activities that smokers engage in or, if their levels of pleasant activities are already high, to maintain this high rate of pleasant activities throughout the process of quitting smoking. It is generally helpful for smokers to schedule pleasant activities on a weekly basis or to contract to increase pleasant activities and use rewards or both. An example of the Contract for Increasing Pleasant Activities (with a Weekly Plan for Pleasant Activities) is shown in Table 6.13. If the contract is used, smokers should be cautioned to keep goals at modest levels and to be sure

TABLE 6.13. Contract for Increasing Pleasant Activities

My goal for the next week is to bring my total pleasant activity count up to 21 .

This means that I will try to engage in 3 pleasant activities each day.

I will also try to keep my pleasant activities level from falling below 2 on any given day.

If my daily total is 3, I will reward myself by putting aside $2 toward a CD .

If my total for the week is 21 , I will reward myself by going out to dinner .

Signed: _____   Date: 5/28

Weekly Plan for Pleasant Activities

Time	Monday	Tuesday	Wednesday	Thursday	Friday	Saturday	Sunday
8:00 a.m.	Read paper	Read paper	Read paper	Read paper	Read paper	Haircut	Sunday paper
9:00						Work on car	
10:00							
11:00							
12:00	Go for a walk	Go for a walk		Go for a walk	Lunch w/Pam		Go to the beach
1:00						Shopping	
2:00							
3:00							
4:00							
5:00	Tennis		Tennis	Listen to music			Ice cream
6:00							
7:00				Out to dinner	Movie		
8:00							
9:00						Dancing	
10:00 p.m.							

that goals are realistic and achievable. Although no goal is too small, an overly ambitious goal that is not accomplished may discourage them. Once a small achievable goal is reached, it can be increased a modest amount on the next try. In this way, smokers will experience continued success and will be likely to continue to engage in the goal-setting process to increase pleasant activities.

The Weekly Plan may be useful for smokers who are committed to the idea of increasing their pleasurable activities, but who may have difficulty finding the time in their busy week. Scheduling pleasant activities as one would a business appointment increases the likelihood of fitting these activities into an otherwise busy lifestyle. The goal is for smokers to maintain or increase pleasant activities in their daily lives at a time when they are choosing to give up a major source of positive reinforcement and are at risk for feeling deprived and even depressed. Maintaining a focus on pleasant activities can help them to prevent or to keep these negative feelings under control and, in turn, should increase the likelihood of successfully quitting smoking.

4. *Review ABC(D) method and worksheet homework.* Facilitators can review the idea that nonconstructive beliefs at <u>B</u> can be argued against or disputed at <u>D</u> and that, if this is done effectively, smokers can change the emotional consequence, <u>C</u>, and end up feeling less upset. For homework, smokers were to have completed an ABC(D) Worksheet exercise for one upsetting situation that occurred since the previous session. Facilitators should carefully review, in session, as many examples as time allows. Smokers will learn this technique by hearing multiple examples identifying key nonconstructive beliefs that match the emotional reactions reported. Effectively disputing beliefs is easier when the important nonconstructive aspect is "fleshed out." A common problem is that smokers will identify surface-level nonconstructive beliefs that do not really match the levels of their emotional reactions. For example, a smoker reports that at point <u>A</u>, her husband did not help her with a weekend project as he had promised, and at <u>C</u> she is extremely angry, almost furious. At <u>B</u>, she identifies her beliefs as (a) "I really could have used his help" and (b) "I wish I had a more cooperative husband." The facilitator notices that these thoughts don't quite match the level of anger that she reported feeling at <u>C</u>. On further reflection, the smoker is able to identify these additional thoughts: (c) "All he ever cares about is himself—he doesn't give a damn about me," (d) "I never get my needs met in this relationship, and (e) "If he loved me, he would have helped me with the project." It can be readily seen that the latter three thoughts were the ones driving the smoker's anger, and disputing (<u>D</u>) these thoughts, rather than the first two, is more likely to have a significant impact on the smoker's emotional reaction.

The ABC(D) method is also relevant to the discussion of the Abstinence Violation Effect (AVE). The two concepts can be integrated to strengthen smokers' coping skills in the event of a slip. Facilitators can provide smokers with the following example of how the ABC(D) method can be used to help them deal with a possible AVE:

<u>A</u> Joan smokes a cigarette while at a party with friends

<u>B</u> "What an idiot I am."

"I have absolutely no willpower, I'll never quit smoking."

"I should have known better than to go to a party right after quitting."

"I worked so hard, and now it's all for nothing."

<u>C</u> Depressed, discouraged, feels like giving up.

Joan has done an excellent job identifying the nonconstructive beliefs at *B* that will probably lead her to continue smoking and eventually to relapse if they go undisputed. However, Joan is able to develop the following disputing statements:

<u>D</u> "I'm *not* an idiot, I'm human. I had a slip. I made a mistake."

"I *can* quit smoking if I keep working hard."

"I'm proud that I didn't smoke any more cigarettes after that first one."

"It would have been better if I'd avoided the party, but I can't change it now."

"It's *not* for nothing. I just have to go on from here and stay determined."

As a result of this exercise, Joan feels much less depressed and much more encouraged about her prospects for quitting smoking. Joan's chances of a slip turning into a relapse are considerably reduced if she can keep these disputing thoughts (<u>D</u>) firmly in mind, rather than dwelling on the nonconstructive beliefs at <u>B</u>.

Facilitators should assign smokers the homework, which is to complete the ABC(D) Worksheet for at least one upsetting situation again this week. Smokers can be reminded that acquiring skill at the approach takes time and practice.

5. *Review Positive and Negative Thoughts Method and Worksheet Homework.* Facilitators can review the idea that once smokers have identified their own positive and negative thoughts, they can use specific techniques outlined in Session 2 to increase positive and decrease negative thoughts in order to improve their ratio of positive to negative thoughts. Homework for today was to continue using the Positive and Negative Thoughts Worksheet and to use one specific technique to actively increase positive thoughts and one technique to decrease negative thoughts. Facilitators should ask smokers about their experiences and reactions to this assignment. What are some examples of positive and negative thoughts? Which techniques did smokers use to change positive and negative thoughts? As with other content presented, much of the learning for smokers results from hearing about others' use of the techniques. In a similar vein, many of the suggestions that are most valued by smokers as they share and discuss their own problems with the group come from other group members. Following are some examples of specific areas that facilitators may want to question and help smokers with solving:

a. What thoughts are smokers using with the priming approach? What cues are smokers finding useful to help them remember to focus on positive thoughts?

b. What things are smokers giving themselves credit for? Do they notice a difference in their moods when they focus on these positive thoughts?

c. Has anyone used time projection? Have they found it useful?

d. Has anyone used thought interruption successfully? Have smokers found it useful in response to negative thoughts about quitting smoking?

e. For smokers who have tried worrying time, did they remember to end the "session" after one half-hour? Was it useful in putting off worrisome thoughts throughout the day?

f. Can anyone give an example of how they used the blow-up strategy? Did they blow up the thought to be ridiculous or to seriously consider the "worst that could happen" and then deal with it? Was it helpful?

Facilitators can show smokers how the positive and negative thoughts method has the same relevance in the event of a slip (i.e., in relation to the abstinence violation effect) as does the ABC(D) method and is, in fact, not very different. To use the same example, Joan smokes a cigarette while at a party with friends. She then writes down her *negative thoughts* (B) about the slip:

"What an idiot I am."

"I have absolutely no willpower—I'll never quit smoking."

"I should have known better than to go to a party right after quitting smoking."

"I worked so hard, and now it's all for nothing."

Joan might then use any of several techniques to combat these negative thoughts. For example, she could use thought interruption to stop the negative thoughts and replace them with the following *positive thoughts*:

"I'm *not* an idiot, I'm human—I had a slip; I made a mistake."

"I *can* quit smoking if I keep working hard—I'm proud of myself that I didn't smoke any more cigarettes after having that first one."

"It would have been better if I'd avoided the party, but I can't change it now."

"It's *not* for nothing—I just have to go on from here and stay determined."

Or the positive thoughts could be written on 3" × 5" file cards and used for priming. Thus it can be shown that, in some respects, the two thought-changing techniques are not dramatically different, and smokers can adopt elements of each.

Prior to next session, smokers should continue to monitor their positive and negative thoughts and to practice using techniques for increasing positive thoughts and decreasing negative thoughts. Smokers can continue to use the Positive and Negative Thoughts Worksheet to monitor their positive and negative thoughts and to indicate which techniques they have used, how effective they were, and what they might do differently next time to make them more useful. Facilitators can remind smokers that these techniques will take practice to learn but that improving their ability to change their thoughts will undoubtedly have a positive impact on their moods and on their ability to quit smoking and remain abstinent.

6. *Review mood component homework assignments for next session.* Facilitators should confirm the date and time of the next session, review assignments to be completed before the next session, and answer any questions that smokers might have about the assignments.

Prior to Session 5

Do for the first time:

1. Complete the Contract for Increasing Pleasant Activities and the Weekly Plan for Pleasant Activities.

Continue to do:

2. Based on whichever method for changing thoughts was chosen, complete the corresponding assignment. If the ABC(D) method was chosen, complete ABC(D) Worksheet: Changing Faulty Thinking for an upsetting situation this week. If the Positive and Negative Thoughts method was chosen, complete the Positive and Negative Thoughts Worksheet for an upsetting situation.

3. Complete the Daily Mood Rating Form at the end of each day.

COMORBIDITY MODULE SESSION 5: QUIT DAY

Integrated Session 5 Objectives

1. To discuss with smokers their quit day experiences (smokers were to quit smoking as of the morning of today's session).
2. To review the homework assignment to identify and develop coping strategies for dealing with high-risk situations for relapse.
3. To review the concept of the abstinence violation effect and how to cope with a possible slip, should it occur (as well as applying it to any slips that may have already occurred).
   a. **To review self-monitoring of daily mood (Daily Mood Rating Form) assignment with regard to quitting.**
   b. **To review smokers' progress in making active plans to increase pleasant activities using the Contract for Increasing Pleasant Activities and the Weekly Plan for Pleasant Activities.**
   c. **To review smokers' progress in their use of disputing (D) nonconstructive beliefs to change negative ways of thinking, using the ABC(D) Worksheet.**
   d. **To review smokers' progress in the active use of strategies for increasing positive and decreasing negative thoughts to change negative ways of thinking, using the Positive and Negative Thoughts Worksheet.**
   e. **To discuss how smokers can apply thought-changing techniques to stay abstinent following quit day.**
   f. **To preview basic concepts regarding social skills and assertiveness.**
4. To review smokers' progress regarding making broader lifestyle changes that support quitting smoking.
5. To introduce the concept of social support for nonsmoking and to assist smokers in maximizing their social support for quitting smoking.
6. To review smokers' final experiences with nicotine fading prior to quitting.
7. To assist smokers in making specific plans for maintaining abstinence over the next several days (prior to the next session).
8. To preview the homework assignments to be completed prior to Session 6.
   a. **Includes homework for managing negative mood.**

Session 5 Handouts and Worksheets

1. Social Support for Nonsmoking Worksheet
2. Coping with High-Risk Situations Worksheet
3. Nonsmoking Game Plan: Lifestyle Change Worksheet
4. **Daily Mood Rating Form (Table 6.2)**
5. **Contract for Increasing Pleasant Activities and Weekly Plan for Pleasant Activities (Table 6.13)**
6. **ABC(D) Worksheet (Table 6.9)**
7. **Positive and Negative Thoughts Worksheet (Table 6.10)**

Session 5 Comorbidity Treatment Content

1. *Review daily mood monitoring.* Facilitators should ask smokers about their experiences rating their moods since the previous session. It is very possible that smokers are now noticing increased depressed, irritable, angry, or anxious moods related to quitting, despite their use of coping skills to ameliorate these negative moods. If this occurs, it is important for smokers to react with an increased focus on thoughts and pleasant activities. That is, they should identify negative thoughts and counteract them, increase positive thoughts, and make a special effort to do more pleasant activities. It is important that smokers understand that this does not represent a "failure" in their use of the coping skills but rather a fairly typical type of emotional reaction to quitting smoking. Smokers should also continue to rate their moods between now and the next session using the Daily Mood Rating Form and to use all three mood dimensions each day.

2. *Review progress in increasing pleasant activities.* Facilitators should reiterate the rationale for increasing pleasant activities and then review homework. For homework, smokers were to increase their number of daily or weekly pleasant activities or, if their levels of pleasant activities were already high, to maintain their high rates of pleasant activities. Smokers were to do this by using their Top 20 list and either scheduling pleasant activities on the Weekly Plan for Pleasant Activities or contracting to increase pleasant activities and rewards on the Contract for Increasing Pleasant Activities or both. If a contract is being used, smokers should be reminded to keep goals at modest levels and to be sure that the goals are realistic and achievable. If using the weekly plan, smokers should be reminded that it is important to follow through with the pleasant activity once it has been scheduled, just as one would keep any other important appointment. Facilitators can now review smokers' experiences in attempting to increase pleasant activities. Some questions that might be posed to smokers include: What activities did people do? Was the weekly plan useful? Was the contract useful? Did smokers deliver the rewards, if earned? Did smokers find there were obstacles to increasing pleasant activities? Do smokers need to decrease time spent in Type A, or "should," activities?

   Smokers should continue to work on pleasant activities during the coming week. As before, they should use either the contract or the weekly plan. If using the contract, are they ready to increase their goals to the next small step up? If they didn't meet their goals, they should set a new, slightly reduced goal. In all cases, the overall aim is to maintain or increase pleasant activities in their daily lives at a time when they are choosing to give up a major source of positive reinforcement and are at risk for feeling deprived and even depressed. Pleasant activities can help prevent or to keep negative feelings under control and, in turn, should increase the likelihood of successfully quitting smoking.

3. *Review ABC(D) method and worksheet homework.* For homework, smokers who chose this method for changing thoughts were to have completed an ABC(D) exercise for one upsetting situation that occurred since the previous session. Facilitators should carefully review as many examples as time allows. As before, the emphasis should be on making sure that smokers have identified the key nonconstructive beliefs at <u>B</u> that match the emotional reactions reported at <u>C</u>. Smokers can be engaged in a discussion of whether the use of the ABC(D) method has had an impact on reducing their smoking, as well as whether they be-

lieve it will help them avoid smoking in high-risk, negative-mood situations. For homework, smokers should continue to use the ABC(D) method for at least one upsetting situation. They should also actively use the technique in any high-risk (for smoking) negative-mood situation or, in the case of a slip, for coping with possible abstinence violation effects.

4. *Review positive and negative thoughts method and worksheet homework*. Facilitators can ask smokers how they are doing in their use of the positive and negative thoughts method. For homework, smokers who chose this method were to have continued monitoring their positive and negative thoughts and to have practiced using techniques for increasing positive thoughts and decreasing negative thoughts. Smokers can be asked to share with the group some current positive and negative thoughts and how they are faring with the different techniques they are using to increase positive and decrease negative thoughts. Are they having any particular successes and/or difficulties with the use of any of the approaches? Successes can be shared with the group, and difficulties can be discussed by the facilitators and group members.

Smokers should be reminded that actually writing down thoughts in complete sentences is a critical step in using this approach. After considerable practice with written thoughts, smokers may begin to identify and work with the thoughts mentally. For homework, smokers should continue to monitor their thoughts and to use the thought-changing techniques. Now that they have quit smoking, they should actively use the techniques to keep their moods reasonably positive or, in the event of a slip, to combat possible abstinence violation effects.

5. *Applying "changing thoughts" techniques to the quitting experience*. Exploration of smokers' thoughts about the quitting experience, both positive and negative, can be a useful experience. Begin by asking smokers what their specific thoughts are about quitting smoking. As they are responding, a facilitator can make a positive-thought list and a negative-thought list on the board or flip chart.

Smokers may be reluctant to offer negative thoughts about quitting. They may have to be told that it is all right to have negative thoughts about quitting. For most people, it is better to identify and deal with (e.g., dispute or counteract) negative thoughts than to deny that they exist. Facilitators can prompt for negative thoughts about fears of failing ("I can't do it"), problems and obstacles they may face ("If I get upset about something, I'll have to smoke"), or urges ("These urges are killing me—I can't deal with this—they'll keep getting worse until I smoke"). Facilitators can use the cognitive distortion list and group input to help people counteract negative thoughts about quitting (e.g., "Urges are discrete and only last 5 minutes or so; they gradually become fewer and less intense over time. Distracting myself and getting busy can help me not to focus on them").

As far as positive thoughts are concerned, facilitators should prompt group members to compile a list of as many as possible. "Benefits of quitting" thoughts (e.g., "when I quit smoking I'll be able to breathe better") can be added to the list and serve a useful purpose at this critical juncture. Smokers should be encouraged to adopt as many positive thoughts as possible for themselves. If time allows, facilitators might review with smokers the type of distorted thoughts that they might have if they were to experience the abstinence violation effect following a slip.

6. *Introduce social skills and assertiveness skills.* Another important way to manage mood is by improving specific social skills that will allow smokers to feel better about their interactions with others. Facilitators can define social skills as the ability to interact with others in a way that allows them to achieve their personal goals in social situations. Assertiveness is the ability to express one's thoughts and feelings openly and directly to others without "turning off" other people or alienating them. Both social and assertiveness skills represent behaviors that can be learned, practiced, and improved.

Assertiveness also means that people have the *right* to decide what to do in any situation (instead of doing what someone else expects or asks). It also means that people recognize that others they deal with *also* have rights. Facilitators can provide smokers with the following example of what is meant by "rights":

a. People have a *right* to make their feelings known in a way that does not hurt others.

b. People have the *right* to make their opinions known to others.

c. People have the *right* to request that another person change behavior that affects them.

d. People have the *right* to accept or reject anything that someone else says to them or requests from them.

Facilitators can inform smokers that they will be working on improving these skills over the next few sessions. It can be pointed out to smokers that these skills also fit nicely with the discussion about social support for quitting smoking covered in this session.

7. *Review mood component homework assignments for next session.* Facilitators should confirm the date and time of the next session, review assignments to be completed before the next session, and answer any questions that smokers might have about the assignments.

Prior to Session 6

Continue to do:

1. Complete the Contract for Increasing Pleasant Activities and the Weekly Plan for Pleasant Activities.

2. Based on whichever method for changing thoughts was chosen, complete the corresponding assignment. If the ABC(D) method was chosen, complete ABC(D) Worksheet: Changing Faulty Thinking for an upsetting situation this week. If the positive and negative thoughts method was chosen, complete the Positive and Negative Thoughts Worksheet for an upsetting situation.

3. Complete the Daily Mood Rating Form at the end of each day.

COMORBIDITY MODULE SESSION 6

Integrated Session 6 Objectives

1. To discuss with smokers their quitting experiences **and the use of mood management techniques while quitting.**
   a. **To review self-monitoring of daily mood (Daily Mood Rating Form) assignment.**
   b. **To review smokers' progress in making active plans to increase pleasant activities**

    using the Contract for Increasing Pleasant Activities and the Weekly Plan for Pleasant Activities.

  c. To discuss how smokers can increase their social skills and assertiveness and to preview specific homework assignments designed to help them enhance the development of these skills.

  d. To discuss how smokers can use the thought-changing techniques to apply to their experiences in quitting smoking.

  e. To review smokers' progress in their use of thought-changing techniques to change negative ways of thinking.

2. To review the concept of the abstinence violation effect and how to cope with a possible slip should it occur (as well as applying it to any slips that may have already occurred).

3. To introduce new strategies for coping with urges to smoke.

4. To review the homework assignment to identify and develop coping strategies for situations high in risk for relapse.

5. To review smokers' experiences in attempting to maximize social support for quitting smoking.

6. To review smokers' progress regarding making broader lifestyle changes that support quitting smoking.

7. To assist smokers in making specific plans for maintaining abstinence over the next several days (prior to the next session).

8. To preview the homework assignments to be completed prior to Session 7.

  a. Includes homework for managing negative mood.

Session 6 Handouts and Worksheets

1. Coping with High-Risk Situations Worksheet
2. Social Support for Nonsmoking Worksheet
3. Nonsmoking Game Plan: Lifestyle Change Worksheet
4. **A Plan for Assertiveness (Table 6.14)**
5. **Assertiveness Worksheet (Table 6.15)**
6. **Daily Mood Rating Form—blank (Table 6.2)**
7. **ABC(D) Method Worksheets (Tables 6.6 and 6.9)**
8. **Positive and Negative Thoughts Worksheet (Table 6.10)**
9. **Contract for Increasing Pleasant Activities (Table 6.13)**

Session 6 Comorbidity Treatment Content

1. *Review daily mood monitoring.* Facilitators should briefly review with smokers their mood ratings since the previous session. Facilitators should acknowledge the possibility of more depressed, irritable, angry, or anxious moods related to quitting. It is important for smokers to react to increases in negative moods with an increased focus on thoughts and pleasant activities. Identifying negative thoughts and counteracting them, increasing positive thoughts, and making a concerted effort to do more pleasant activities will all be helpful.

Smokers can also begin to focus on assertiveness. Smokers should also be asked to continue to rate their moods between now and the next session on the Daily Mood Rating Form and to use all three mood dimensions each day.

2. *Review increasing pleasant activities and worksheet homework*. The rationale for pleasant activities should now be familiar to smokers. Smokers have been working on increasing their number of daily or weekly pleasant activities or maintaining their already high rate of pleasant activities. Facilitators can now lead smokers in a discussion of their experiences with questions such as: What activities did people do? Was the weekly plan useful? Was the contract useful? Did smokers deliver rewards, if earned? Did smokers find there were obstacles to increasing pleasant activities? Do smokers need to decrease time spent in Type A, or "should," activities?

   Smokers should continue to work on pleasant activities during the coming week. If using the contract, they should increase their goals the next small step. If they did not meet their goals, they should set a new, slightly reduced goal. In all cases, the overall aim is to maintain or increase pleasant activities in their daily lives at a time when they are at risk for feeling deprived and even depressed due to quitting smoking.

3. *Discuss social skills and assertiveness*. As previewed in the previous session, an important way for smokers to manage their moods is to improve specific social skills. This will allow them to feel better about their interactions with others. Social skills have been defined as the ability to interact with others in a way that allows individuals to achieve their personal goals in social situations. Assertiveness is the ability to express one's thoughts and feelings openly and directly to others without "turning off" other people or alienating them. Both of these skills can be learned and improved on with practice.

   Facilitators can review the notion that assertiveness also means that people have *rights*, including the right to decide what to do in any situation (instead of doing what someone else expects or asks). It is also the recognition that others *also* have rights.

   a. People have a *right* to make their feelings known in a way that does not hurt others.

   b. People have the *right* to make their opinions known to others.

   c. People have the *right* to request that another person change behavior that affects them.

   d. People have the *right* to accept or reject anything that someone else says to them or requests from them.

   An assertive style of interacting is best explained by contrasting it with two other common styles, as follows:

   a. *Passive style*. When people act passively, they almost always give up their rights if there appears to be a conflict between what they want and what someone else wants. When they have thoughts and feelings, they do not let the other person know about them. The passive person will often not get what he/she wants and will feel angry at others or depressed by his/her lack of assertiveness.

   b. *Aggressive style*. When people act aggressively, they will usually act on their own rights but will ignore the other person's rights. They meet their immediate short-term goals, but their long-term results are more negative. Because they achieve their goals at someone else's expense, they make enemies. Other people tend to get angry and resentful toward them.

   c. *Assertive style*. When people act assertively, they will decide what their goals are, will plan the most effective way to deal with the people involved, and will act on their plan. The assertive person will act in a way that *best fits the situation*, not always in the same programmed and automatic way. The assertive person generally feels better about his or her actions and *is well thought of by others*.

Facilitators can inform smokers that although there may be situations in which they choose to respond passively or aggressively, most often an assertive response will be most effective. Facilitators should ask smokers to read A Plan for Assertiveness (Table 6.14) for homework. To begin working on assertiveness, smokers should identify situations in which they would like to become more assertive. These situations are likely to fit the following pattern: (a) the person has not been assertive in the past; (b) the situation occurs regularly (at least once a month); (c) the situation is troubling to the person; and (d) the situation is not too specific or too general.

Once smokers have identified these situations, they can work on developing assertive responses, one situation at a time. Using the following steps may be helpful:

a. *Step 1*. Describe the other person's behavior *accurately in neutral terms* so that they (or anyone else) cannot argue.

    Example: "*When you offered me a cigarette despite knowing that I had just quit smoking. . . .* "

b. *Step 2*. Use "I feel" statements to describe your feeling about what has happened. These statements will let the other person know that you are responsible for your *own* feelings and that you are not blaming them. Avoid *"you" statements* that are hostile or blaming.

    Example: "*I felt angry. . . .* "

c. *Step 3*. Let the person know what you want. Request a specific behavior change on his or her part.

    Example: "*In the future, I'd appreciate it if you would be more supportive of my effort to quit smoking. Please don't offer me a cigarette when you know that I've quit smoking.*"

Facilitators should inform smokers that using these steps can help them to be assertive in specific situations and improve communication with others. However, smokers should be cautioned that the other person might not change his or her behavior in response to an assertive request. Even so, the assertive individual is likely to feel better about him/herself and is more likely to get what he/she wanted than if he/she used a passive or aggressive style.

Facilitators can offer several other helpful tips when using assertiveness. Before approaching a person in a given situation, it is best to *practice* what one intends to say. This can be done through the use of what is called *assertive imagery*. The steps to follow in this process are detailed in the Assertiveness Worksheet (Table 6.15), which smokers are to complete for homework. Facilitators can suggest that smokers practice assertive imagery for at least 15 minutes per day. Smokers should begin by using two easy situations or two situations that are most likely to occur. Smokers should create a mental picture in their imagination of: (a) the entire scene, (b) themselves making the assertive statement, and (c) how the other person responds. Smokers can be encouraged to change the details of the

TABLE 6.14. A Plan for Assertiveness

Think of situations in which you would like to be more assertive. You probably don't feel very positive about these situations and would like to change your feelings in the future. The first step in acting more assertively is to identify situations that fit the following pattern:

1. You have not been assertive in the past.
2. The situation occurs regularly in your life (at least once a month).
3. The situation is troubling you.
4. The situation is not too specific or too general.

Once you have identified these situations, work on developing assertive responses one situation at a time. Use the following steps to help you.

Step 1: Describe the other person's behavior *accurately in neutral terms* so that they (or anyone else) cannot argue.

> Example: "When you asked me a question while I was talking to your sister on the telephone . . . "

Step 2: Use "I feel" statements to describe your feeling about what has happened. These statements will let the other person know you are responsible for your *own* feelings and that you are not blaming him/her. Avoid "*you*" statements that are hostile or blaming.

> Example: "I felt angry . . . "

Step 3: Let the person know what you want. Request a specific behavior change on his or her part.

> Example: "In the future, I'd appreciate it if you would wait until I'm off the phone before asking me questions."

Using these steps can help you to be assertive in specific situations and to improve communication with others. Recognize that a person may not change his or her behavior because of your request. By being assertive, you have the best chance of getting what you want, and you will feel better about yourself for stating your request assertively.

Other Helpful Tips When Using Assertiveness

1. Before approaching a person, *practice* what you will say. Use assertive imagery. Imagine the following:
   a. The entire scene
   b. Your assertive statement
   c. How the other person responds
   You can change the details of the scene and practice again. Imagine the person responding positively. After several practices, imagine the person responding more negatively.
2. *Listen* to the other person's answer. Acknowledge and accept his or her feelings.
3. *Avoid "you" statements* that are hostile or judgmental (such as "When you acted like a jerk . . . ").
4. End the conversation on a *positive note* . . . even if it means you agree to disagree.
5. Praise and *reward yourself* for practicing assertiveness.

TABLE 6.15. Assertiveness Worksheet

1. Situation you want to respond to (what happened):
   <u>Coworker offered me a cigarette, knowing I had just quit smoking</u>

2. Developing the assertive response:
   Step 1: "WHEN YOU <u>offered me a cigarette ...</u>

                                                 (Describe his or her behavior in neutral terms.)

   Step 2: "I FELT <u>angry</u>

                                         (Describe your emotional reaction.)

   Step 3: "I WOULD LIKE YOU <u>to support my quitting and not offer me cigarettes</u>

                                    (Request specific behavior change.)

3. Assertive imagery practice:

   Before practicing, rate your comfort with assertiveness and your level of assertiveness skill on a scale of 0–10, where 0 = very low and 10 = very high.

   Level of Comfort: <u>2</u>   Level of Skill: <u>3</u>

   > NOW PRACTICE:
   > Step 1: Imagine the scene.
   > Step 2: Practice your assertive statement. Say it out loud.
   > Step 3: Imagine how the other person will respond.

   After practicing, rate your comfort with assertiveness and your level of assertiveness skill on a scale of 0–10, where 0 = very low and 10 = very high.

   Level of Comfort: <u>6</u>   Level of Skill: <u>7</u>

4. Using assertiveness skills in actual situations.

   Try out the assertiveness technique in a real situation. After practicing, rate your comfort with assertiveness and your level of assertiveness skill on a scale of 0–10 points, where 0 = very low and 10 = very high.

   Level of Comfort: <u>6</u>   Level of Skill: <u>6</u>

---

scene and practice again several times in imagery. They might first imagine the other person responding positively. After several practices, they might imagine the person responding more negatively and then practice in imagery how they might react to this more negative response. In this way, the smoker will be prepared for all eventualities.

Before practicing assertive imagery, smokers should rate their comfort with assertiveness and their perceived level of assertiveness skill using a 0- to 10-point rating scale (0 = very low; 10 = very high). After practicing the assertive imagery, smokers should again rate their comfort and skill levels on this same 10-point scale:

    Before assertive imagery practice: *Level of Comfort:* ____   *Level of Skill:* ____
    After assertive imagery practice: *Level of Comfort:* ____   *Level of Skill:* ____
    (For all ratings: "0" = very low; "10" = very high)

Smokers can be advised that, when transferring their assertiveness skills from imagery to real life, they should start with an easy situation, plan the situation, practice the assertive response, and evaluate their progress afterward. When actually using assertiveness in real life, smokers should *listen* carefully to the other person's answer and should be prepared to acknowledge and accept his or her feelings. It is important to avoid "you" statements that are hostile or judgmental (e.g., "When you acted like a jerk . . . "). Whenever possible, it is advisable to end a conversation on a *positive note*, even if it means agreeing to disagree. Finally, smokers should realize that it is difficult to be assertive and that they should praise and reward themselves for practicing assertiveness. After trying out the assertiveness technique in a real situation, smokers should rate their comfort with assertiveness and their level of assertiveness skill, as before:

> *After actual use of assertion:*   *Level of Comfort:* ____   *Level of Skill:* ____
> *(For all ratings: "0" = very low; "10" = very high)*

4. *Applying "changing thoughts" techniques to the quitting experience.* As they did at the last session, facilitators can use this time to focus on specific thoughts, both positive and negative, that smokers are having about quitting smoking by making two lists on the board. Facilitators can focus on how smokers may have challenged negative thoughts or utilized positive thoughts offered last session, and they should attempt to elicit new thoughts that have emerged now that it is several days after quit day. Smokers can be reminded that it is better to identify negative thoughts about quitting and dispute or counter them rather than to try to suppress them and make believe they do not exist. The group can spend time collectively trying to dispute the negative thoughts offered by group members, with the help of facilitators and the cognitive distortion list.

5. *Review ABC(D) and positive and negative thoughts methods.* At this point in the treatment, facilitators can initiate a more general discussion of how smokers are doing with their use of the thought-changing approaches. Smokers have sat through several reviews of both approaches and have probably begun to see a number of similarities between the two. In truth, smokers often do not follow the techniques to the "letter of the law" anyway, and therefore they will often focus on upsetting situations or their difficulties with quitting smoking. The task of the facilitators is to focus the smokers on the thoughts that accompany their experiences and on the means of counteracting negative thoughts. The other side of the coin, of course, is merely to continue to encourage an active effort to promote positive thoughts on a regular basis. During the course of the discussion, facilitators can make specific reference to particular approaches that seem to be indicated. For instance, if someone is discussing a specific upsetting situation, the ABC(D) model might be invoked. If persistent doubts about quitting smoking are at issue, thought interruption might be most appropriate. In general, discussing different situations or circumstances and bringing the thought-changing approaches to the situations (rather than vice versa) may help to promote the more flexible use of these skills in the everyday environment.

6. *Review mood component homework assignments for next session.* Facilitators should confirm the date and time of the next session, review assignments to be completed before the next session, and answer any questions that smokers might have about the assignments.

Prior to Session 7

Do for the first time:

1. Read A Plan for Assertiveness.
2. Complete Assertiveness Worksheet.

Continue to do:

3. Complete the Contract for Increasing Pleasant Activities and the Weekly Plan for Pleasant Activities.
4. Based on whichever method for changing thoughts was chosen, complete the corresponding assignment. If the ABC(D) method was chosen, complete ABC(D) Worksheet for an upsetting situation this week. If the positive and negative thoughts method was chosen, complete Positive and Negative Thoughts Worksheet for an upsetting situation.
5. Complete Daily Mood Rating Form at the end of each day.

COMORBIDITY MODULE SESSION 7

Integrated Session 7 Objectives

1. To discuss with smokers their quitting experiences **and the use of mood management techniques while quitting.**
   a. **To review self-monitoring of daily mood (Daily Mood Rating Form) assignment.**
   b. **To review general concepts regarding social skills and assertiveness and to review smokers' experiences with the homework involving formulating assertive responses and practicing assertiveness (in imagery and real-life situations) using the Assertiveness Worksheet.**
   c. **To review smokers' progress in making active plans to increase pleasant activities using the Contract for Increasing Pleasant Activities and the Weekly Plan for Pleasant Activities.**
   d. **To review smokers' progress in their use of thought-changing techniques to change negative ways of thinking.**

2. To review the concept of the abstinence violation effect and how to cope with a possible slip should it occur (as well as applying it to any slips that may have already occurred).
3. To introduce new strategies for managing thoughts that can encourage relapse.
4. To review the use of strategies for coping with urges to smoke.
5. To review the homework assignment to identify and develop coping strategies for dealing with high-risk situations for relapse.
6. To review smokers' experiences in attempting to maximize social support for quitting smoking.

7. To assist smokers in making specific plans for maintaining abstinence over the next week (prior to the next session).
8. To preview the homework assignments to be completed prior to Session 8.
   a. **Includes homework for managing negative mood.**

Session 7 Handouts and Worksheets

1. Strategies for Identifying and Counteracting Resumption Thoughts handout
2. Coping with High Risk Situations Worksheet
3. Social Support for Nonsmoking Worksheet
4. Nonsmoking Game Plan: Lifestyle Change Worksheet
5. **Assertiveness Worksheet (Table 6.15)**
6. **Contract for Increasing Pleasant Activities (Table 6.13)**
7. **ABC(D) Worksheet: Changing Faulty Thinking (Table 6.9)**
8. **Positive and Negative Thoughts Worksheet (Table 6.10)**
9. **Daily Mood Rating Form (Table 6.2)**

Session 7 Comorbidity Treatment Content

1. *Review daily mood monitoring.* Facilitators should briefly review smokers' experiences in rating their moods since the previous session. It is important for smokers to react to more depressed, irritable, angry, or anxious moods with an increased focus on thoughts and pleasant activities. Smokers can also begin to focus on assertiveness. All smokers should be asked to continue to rate their moods between now and the next session on the Daily Mood Rating Form, using all three mood dimensions each day.
2. *Review social skills and assertiveness and homework.* Facilitators can review, from previous sessions, the definition of assertiveness, the descriptions of passive, aggressive, and assertive styles of interacting, and the three steps for assertive communication.

   For homework, smokers were to identify two situations in which they would like to become more assertive and then to practice assertive imagery for at least 15 minutes per day, rating their comfort level and perceived level of skill both before and after the practice. Facilitators should ask smokers how they did in using the assertive imagery. What situations did they use for imagery practice? How were their comfort and skill ratings? Did the ratings improve with practice? Did any smokers use assertiveness skills in conjunction with the social support for nonsmoking exercise? Finally, did any smokers begin to transfer the assertiveness skills to real-life situations? If so, how did they do in asserting themselves? Did they feel better about themselves for having been assertive? Facilitators should elicit discussion from several group members. Smokers will gain much from listening to other smokers' experiences.

   Smokers can be reminded that they should start with an easy situation, plan the situation, practice the assertive response, and evaluate their progress afterward. When actually practicing assertiveness in real life, smokers should *listen* carefully to the other person's answer and should be prepared to acknowledge and accept his or her feelings. Whenever possible, it is advisable to end a conversation on a *positive note*, even if it means agreeing to disagree. Finally, smokers should realize that it is difficult to be assertive and that they should praise and reward themselves for practicing assertiveness.

3. *Review increasing pleasant activities and homework*. Smokers have been either scheduling pleasant activities on the Weekly Plan for Pleasant Activities or contracting to increase pleasant activities and rewards using the Contract for Increasing Pleasant Activities or both. As in previous sessions, facilitators can ask about their experiences. What activities did people do? Was the weekly plan or contract useful? Did smokers deliver rewards, if earned? Did smokers find there were obstacles to increasing pleasant activities?

   Smokers should continue to work on pleasant activities prior to the next session. If using the contract, they should increase their goals the next small step. If they did not meet their goals, they should set a new, slightly reduced goal. In all cases, the overall aim is to maintain or increase pleasant activities in their daily lives at a time when they are at risk for feeling deprived and even depressed due to quitting smoking.

4. *Review thought-changing techniques and homework*. As they did in the previous session, facilitators can lead a more general discussion of how smokers are doing with their use of the thought-changing approaches. The task of the facilitators is to focus the smokers on the thoughts that accompany their negative moods and on the means of counteracting negative thoughts. In addition, they should continue to encourage an active effort to promote positive thoughts on a regular basis. During the course of the discussion, facilitators can make specific reference to particular approaches that seem to be indicated. For instance, if someone is discussing a specific upsetting situation, the ABC(D) model might be invoked. If persistent doubts about quitting smoking are at issue, thought interruption might be most appropriate. In general, discussing different situations or circumstances and bringing the thought-changing approaches to the situations (rather than vice versa) may help to promote the more flexible use of these skills in the everyday environment. Several examples of how smokers are using the thought-changing techniques should be solicited.

5. *Review mood component homework assignments for next session*.

Prior to Session 8

Continue to do:

1. Complete Assertiveness Worksheet.
2. Complete the Contract for Increasing Pleasant Activities and the Weekly Plan for Pleasant Activities.
3. Based on whichever method for changing thoughts was chosen, complete the corresponding assignment. If the ABC(D) method was chosen, complete the ABC(D) Worksheet: Changing Faulty Thinking for an upsetting situation this week. If the positive and negative thoughts method was chosen, complete the Positive and Negative Thoughts Worksheet for an upsetting situation.
4. Complete the Daily Mood Rating Form at the end of each day.

COMORBIDITY TREATMENT SESSION 8

Integrated Session 8 Objectives

1. To discuss with smokers their quitting experiences **and review strategies for managing mood**.
   a. **To review mood management strategies, assist smokers in deciding which strategies were helpful and that they plan to continue using, and provide an opportunity for questions or comments.**
   b. **To help smokers to anticipate upcoming situations that might involve negative mood and to develop an active coping plan.**
2. To review the concept of the abstinence violation effect and how to cope with a possible slip should it occur (as well as applying it to any slips that may have already occurred).
3. To review the use of strategies for managing thoughts that can encourage relapse.
4. To review the homework assignment to identify and develop coping strategies for dealing with high-risk situations for relapse.
5. To review smokers' progress regarding making broader lifestyle changes that support quitting smoking.
6. To offer some final remarks and observations about planning for the future.

Session 8 Comorbidity Treatment Content

1. *Reviewing mood management strategies.* Facilitators should review the different mood management strategies presented in the program and ask smokers to decide which strategy or strategies have worked the best for them. What would they like to continue to do to maintain their use of that strategy? The review also provides smokers with a final opportunity to ask any questions or make any comments about a particular strategy.
   a. *Daily mood monitoring.* Facilitators can lead smokers in a brief discussion of how they are doing with rating their moods. If smokers have noticed increased depressed, angry, irritable, or anxious moods, it is particularly important to react to this with an increased focus on thoughts, pleasant activities, and assertiveness. In general, rating one's mood is akin to taking one's temperature. If an individual is feeling well, there is really no need to take a temperature or rate moods. However, as one begins to feel a bit "down," anxious, or irritable, keeping track of one's moods may help to determine when more coping efforts are needed (just as knowing one's temperature helps determine when medicine or medical care is needed). Smokers should be encouraged to continue to maintain an awareness of their mood levels and to consider resuming daily mood monitoring during any period in which they find themselves beginning to experience negative moods.
   b. *ABC method.* Facilitators can remind smokers that the ABC(D) method promotes the idea that "it's not what happens to us that makes us upset, but rather what we tell ourselves about the situations or circumstances." Using the ABC method, smokers have learned to identify faulty thinking patterns (nonconstructive beliefs or thoughts that

lead to emotional upset). The next step was to change these beliefs or self-talk in order to reduce or avoid emotional overreactions. To change their emotional <u>Consequences</u> (<u>C</u>), smokers learned to <u>Dispute</u> (<u>D</u>) their <u>Beliefs</u> (<u>B</u>) about <u>Activating</u> events (<u>A</u>).

Facilitators can engage smokers in discussion of how they fared using the ABC method. Several recent examples of the use of the approach may be solicited. Smokers should be encouraged to continue to use this approach to the extent that they found it helpful.

c. *Positive and negative thoughts method.* Facilitators can remind smokers that the positive and negative thoughts method promotes the idea that mood is related to balance between positive and negative thoughts. When negative thoughts far outweigh positive thoughts, this imbalance results in a depressive, anxious, angry, or otherwise negative mood in which smoking becomes a reliable and familiar coping strategy.

The first step for smokers who used this method was to identify both types of thoughts, positive and negative, using their Inventory of Thoughts form. Once smokers gained experience in writing down positive and negative thoughts, they began to use *specific strategies* to increase positive thoughts and decrease negative thoughts. Facilitators can remind smokers of the need to work at both increasing positive and decreasing negative thoughts.

Facilitators can engage smokers in discussion of how they made out using the positive and negative thoughts method. Several recent examples of the use of the approach may be solicited from group members, and members can continue to actively use this approach to both increase positive thoughts and decrease negative thoughts.

d. *Increasing pleasant activities.* Facilitators should review the rationale for increasing pleasant activities: People often feel deprived when they quit smoking; therefore, it is important to add positive activities and experiences at a time when they are taking away an important source of positive reinforcement.

After creating a Top 20 Pleasant Events list, smokers were to increase or maintain (if already high) their number of daily or weekly pleasant activities. They were to do this either by scheduling on the Weekly Plan for Pleasant Activities or by using the Contract for Increasing Pleasant Activities or both. Facilitators can lead smokers in a discussion of how they did with the approach of increasing pleasant activities.

e. *Social skills and assertiveness.* Improving specific social skills allows people to feel better about their interactions with others. Social skills and assertiveness can be learned, practiced, and improved. Facilitators can initiate a discussion of how smokers did at using assertiveness skills. Discussion could focus at one of four points in the process: (1) how well smokers did at identifying specific situations in which they wanted to be more assertive, (2) how well smokers did at formulating an effective assertive response, (3) how comfortable and skillful smokers were in practicing this response using assertive imagery, and (4) how comfortable and skillful smokers were in applying the assertive response in a real-life situation. Smokers should continue to practice and develop their assertiveness skills if they think it will be helpful or if they find that they are experiencing negative moods related to interpersonal conflict or a lack of assertiveness or both.

2. *Planning for the future.* Negative moods and negative mood situations will continue to represent high-risk situations for smoking relapse in the future. In our long-term follow-up in cessation trials, smokers who have relapsed even after maintaining abstinence for 6 months or more often tell us a similar story, "Something happened and I became very upset and reached for a cigarette." Sometimes the precipitating events are unexpected, like an accident or a death in the family, and do not allow much time for planning. Other times the events could have been anticipated, such as having difficulty finding a job after graduation or having continuing conflict with a teenage son or daughter. Facilitators should encourage smokers to continue to practice and use the negative-mood coping skills learned during these sessions and to try to incorporate them into their everyday activities. At the same time, smokers should try to anticipate future situations that might involve undue stress, depression, anger, or some other negative mood state and develop a plan to reinstate their use of these coping skills in anticipation of these events. Developing skills for identifying one's own moods and the factors that affect them, as well as developing a strong repertoire of coping skills to deal with negative moods and negative mood situations, can, for many smokers, be their best defense against relapse to smoking.

7

Pharmacotherapy for Smoking Cessation

Michael G. Goldstein

Before the mid-1980s, no pharmacotherapies had been approved by the United States Food and Drug Administration (FDA) for smoking cessation. However, since nicotine gum, the first form of nicotine replacement therapy (NRT), the number of available pharmacological agents has increased rapidly. By 1998, four forms of NRT (gum, transdermal patch, nasal spray, and inhaler) and one antidepressant (bupropion sustained release, SR) had been approved by the FDA as treatments for smoking cessation. All five of these pharmacotherapies are recommended as first-line agents for treating tobacco addiction by the PHS Clinical Practice Guideline (Fiore et al., 2000). Evidence reviewed in the PHS guideline indicates that use of NRT or bupropion SR roughly doubles cessation rates (compared with placebo) independent of the type and intensity of accompanying treatment. The PHS guideline also recommends two agents, clonidine hydrocloride and nortriptyline, as second-line pharmacological agents to be considered by clinicians when first-line treatments are ineffective (Fiore et al., 2000).

Thus, based on the evidence available from clinical trials, all treatment plans for smokers who are ready to quit in the next 30 days should include a recommendation for pharmacotherapy with either NRT or bupropion (American Psychiatric Association Work Group on Nicotine Dependence, 1996; Fiore et al., 2000; J. R. Hughes, Goldstein, et al., 1999; see also Chapters 1 and 2). Some smokers may prefer to attempt cessation without pharmacotherapy. Decisions about the use of pharmacotherapy and the choice of a specific agent should be made collaboratively with the smoker (see Chapter 2). The pros and cons for using specific pharmacological agents are discussed in this chapter.

Because both transdermal nicotine and nicotine gum are now available over the counter (OTC), smokers who want to quit can obtain them without a physician's prescription. At least three placebo-controlled trials have demonstrated the efficacy of OTC NRT (American Psychiatric Association Work Group on Nicotine Dependence, 1996; J. R. Hughes, Goldstein, et

230

al., 1999). The availability of OTC NRT has further increased the need for smoking cessation specialists and health care providers to become fully informed about the use of pharmacotherapy in smoking cessation. In developing a treatment plan, you should assess prior use of pharmacotherapy for smoking cessation, as well as the smokers' attitudes and beliefs about pharmacotherapy. This information will help you correct misperceptions, address concerns about pharmacotherapy, and tailor the treatment plan to best meet the smokers' needs and preferences.

This chapter reviews (1) the rationale for pharmacological treatment of smokers; (2) the use of all four currently approved forms of NRT (nicotine gum, nicotine transdermal patches, nicotine nasal spray, and nicotine inhaler); (3) the use of bupropion SR; (4) use of clonidine, nortriptyline, other promising pharmacotherapies; and (5) strategies for tailoring pharmacotherapy for specific populations. Pharmacotherapy for smoking cessation should, if possible, be integrated into brief behavior treatment (Chapter 4) or intensive treatment (Chapters 5 and 6).

RATIONALE FOR PHARMACOTHERAPY FOR NICOTINE DEPENDENCE

The rationale for the use of pharmacotherapy for smoking cessation is based on the pharmacological actions of nicotine and the role of nicotine in promoting and maintaining nicotine dependence (N. Benowitz, 1998b; Henningfield, Cohen, & Pickworth, 1993; U.S. Department of Health and Human Services, 1988). The discussion that follows will assist you to understand the role of NRT, bupropion, and other pharmacological agents in treating smoking and help you to educate smokers and physicians about the mechanism and potential benefits of pharmacotherapy.

Cigarettes are an extremely efficient device for delivering nicotine. Nicotine is carried on tar droplets that are inhaled and deposited deep within the lung where nicotine is absorbed rapidly and efficiently (N. Benowitz, 1998a). From the lung, nicotine is carried directly to the left side of the heart, where it is pumped throughout the brain and body, creating a bolus effect that is greater than a direct injection of nicotine into a peripheral vein (Benowitz, 1998a). Nicotine rapidly accumulates in the brain after cigarette smoking and produces maximum brain concentrations within seconds (Henningfield et al., 1993).

The rapid accumulation of nicotine in the brain after cigarette smoking, in combination with nicotine's effects on brain activity and function, provide optimal conditions for the development of drug dependence (Henningfield et al., 1993; U.S. Department of Health and Human Services, 1988). Acute and chronic tolerance to many effects of nicotine contributes to an increase in cigarette consumption, as individuals smoke more to obtain desired effects of nicotine. Nicotine delivered in a cigarette is an ideal drug for "self-medication" to improve biobehavioral functioning (see Chapter 1).

Nicotine's wide variety of stimulant and depressant effects contribute to positive reinforcement and nicotine self-administration (N. Benowitz, 1998a; Henningfield et al., 1993; U.S. Department of Health and Human Services, 1988). The rewarding properties of nicotine appear to be related to nicotine's stimulatory effects on dopaminergic pathways in the mesolimbic system of the brain, an area known to be involved in reinforcement for several drugs of abuse (N. Benowitz, 1998a; Koob & LeMoal, 2001). Nicotine has stimulating effects similar to those of the psychostimulants amphetamine and methylphenidate and has been shown to increase attention, memory, the speed of information processing, and learning in smokers, especially in the setting of low environmental demand, when stimulation is most desirable (e.g., a blue-collar worker performing repetitive tasks on an assembly line; N. Benowitz, 1998a). Because nicotine also has antianxiety, antipain, and antidepressant effects, smokers are more apt to use cigarettes during stressful situations or in situations involving negative mood. There is a strong association between a history of clinical depression, the presence of depressive symptoms, and subsequent difficulty in quitting smoking (N. Benowitz, 1998a; Glassman, 1997).

Nicotine's metabolic effects include both increased metabolic rate and decreased appetite. Smoking cessation is associated with an increase in appetite and caloric intake, particularly of sweet foods, resulting in an increased body weight of 4 kg, on average, after cessation (N. Benowitz, 1998a). These effects on appetite and weight are important for the many smokers who smoke to reduce appetite and prevent weight gain. Considerable variability exists in nicotine's effects between and within individuals over time. From this discussion of the multiple reinforcing and rewarding effects of nicotine, it is easy to understand how nicotine, especially when delivered so rapidly and efficiently via smoking cigarettes, is highly reinforcing and addictive and how many smokers appear to use nicotine to "self-medicate" to improve mood, attention, and performance and to control weight (see also Chapter 1).

The characteristics and patterns of chronic nicotine use have much in common with the use of other psychotropic drugs. Nicotine is included among the drugs that may produce psychoactive substance dependence (see Table 7.1) in the fourth edition of the American Psychiatric Association's *Diagnostic and Statistical Manual of Mental Disorders* (DSM-IV; American Psychiatric Association, 1994). One of the principal rationales for the use of pharmacotherapy in

TABLE 7.1. Diagnostic Criteria for Nicotine Dependence

A maladaptive pattern of substance use, leading to clinically significant impairment or distress, as manifested by three (or more) of the following, occurring at any time in the same 12-month period:

1. Tolerance, as defined by either:
   - a need for markedly increased amounts of the substance to achieve desired effect
   - markedly diminished effect with continued use of the same amount of substance
2. Withdrawal, as manifested by either:
   - the characteristic withdrawal syndrome for the substance
   - the substance is taken to relieve or avoid withdrawal symptoms
3. The substance is often taken in larger amounts or over a longer period than was intended.
4. There is persistent desire or unsuccessful effort to cut down substance use.
5. A great deal of time is spent in activities necessary to obtain the substance or use the substance.
6. Important social, occupational, or recreational activities are given up or reduced because of substance abuse.
7. The substance use is continued despite knowledge of having a persistent or recurrent physical or psychological problem that is likely to have been caused or exacerbated by the substance.

Note. Reprinted with permission from the *Diagnostic and Statistical Manual of Mental Disorders*, Fourth Edition, Text Revision. Copyright 2000 American Psychiatric Association.

TABLE 7.2. Diagnostic Criteria for Nicotine Withdrawal

A. Daily use of nicotine for at least several weeks.
B. Abrupt cessation of nicotine use, or reduction in the amount of nicotine used, followed within 24 hours by four (or more) of the following signs:
   1. dysphoric or depressed mood
   2. insomnia
   3. irritability, frustration, or anger
   4. anxiety
   5. difficulty concentrating
   6. restlessness
   7. decreased heart rate
   8. increased appetite or weight gain
C. The symptoms in Criterion B cause clinically significant distress or impairment in social, occupational, or other important areas of functioning.
D. The symptoms are not due to a general medical condition and are not better accounted for by another mental disorder.

Note. Reprinted with permission from the *Diagnostic and Statistical Manual of Mental Disorders*, Fourth Edition, Text Revision. Copyright 2000 American Psychiatric Association.

smoking cessation is an attempt to attenuate the nicotine withdrawal syndrome (see Table 7.2 for the DSM-IV criteria), which is experienced by approximately 50% of smokers who make a serious attempt to quit smoking without pharmacological assistance (American Psychiatric Association, 1994). The signs and symptoms of the nicotine withdrawal syndrome can appear within 2 hours after the last use of tobacco, usually peak between 24 and 48 hours after cessation, and usually last from a few days to 4 weeks, though craving and subclinical symptoms (e.g., malaise, low energy, difficulty concentrating) can persist for months (J. Hughes & Hatsukami, 1992). The average decrease in heart rate is eight beats per minute, and the average weight gain is 4 kg (N. Benowitz, 1998a; J. Hughes & Hatsukami, 1992). Weight gain and fear of weight gain are important deterrents to smoking cessation, particularly among women (Perkins et al., 2001; Pomerleau & Kurth, 1996). The role of specific pharmacological agents in addressing weight concerns during smoking cessation treatment is discussed later in this chapter.

PHARMACOLOGICAL TREATMENT OPTIONS FOR SMOKING CESSATION

Now that I have briefly reviewed the pharmacological properties of nicotine, including its rapid absorption and delivery to the brain, its multiple reinforcing effects, and the nature of nicotine dependence and withdrawal, I consider specific pharmacological treatments for smoking. Pharmacological treatments can be characterized using the same typology that has been developed for treating other forms of drug dependence (Jarvik & Henningfield, 1988): nicotine replacement therapy (NRT); nonspecific pharmacotherapy (i.e., antidepressants, anxiolytics, treatment of weight gain); blockade therapy (i.e., mecamylamine); and deterrents (i.e., silver acetate). At present, only agents from the first two categories have been approved by the FDA for smoking cessation or recommended by clinical practice guidelines (American

Psychiatric Association Work Group on Nicotine Dependence, 1996; Fiore et al., 2000). Recommendations for use of NRT and nonspecific pharmacotherapy are described in detail in the sections that follow, using specific agents as examples.

Nicotine Replacement Therapy

The principle of replacement therapy is to provide the smoker with a more manageable and safer form of the drug, in this case nicotine, to ameliorate withdrawal symptoms and allow the smoker to gradually discontinue use of the drug. Replacement therapy also provides an opportunity to develop strategies to deal with behavioral or learned components of the drug dependence while controlling the physiological "need" for the drug. Moreover, if the method of administration of the replacement drug is sufficiently different from the method associated with the development of drug dependence, the learned associations between cues associated with drug administration and physiological effect can be broken (see Chapter 1 for more details on learning theory).

Forms of Nicotine Replacement Therapy

As mentioned earlier, four forms of NRT have been approved by the FDA for use as aids to smoking cessation: nicotine gum (2 and 4 mg), transdermal nicotine, nicotine nasal spray, and nicotine inhaler. The PHS Clinical Practice Guideline (Fiore et al., 2000) concluded that all four forms of NRT were efficacious as smoking cessation interventions across a variety of diverse settings and populations and even when administered with minimal adjuvant behavioral and psychosocial interventions. Nicotine gum and nicotine transdermal patches are effective when used OTC (American Psychiatric Association Work Group on Nicotine Dependence, 1996; Fiore et al., 2000; J. R. Hughes, Goldstein, et al., 1999). Though nicotine nasal spray and nicotine inhaler are currently not available OTC and less evidence exists regarding their efficacy in minimal contact settings, there is no reason to believe that they will perform differently from transdermal nicotine or nicotine gum with minimal adjunctive treatment. However, absolute smoking cessation rates are clearly enhanced when more intensive behavioral treatment is provided along with NRT (American Psychiatric Association Work Group on Nicotine Dependence, 1996; J. R. Hughes, Goldstein, et al., 1999; Fiore et al., 2000).

We recommend that smoker preferences guide the choice of type of NRT. This conclusion is based on the following evidence: (1) three of the four forms of NRT (i.e., transdermal patches, nasal spray, and inhaler) have very similar efficacies (i.e., each approximately doubles smoking cessation rate over placebo controls); (2) though the efficacy of nicotine gum is slightly lower than the other three, this difference may be due to decreased adherence to treatment recommendations for gum use, as well as improper chewing technique; (3) direct comparisons of different forms of NRT have found no evidence of differential efficacy (Hajek et al., 1999); and (4) there is no evidence to suggest that specific forms of NRT are more effective with subgroups of smokers. However, highly dependent smokers, as measured by the Fagerstrom Tolerance Questionnaire (FTQ; Fagerstrom & Schneider, 1989), and smokers who smoke more than 25 cigarettes per day benefit more from the 4-mg dosage than from the

2-mg gum (Fiore et al., 2000; J. R. Hughes, Goldstein, et al., 1999). Thus we recommend the use of the 4-mg dose of nicotine gum when highly dependent smokers choose gum as their preferred form of NRT.

Smoker preference for a specific form of NRT is affected by a number of factors, including past experiences with NRT, the relative number and severity of side effects, ease and convenience of use, relative impact on weight gain associated with smoking cessation, and effect on craving for cigarettes. The following sections of this chapter provide detailed information about each of the four forms of NRT to assist clinicians in tailoring treatment to smoker preferences.

Transdermal Nicotine

Transdermal nicotine, compared with placebo, doubles 6-month to 1-year quit rates (Fiore et al., 2000). Absolute 6-month quit rates range from 9% in OTC studies to more than 50% in clinic-based studies that provided group-based behavioral therapy. Though smokers with high levels of nicotine dependence (as measured with the FTQ; see Chapter 2) are less likely to be successful in quitting smoking, both high- and low-dependent smokers benefit from the use of transdermal nicotine (American Psychiatric Association Work Group on Nicotine Dependence, 1996; Fiore et al., 2000).

Many smokers prefer transdermal patches to other forms of NRT because of ease of use (e.g., one application per day) and more tolerable side effects (Fiore et al., 2000). The OTC availability of nicotine patches simplifies access. The downside of patch use for some is that patches, unlike other forms of NRT, cannot be used to mollify specific episodes of craving or as behavioral (oral) substitutes for cigarettes. For smokers concerned about weight gain, nicotine gum and bupropion may be preferable, as these agents appear to delay weight gain during active treatment (Fiore et al., 2000; Gross, Stitzer, & Maldonadok, 1989; Jorenby et al., 1999). Some smokers prefer non-nicotine pharmacotherapy and wish to avoid all forms of NRT. They may benefit from gradually cutting down on nicotine exposure prior to quitting, using either brand or rate fading (see Chapter 5 for details; Foxx & Brown, 1979).

Dose selection is based primarily on rate of smoking. The PHS guideline recommends that smokers who smoke more than 10 cigarettes per day use the highest dose nicotine transdermal patch (i.e., 21- or 22-mg 24-hour patches; 15-mg 16-hour patches). Those smoking fewer than 10 cigarettes per day can be started on the middle dose patch. Higher dose patches (higher than 22 mg) or use of more than one nicotine transdermal patch have not been demonstrated to enhance quit rates in controlled clinical trials. Patch use may be discontinued after 8 weeks by tapering the dose. Most of the clinical trials utilized protocols that tapered dose of the patch over several weeks. We recommend that the initial dose patch be continued for 2 to 4 weeks before stepping down to the intermediate and lowest doses of patches for 2 weeks each. There does not appear to be any benefit to use of transdermal patches beyond 8 weeks (Fiore et al., 2000).

The choice of 16-hour versus 24-hour patches is also based on smoker preference. The 24-hour patch appears to be more likely to cause sleep disturbance or vivid dreams, whereas use of the 16-hour patch (and the absence of nicotine delivery overnight) may lead to early-morning withdrawal symptoms (Leischow et al., 1997). Insomnia and dreams related to 24-

hour patches usually improve over time with continued use. Twenty-four hour patches may also be removed at bedtime if significant sleep problems arise. We recommend providing smokers with information about the benefits and problems related to duration of action and allowing them to choose the patch they prefer. Nicotine transdermal patches should be avoided during pregnancy and by women who are breastfeeding because of potential adverse effects on the developing fetus and newborn (Fiore et al., 2000; Slotkin, 1998). Patches may not be tolerable for smokers with allergies to adhesive or generalized skin diseases. Transdermal nicotine's most frequent adverse effects are skin reactions, insomnia, and vivid dreams (American Psychiatric Association Work Group on Nicotine Dependence, 1996). The safety of nicotine transdermal patches and nicotine gum in smokers with cardiovascular disease is discussed later in this section.

Providers should instruct smokers to apply their first patch as soon as they arise on their quit day (see the preceding discussion for dosing recommendations). Quitters may experience some withdrawal discomfort the first few hours after applying their first patch, because nicotine levels will not reach steady state for several hours. Patches should be applied to a relatively hairless, though unshaven, clean and dry skin location, preferably above the waist. New patches should be reapplied at approximately the same time each day. Patch sites should be rotated to limit skin irritation. Should minor skin irritation or itching occur, hydrocortisone cream, available OTC, may provide relief. It is not necessary to limit activity while wearing the patch. If a patch falls off, it is best to apply a fresh patch. Quitters should not smoke while on the patch and should discontinue patch use if they smoke more than five cigarettes per day for several consecutive days. Patch use may be resumed if the smoker sets and keeps a new quit day. Table 7.3 provides a summary of recommendations for patch use.

TABLE 7.3. Suggestions for Use of Nicotine Transdermal Patches

Selection of smokers:	Avoid during pregnancy and breastfeeding, in the presence of unstable angina or other unstable vascular disease. Smokers with an allergy to adhesive or generalized skin diseases may be unable to use patches.
Dosage and duration:	Initially, use highest dose patch *unless* smoking less than 10 cigarettes per day or if the smoker weighs less than 100 pounds. After 4 weeks at initial dose, taper to intermediate dose for 2 weeks and lowest dose for 2 weeks. Consider supplementing with nicotine gum if breakthrough craving or withdrawal occur. Use of more than one patch at a time can be considered for smokers with significant withdrawal symptoms on single patch.
16- vs. 24-hour patches:	Based on smoker preference. Twenty-four hour patch is more likely to cause sleep disturbance or vivid dreams, whereas 16-hour patch may be associated with early-morning withdrawal symptoms.
Instructions for use:	Apply first patch after awakening on quit day. Apply patches to a relatively hairless, though unshaven, clean, and dry skin location, preferably above the waist. Apply new patches at the same time each day. Rotate patch sites to limit skin irritation. Instruct smokers not to smoke while on patch and to discontinue patch if they smoke more than five cigarettes per day for several consecutive days.

Note. Adapted from the "Practice Guideline for the Treatment of Patients with Nicotine Dependence," by the American Psychiatric Association Work Group on Nicotine Dependence, 1996, *American Journal of Psychiatry, 153*(10, Suppl.), 1–31. Adapted with permission from the American Psychiatric Association (*www.appi.org*).

Nicotine Gum

Major meta-analyses of research studies have demonstrated that nicotine gum is efficacious and increases smoking cessation rates by about 40% to 60% when compared to placebo or controlled interventions (Fiore et al., 2000). Some smokers prefer nicotine gum because they have control over the dosing of gum and can use the gum as needed to control craving or as an oral substitute for a cigarette. Recent research suggests that nicotine gum may be uniquely effective in helping those smokers who experience more frequent or severe acute cigarette cravings (Shiffman et al., in press). Nicotine gum also appears to be more effective at limiting or delaying postcessation weight gain, and there appears to be a dose–response relationship between nicotine gum use and weight gain suppression (Fiore et al., 2000). The OTC availability of nicotine gum simplifies access to this form of NRT. Negative aspects of gum use that may influence smoker preferences include the frequency and type of side effects (e.g., oral and jaw soreness, dental problems, nausea, belching, stomach upset), the need to take multiple doses per day, the inconvenience of having to carry gum, and the need to chew gum in public, which may be a particular problem in some occupational or social settings.

The choice of dose of nicotine gum is based on smokers' level of nicotine dependence. Highly dependent smokers are more likely to benefit from the use of the 4-mg nicotine gum than the 2-mg nicotine gum (American Psychiatric Association Work Group on Nicotine Dependence, 1996; Fiore et al., 2000). Therefore, we recommend that the following subgroups of smokers initiate treatment with 4-mg nicotine gum: (1) smokers scoring 7 or greater on the FTQ (see Chapter 2); (2) smokers who smoke more than 25 cigarettes per day; and (3) smokers who have had significant withdrawal symptoms or who have failed to achieve long-term abstinence using 2-mg gum. Smokers, especially highly dependent smokers, appear to derive the most benefit from nicotine gum when they chew at least one piece every 1–2 hours on a fixed schedule for the first few weeks (Fiore et al., 2000; Goldstein et al., 1989; J. R. Hughes, Goldstein et al., 1999).

Because the effectiveness of nicotine gum depends on whether the gum is chewed correctly, all nicotine gum users should receive careful and detailed instructions for proper use (see Table 7.4). Nicotine gum is buffered, as absorption is most efficient at higher pHs. Thus

TABLE 7.4. Suggestions for Use of Nicotine Gum

Selection of smokers:	Avoid during pregnancy and breastfeeding, in the presence of unstable angina or other unstable vascular disease. Smokers with jaw pain, gum disease, poor dentition, or peptic ulcer disease may be unable to use due to side effects.
Dosage and duration:	Smokers with high levels of nicotine dependence (more than 25 cigarettes per day, smoking within 30 minutes after awakening) should use 4-mg gum. Initially, smokers should chew at least 1 piece per hour for several weeks, then taper gradually. Maximum is 30 pieces per day for 2 mg, 20 pieces per day for 4 mg.
Instruct	Smoker not to smoke while using gum. Gum must be chewed properly to get benefit and avoid side effects. Chew slowly until taste emerges, then "park" between gum and cheek to facilitate absorption. Alternate chewing and parking for 20–30 minutes. Acidic beverages must be avoided before and during gum use.

Note. Adapted with permission from the American Psychiatric Association (*www.appi.org*) from the "Practice Guideline for the Treatment of Patients with Nicotine Dependence," by the American Psychiatric Association Work Group on Nicotine Dependence, 1996, *American Journal of Psychiatry, 153*(10, Suppl.), 1–31; and with permission from Springer-Verlag from "Nicotine Gum: Pharmacological and Clinical Aspects," by M. G. Goldstein and R. S. Niaura, 1991, in J. A. Cocores (Ed.), *Clinical Management of Nicotine Dependence* (pp. 181–195), New York: Springer-Verlag.

it is important for users to learn to chew slowly for several seconds and then "park" the gum between the cheek and gums. Acidic beverages (e.g., coffee, tea, citrus juices) should be avoided before or during gum use. Fast or vigorous chewing will lead to inefficient absorption, lower blood nicotine levels, less benefit, and more side effects in the mouth, pharynx, and gastrointestinal tract. We recommend having samples of gum available at treatment visits so that smokers can be taught to use the gum correctly and given feedback if chewing technique is faulty.

Nicotine Nasal Spray

Nicotine nasal spray was approved by the FDA in 1996 and was included as an effective first-line agent for smoking cessation in the PHS guideline (Fiore et al., 2000). As with nicotine gum, some smokers prefer nicotine nasal spray to transdermal patches because they have control over the dosing of nasal spray and can use it as needed to control craving. The nasal spray provides a more rapid rise in nicotine levels than either transdermal or gum products, with peak levels of nicotine occurring within 10 minutes (American Psychiatric Association Work Group on Nicotine Dependence, 1996). However, in weighing the pros and cons of choosing nicotine nasal spray, smokers need to know that the nasal spray has considerably more side effects than other forms of NRT. These include nasal and throat irritation, rhinitis, sneezing, coughing, and watering eyes, though tolerance develops to these effects (American Psychiatric Association Work Group on Nicotine Dependence, 1996; Hurt et al., 1998). Nicotine nasal spray may also have greater dependence liability, which may be related to the spray's rapid onset of action (American Psychiatric Association Work Group on Nicotine Dependence, 1996). The side effects associated with nicotine nasal spray may limit abuse liability. Another downside from the user's point of view is the need to obtain a physician's prescription for nicotine nasal spray.

In our opinion, nicotine nasal spray seems best suited for those who are highly dependent (based on numbers of cigarettes smoked per day, FTQ score, or previous withdrawal symptoms) or those who have failed other forms of NRT. However, only one study (Sutherland et al., 1992) reported that nicotine nasal spray was more beneficial for highly dependent smokers. Quitters using nicotine nasal spray are instructed to use 1–2 doses per hour for 3 months. Maximum recommended use is 5 doses per hour or 40 doses in 24 hours. Before administering the spray, quitters are instructed to blow their noses, tilt their heads back slightly, and insert the tip of the spray bottle into one nostril as far as is comfortable. Users should continue to breathe through the mouth while spraying once in each nostril, being careful not to sniff or inhale while spraying. If the nose runs, users may gently sniff but should avoid blowing their noses for 2 to 3 minutes.

Nicotine Inhalers

Nicotine inhalers produce a nicotine vapor when air is drawn into the mouth and throat through a plastic tube containing a nicotine plug. Nicotine is absorbed through the cheeks, and significant amounts of nicotine vapor do not reach the lungs. Peak plasma nicotine levels occur after 15 to 20 minutes of almost continuous puffing (i.e., 80 deep draws over 20 minutes). Inhalers were approved by the FDA in 1997 and became available as a prescription product in the United States in the spring of 1998. Inhalers were included as first-line treatments for effective smoking cessation in the PHS guideline (Fiore et al., 2000).

Use of the inhaler substitutes for some of the behavioral components of smoking (e.g., puffing, handling), which may be a particularly attractive feature for some smokers. Nicotine inhalers share with nicotine gum the feature of oral substitution. The availability of an oral substitute during the quitting process may help some smokers manage oral cravings and provide a behavioral strategy for managing increased caloric intake and associated weight gain after quitting. Because of slow absorption and few subjective effects, dependence liability appears to be quite low. Negative aspects of inhaler use include the need to continuously use the inhaler for 15 to 20 minutes and the inconvenience of having to carry the inhaler and use it in public or social situations. As with nicotine nasal spray, another negative aspect from the user's point of view is the need to obtain a physician's prescription for the inhaler.

Successful quitters in the research clinical trials used between 6 and 16 cartridges a day (each cartridge contains 4 mg of nicotine). The recommended treatment is up to 3 months, followed by gradual reduction over the next 6–12 weeks. Total treatment should not exceed 6 months. Side effects are quite mild and include coughing and throat irritation. The nicotine inhaler loses significant bioavailability at ambient temperatures below 50 degrees Fahrenheit (J. R. Hughes, Goldstein, et al., 1999). As with nicotine gum, acidic beverages should be avoided for 15 minutes before and after inhalation, as they interfere with absorption of nicotine in the mouth (Fiore et al., 2000).

Combination Nicotine Replacement Therapy

Smokers who do not succeed with a single form of NRT may benefit from the combination of nicotine patches with either nicotine gum or nicotine spray (American Psychiatric Association Work Group on Nicotine Dependence, 1996; Fiore et al., 2000; J. R. Hughes, Goldstein, et al., 1999). The combination of transdermal nicotine and an ad libitum form of NRT (e.g., gum or spray) may be particularly useful for quitters who continue to have significant cravings while on the nicotine patch alone. We recommend consideration of this combination when quitters have failed either form of NRT alone. When combining patch and gum, the dose of transdermal nicotine should be the highest available dose, whereas the dose of nicotine gum is usually 2 mg, even for heavy smokers who would normally be advised to use 4-mg nicotine gum.

Use of NRT in Smokers with Cardiovascular Disease

Because of anecdotal reports of myocardial infarctions in users who smoked cigarettes while using transdermal nicotine, the safety of NRT for smokers with cardiovascular disease was questioned. However, transdermal nicotine produces considerably lower peak plasma nicotine levels than cigarette smoking, even if the smoker continues to smoke during treatment (Joseph et al., 1996), and two studies of transdermal nicotine in smokers with cardiovascular disease found no increase in angina, arrhythmias, ischemia, or cardiac events (Joseph et al., 1996; Working Group for the Study of Transdermal Nicotine in Patients with Coronary Artery Disease, 1994). Moreover, nicotine gum use was not associated with any cardiovascular illness or events in more than 3,000 participants in the Lung Health Study (R. P. Murray et al., 1996). To our knowledge, the safety of nicotine nasal spray and nicotine inhaler therapy has not been specifically tested in smokers with cardiovascular disease.

Non-Nicotine Pharmacotherapy

Bupropion

Because of the relationship between nicotine dependence and mood disorders (Glassman, 1997), researchers have considered antidepressants as potential treatments for smoking cessation. Bupropion is an antidepressant that exhibits both noradrenergic and dopaminergic activity (Ascher et al., 1995). Bupropion's dopaminergic effects may be especially relevant given nicotine's stimulatory effects on dopaminergic pathways in the mesolimbic system of the brain.

Based on the results of two large multicenter randomized controlled trials, the PHS guideline (Fiore et al., 2000) recommends bupropion as a first-line pharmacological treatment for smoking cessation. Results from a randomized controlled trial comparing transdermal nicotine, bupropion, and a double placebo found that treatment with bupropion alone or in combination with a transdermal nicotine resulted in significantly higher 12-month cessation rates (30% for bupropion, 35% for the combination of bupropion and transdermal nicotine) than use of either the nicotine patch alone (16%) or placebo (16%; Jorenby et al., 1999). These results suggest that bupropion is at least as effective as transdermal nicotine.

As noted previously, choice of pharmacotherapy is based primarily on smoker preferences. Some prefer to use a non-nicotine treatment, and others prefer a pill over patches, gum, inhalers, and nasal spray. Bupropion SR, like nicotine gum, also appears to delay weight gain after smoking cessation (Jorenby et al., 1999). A downside of bupropion use is that, like transdermal patches, bupropion cannot be used to ameliorate specific episodes of craving or as behavioral substitutes for cigarettes. Bupropion also has frequent side effects, and some side effects are considerably more serious than those seen with NRT. In clinical trials, the 300-mg dose of bupropion SR produced 8–12% discontinuation rates due to adverse events. The most common reasons for discontinuation were tremor, rash, headache, and urticaria. Only insomnia and dry mouth were significantly more likely to occur in active treatment than in placebo. Because bupropion may lower the threshold for seizures, it is contraindicated in smokers with a history of seizures and should be used with caution in smokers with a personal or family history of seizures, active alcohol or other substance abuse, a history of anorexia or bulimia, or a history of head injury. However, no seizures were reported in any of the bupropion SR smoking cessation trials, which included a total of 1,828 smokers. Other, less common but potentially important adverse effects of bupropion, include agitation, exacerbation of high blood pressure, and liver function abnormalities. Thus quitters who have a predisposition to these adverse effects or those who wish to minimize the risk of serious side effects may choose NRT over bupropion.

Another reason for choosing bupropion over NRT relates to its antidepressant effects. Though bupropion's efficacy as an aid for smoking cessation appears to be independent of its antidepressant effects (Hayford et al., 1999), emerging evidence indicates that antidepressants may be particularly helpful as a smoking cessation treatment for those with coexisting depressive symptoms (Dalack, Glassman, Rivelli, Covey, & Stetner, 1995; Niaura et al., 1995). When smokers with a history of recurrent depression or dysthymia present for smoking cessation, bupropion may be the pharmacological treatment of choice. Antidepressants may be useful for treating nicotine dependence for several reasons: a history of depression is associated with increased difficulty in smoking cessation; depressive symptoms commonly occur during nicotine withdrawal, especially when there is a past history of depression; nicotine appears to be a powerful regulator of negative affect; and antidepressants have been useful in ameliorating the withdrawal state associated with other drugs (American Psychiatric Association Work Group on Nicotine Dependence, 1996).

Nortriptyline

Two randomized controlled trials of the tricyclic antidepressant nortriptyline demonstrated the efficacy of this agent as a treatment for smoking cessation (Hall et al., 1998; Prochazka et al., 1998). These studies led the PHS guideline to recommend nortriptyline as a second-line treatment for smoking cessation (Fiore et al., 2000). In smoking cessation trials, the starting dose of nortriptyline was 25 mg. The dose was gradually increased to a target dose of 75–100 mg per day (Fiore et al., 2000). Side effects are common and include sedation, dry mouth, blurred vision, urinary retention, constipation, lightheadedness, and tremor. Nortriptyline should be used with extreme caution in smokers with cardiovascular disease because of its potential to cause heart rhythm and heart muscle abnormalities. See the discussion of tailoring pharmacotherapy for smokers with comorbid depression and anxiety in the following section.

Clonidine Hydrochloride

Clonidine is an alpha-2 agonist that dampens sympathetic activity and attenuates withdrawal symptoms associated with alcohol, opiate, and nicotine abstinence (American Psychiatric Association Work Group on Nicotine Dependence, 1996). The PHS Clinical Practice Guideline panel (Fiore et al., 2000) concluded that clonidine was more effective than placebo in promoting abstinence from smoking. Doses used for smoking cessation are 0.1–0.75 mg per day for 2–6 weeks in oral or transdermal formulations (American Psychiatric Association Work Group on Nicotine Dependence, 1996; Fiore et al., 2000). The most common side effects are sedation, dry mouth, constipation, lightheadedness, and postural hypotension (Gourlay & Benowitz, 1995). The APA Clinical Practice Guideline (American Psychiatric Association Work Group on Nicotine Dependence, 1996) and the PHS guideline (Fiore et al., 2000) both recommend clonidine as an alternative for smokers who prefer not to receive nicotine and for smokers who have failed NRT.

Tailoring Pharmacotherapy for Specific Populations

The following sections of this chapter provide guidelines for tailoring pharmacotherapy for use in specific populations. These populations include smokers with comorbid depression and anxiety, comorbid alcohol and substance abuse, weight concerns, adolescent smokers, and smokers using smokeless tobacco. Because limited empirical evidence exists to guide treatment for these populations, our recommendations are based primarily on our clinical experience and our understanding of the factors contributing to nicotine dependence (see also the discussion of the actions of nicotine earlier in this chapter).

Smokers with Comorbid Depression and Anxiety

As noted earlier in this chapter, nicotine has both stimulant and anxiolytic effects; many smokers use cigarettes during stressful situations or in situations involving negative moods (U.S. Department of Health and Human Services, 1988), and there is a strong association between a history of clinical depression, depressive symptoms, and difficulty in quitting smoking (Glassman, 1997). Also, smokers with a history of depression or bipolar disorder may be at risk for developing a relapse to depression after smoking cessation (American Psychiatric Association Work Group on Nicotine Dependence, 1996). Though the efficacy of bupropion and nortriptyline for treating nicotine dependence appears to be independent of their antidepressant effects (Hall et al., 1998; Hayford et al., 1999), there is some evidence that antidepressants may be particularly helpful as a smoking cessation treatment for smokers with coexisting depressive symptoms (Dalack et al., 1995; Hayford et al., 1999; Niaura et al., 1995).

Smokers with a history of depression or anxiety should be carefully assessed for the presence of depressive or anxiety symptoms when they wish to attempt smoking cessation (see Chapter 2). Smokers on maintenance antidepressant or anxiolytic therapy should have their pharmacotherapy adjusted and psychotherapy intensified to minimize depressive symptoms before smoking cessation is attempted. These smokers can be treated with NRT in addition to their usual antidepressant or anxiolytic medication during an initial treatment attempt. Those smokers who have failed the combination of NRT and their usual antidepressant can be treated with either the combination of bupropion and NRT (substituting bupropion for their maintenance antidepressant) or bupropion in addition to their usual antidepressant (watching carefully for drug interactions). When treating smokers on antidepressants other than bupropion, providers should be aware that some antidepressant levels will increase with smoking cessation (American Psychiatric Association Work Group on Nicotine Dependence, 1996).

We recommend that smokers with a history of depression or who are *not* on maintenance antidepressants be treated with bupropion when they are ready to quit smoking. Those smokers with contraindications to bupropion or significant side effects during previous bupropion treatment can be treated with NRT, nortriptyline, or the combination of NRT and nortriptyline (Hall et al., 1998; Prochazka et al., 1998). Smokers with a history of comorbid anxiety may also be treated with NRT, bupropion, or both, though bupropion may exacerbate anxiety symptoms in some smokers. A trial of the combination of NRT and an antidepressant with anxiolytic properties (e.g., paroxetine, nefazodone) is another option for smokers with an anxiety disorder.

Smokers with Comorbid Alcohol and Substance Abuse

Because it is unlikely that smokers with current alcohol or drug problems will stop smoking without addressing their alcohol and other drug dependencies, alcohol and/or drug abuse should be treated prior to or concurrent with treatment of nicotine dependence (American Psychiatric Association Work Group on Nicotine Dependence, 1996). However, it is not known whether it is more advantageous to stop smoking at the same time one is attempting to abstain from other drugs or after smokers have achieved stable sobriety from other drugs. Frequent monitoring and increased levels of support are wise when smokers with histories of alcohol and substance abuse attempt smoking cessation (American Psychiatric Association Work Group on Nicotine Dependence, 1996).

There is little scientific evidence to guide the choice of pharmacotherapies for smoking cessation in the context of alcohol or other drug abuse. However, because smokers with other drug dependencies may have higher levels of nicotine dependence (American Psychiatric Association Work Group on Nicotine Dependence, 1996), the highest doses of nicotine replacement should always be considered. Treatment of comorbid depression or anxiety may also be needed, as these disorders are also more likely in alcohol and substance abusers.

Smokers with Weight Concerns

Although weight gain occurs among the majority of smokers who quit, most will gain fewer than 10 pounds, and the weight gain that follows smoking cessation is a negligible health threat compared with the risks of continued smoking (American Psychiatric Association Work Group on Nicotine Dependence, 1996). However, perceptions (e.g., expectations) of weight gain can be a powerful factor that undermines smoking cessation (see Perkins et al., 2001). Nicotine gum appears to be effective at limiting postcessation weight gain during nicotine gum use, and there appears to be a dose–response relationship between nicotine gum use and weight gain suppression (Fiore et al., 2000; Gross et al., 1989). A recent study suggests that transdermal nicotine use reduced weight gain compared with placebo (Jorenby et al., 1996). There is also a dose–response relationship between bupropion dose and weight gain suppression during bupropion treatment (Hurt et al., 1997). However, after discontinuing nicotine gum or bupropion, the quitting smoker is likely to gain an amount of weight that is equivalent to the amount he/she would have gained if he/she had not used the drug (Fiore et al., 2000; Hurt et al., 1997). Vigorous exercise programs (see Chapters 1 and 5) also appear to hold some promise in preventing postcessation weight gain (Marcus et al., 1999).

Adolescent Smokers

Adolescent smokers who wish to quit should be considered for pharmacotherapy when there is evidence of nicotine dependence, particularly if nicotine withdrawal symptoms were present on previous efforts to quit smoking (American Psychiatric Association Work Group on

Nicotine Dependence, 1996; Fiore et al., 2000). Adolescents who smoke fewer than 10 cigarettes a day, or whose smoking pattern is variable and inconsistent, should probably not use nicotine replacement as a first-line treatment because of the risk of accelerating the development of nicotine dependence.

Smokeless Tobacco Users

Individuals using smokeless tobacco, such as chewing tobacco and snuff, may become nicotine dependent and may develop a withdrawal syndrome upon cessation (N. L. Benowitz, 1988; U.S. Department of Health and Human Services, 1988). The one study that has evaluated the efficacy of NRT in smokeless tobacco users demonstrated no benefit in cessation outcomes when compared with placebo (Hatsukami & Boyle, 1997). Despite the lack of evidence of the efficacy of pharmacological treatments for smokeless tobacco use, a trial of pharmacotherapy is warranted in those who have failed to quit because of withdrawal symptoms (American Psychiatric Association Work Group on Nicotine Dependence, 1996).

   In previous sections of this chapter, I have reviewed the rationale for pharmacological treatment of nicotine dependence and have provided information on the use of nicotine replacement therapy, bupropion, and other promising pharmacotherapies for smoking cessation. Ideally, selection of a specific pharmacological agent for an individual smoker is based on a thorough assessment, which includes an evaluation of the smoker's nicotine dependence, comorbid medical and psychiatric illnesses, past experience with quitting, and preferences for treatment. Chapter 2 presents a detailed description of the assessment process. The following case examples illustrate our approach to choosing pharmacological agents to help smokers to quit smoking.

CASE EXAMPLES

CASE EXAMPLE: MR. B

Background Information

Mr. B. is a 33-year-old divorced man who is a medical outpatient in a hospital-based family medicine clinic. He has mild hypertension and a chronic cough but no other signs of chronic obstructive pulmonary disease. As Mr. B.'s clinical nurse specialist, you have been working with him for 2 years to increase his motivation to quit smoking, and today Mr. B. has told you that he would like to make a serious attempt to quit smoking. You praise him for his commitment to quitting, and your assessment elicits the following information:

Dependence: Smokes 30 cigarettes per day (1.1 mg nicotine content).
                       Smokes first cigarette immediately on awakening.

Past quit attempts:	Quit three times in the past, but only for 1 or 2 days, most recently 2 years ago. He had moderate nicotine withdrawal symptoms when he tried to quit "cold turkey." Tried nicotine patches during last quit attempt, with good initial control over withdrawal symptoms, but had moderate to severe craving; after 2 days, discontinued patches because he resumed smoking.
Substance abuse:	Currently in recovery for alcohol dependence; attends two AA meetings per week; has been totally abstinent from alcohol for 5 years. Mr. B. also drinks 8 to 10 cups of coffee per day.
Psychiatric history:	Meets criteria for generalized anxiety disorder; on buspirone 5 mg three times a day, with moderate control of symptoms.
Medical history:	Head injury due to a motor vehicle accident when he was 20; no sequelae; hypertension well controlled with a beta blocker. There is no history of or evidence of coronary artery disease.

Mr. B. is very concerned about how he will manage craving and anxiety when he tries to quit. He is also concerned about going to AA meetings, at which smoking is quite prevalent. He is willing to try nicotine replacement again and likes the idea of combining nicotine patches with a more immediate form of nicotine replacement to increase his control over urges. Mr. B. was not aware that blood caffeine levels increase after quitting smoking if caffeine intake is not altered. When told of this effect, he expresses concern that increased caffeine levels might exacerbate his anxiety symptoms. Mr. B. is also willing to increase his dose of buspirone to protect against an exacerbation of his anxiety disorder.

A decision is made to increase the buspirone to 10 mg three times a day and to choose a quit day 2 weeks from today. Mr. B. agrees to purchase 24-hour nicotine patches and to begin using these immediately after awakening on his quit day. He will also purchase 2-mg nicotine gum to supplement the patches whenever he has significant craving. He will monitor gum use and limit use to 10 pieces per day. Mr. B. also agrees to a plan to continue the 21-mg patches for 4 weeks, switch to 14-mg patches for 2 additional weeks, and 2 weeks of 7-mg patches. You review common side effects of transdermal nicotine use with Mr. B. Strategies for managing sleep disturbance and skin reactions are discussed. Though Mr. B. agrees to totally abstain from smoking while using NRT, you inform him that, should a slip occur, he should not immediately discontinue patch use. Instead, he will use problem-solving strategies to prevent further slips and discontinue patch use only if he smokes more than six cigarettes per day. If daily smoking persists for several days, he will call you.

You also carefully instruct Mr. B. regarding nicotine gum use and make sure he understands the importance of chewing slowly, "parking" the gum between his teeth and cheek, and avoiding acidic beverages (e.g., coffee) when he uses the gum. He will reduce his caffeine intake by about 50% to guard against an increase in anxiety symptoms. You also review behavioral strategies for managing anxiety and other triggers for smoking. Presently, he is not willing to attend a smoking cessation group or return for specific visits to learn and practice cognitive-behavioral strategies.

You ask Mr. B. to leave a phone message with you on his quit date to let you know how he is doing and schedule a follow-up clinic visit 1 week after quitting. He will also attend additional AA meetings to help him to remain confident about maintaining his abstinence from alcohol.

Comment

Mr. B.'s high level of nicotine dependence, history of significant withdrawal symptoms after previous quit attempts, comorbid anxiety disorder, and past history of alcohol dependence complicate his treatment and choice of pharmacotherapy. He has never had a prolonged trial of nicotine replacement therapy, and his experience of moderate craving despite use of transdermal nicotine suggest he may benefit from combined patch and gum use. He is not a good candidate for bupropion because the history of a head injury increases the risk of a seizure on this medication. Increasing the dose of buspirone may help prevent an exacerbation of Mr. B.'s anxiety disorder, but we do not recommend using buspirone. Reducing caffeine intake and making sure that Mr. B. is fully informed about nicotine gum use will improve the chances of successful cessation. Presently, he is not willing to invest in behavioral treatments, though he may be more willing to accept these if he relapses again.

Close follow-up of Mr. B. will allow further adjustment of the treatment regimen. If the treatment plan outlined herein is not successful, Mr. B. might need additional support or treatment to manage anxiety. For example, further increases in buspirone or use of other pharmacological and nonpharmacological treatments for anxiety may be warranted. Nicotine nasal spray, a nicotine inhaler, and the use of an antidepressant with antianxiety effects (e.g., an SSRI) are other options to consider if future smoking cessation attempts are needed.

CASE EXAMPLE 2: MS. F.

Background Information

Ms. F. is a 47-year-old married woman with two teenage children who is an outpatient in a community-based mental health center. She has recurrent depressive symptoms and meets criteria for a major depressive disorder. She has recurrent sinus headaches and is moderately obese but has no other chronic or recurrent medical problems. As Ms. F.'s clinical therapist, you have been working with her for 3 months to help her to recover from her latest bout of clinical depression. Your colleague, a psychiatrist, has monitored her response to fluoxetine (Prozac), currently dosed at 40 mg each morning. Depressive symptoms have decreased to mild levels in response to medication and psychotherapy. At her most recent visit, Ms. F. has told you that she would like to make a serious attempt to quit smoking. You praise Ms. F for her commitment to quitting, and your assessment elicits the following information:

Dependence:	Smokes 15–20 cigarettes per day (0.4 mg nicotine content). Smokes first cigarette with coffee, 30 minutes after awakening.
Past quit attempts:	Quit two times in the past, most recently 18 months ago. She utilized nicotine patches and remained abstinent for 5 weeks, relapsing after an argument with her 14-year-old daughter. This quit attempt was associated with a 7-pound weight gain and an increase in depressive symptoms, which persisted to the time of relapse despite continued use of 21-mg nicotine patches.
Substance abuse:	No history of psychoactive substance abuse or dependence. Ms. F. also drinks 2–3 cups of coffee per day.
Psychiatric history:	Meets criteria for major depressive episode, recurrent. No history of suicide attempts. She has had three discrete episodes of depression; the last, of moderate severity, began 6 months ago. She has responded to combined treatment with fluoxetine (40 mg every morning) and cognitive-behavioral psychotherapy and is completing a 3-month course of six sessions of psychotherapy. Her psychiatrist has recommended that she remain on antidepressants to prevent further episodes of depression.
Medical history:	Recurrent sinus infections, currently asymptomatic. She is moderately obese (body mass index = 31) and has no history of or evidence for coronary artery disease or COPD.

Ms. F. is very motivated to quit smoking. Both of her teenage children and her husband are eager for her to quit, especially because Ms. F.'s sister, a smoker, suffered a severe heart attack 6 months ago. However, Ms. F. is very concerned about having a recurrence of depressive symptoms when she tries to quit smoking and is also worried about gaining more weight. She is willing to try nicotine replacement again. When her therapist raises the possibility of switching antidepressants and using bupropion, she is hesitant, as she has had such a good response to fluoxetine. You know from your conversations that her psychiatrist would like Ms. F. to remain on fluoxetine indefinitely.

After further discussion, Ms. F. decides to choose a quit day in 1 week, to purchase 24-hour nicotine patches, and to continue on 40 mg fluoxetine each day. Ms. F will closely monitor depressive symptoms, see her psychiatrist 2 weeks after quitting, and continue to see you for psychotherapy every other week for the next 2 months. Ms. F.'s enlightened managed care organization has approved this plan as well. Because her last relapse occurred 5 weeks after quitting, Ms. F. will continue the 21-mg patches for 6 weeks before switching to the 14-mg dose. You review side effects and other instructions for use of transdermal nicotine use with Ms. F. (see Case 1). You also carefully review the cognitive and behavioral strategies that she has used to manage depression and suggest increased use of these during her quit attempts. You also review strategies that might prevent weight gain postcessation, but you stress the importance of focusing on cessation as the primary goal, offering further assistance with weight management once she has reached several weeks of successful abstinence. You also suggest that continued use of fluoxetine during the time she is quitting may help protect her from weight gain and recommend that she increase her level of physical activity as a dual strategy to combat weight gain and improve smoking cessation success. Though she is not willing to attend a smoking cessation group at present, she agrees to consider this if she is unsuccessful with this current quit attempt.

Comment

Ms. F.'s comorbid depressive disorder, obesity, and past history of weight gain and depressive symptoms postcessation influence your treatment recommendations. Her previous success with quitting (5 weeks of abstinence) with NRT suggests that another course of NRT may be useful again. Clearly, both Ms. F. and her clinicians should closely monitor depressive symptoms during this quit attempt and take steps to prevent relapse to both depression and smoking. Ms. F. is a good candidate for bupropion but chooses to remain on fluoxetine because of her current good response to this agent. If depressive symptoms reemerge postcessation, you and her prescribing physician may elect to increase fluoxetine further or consider switching to bupropion or another antidepressant. Ms. F.'s concern about weight gain also influences the choice of treatment. Nicotine gum may limit weight gain more than transdermal nicotine, but Ms. F.'s previous success with the patch in the past influenced her to choose this form of NRT again. Bupropion has been found to limit weight gain postcessation, though fluoxetine also has effects on appetite and weight that may help to limit weight gain. Ms. F. was satisfied with a treatment approach that focused on cessation and maintenance of euthymia as initial goals. The clinician also provided other recommendations to address weight gain that were consistent with the treatment utilized to manage depression.

Close follow-up of Ms. F. will allow further adjustment of the treatment regimen. If the treatment plan outlined herein is not successful, Ms. F. might need additional support or treatment to manage depression and weight gain.

8

Contextual and Systems Factors
That Support Treatment

Judith D. DePue
Laura A. Linnan

An ounce of prevention requires a pound of office system change. . . .
— ELFORD, JENNETT, BELL, SZAFRAN, AND MEADOWS (1994, p. 142)

To maximize treatment success, it is important to address the context or environment in which the smoker lives, works, and plays, and in which the treatment is delivered. Smokers and ex-smokers are constantly exposed to various temptations: tobacco advertising campaigns, stress, social groups with high smoking rates, free or discounted cigarettes, social norms about smoking at work or at recreational opportunities. Delivery systems factors, including competing professional demands, lack of reimbursement, and organizational barriers, can impede your best efforts as a provider.

Several conceptual frameworks help clarify how you may intervene at multiple levels to achieve maximum impact in tobacco control efforts. In his formulation of social cognitive learning theory, Bandura (1997) introduced the concept of *reciprocal determinism*, in which aspects of the individual and of the environment influence one another simultaneously. A change in one is thought to change the other. For example, a nonsmoking policy in the workplace will limit cues to smoke and, in turn, may reduce a smoker's rate of smoking or may even stimulate a quit attempt. At the same time, if smokers choose not to comply with the policy by smoking more secretively, they will have changed their behavior nevertheless. Social ecological models (Stokols, 1992) posit that health is influenced by a dynamic interplay of person and environment at multiple levels, including the physical setting, families and organizational contexts, and the larger social, cultural, and political climate. These people–environment transactions are also cyclical and reciprocal. For example, parents who smoke often influence their children to take up smoking. Teaching children about the effects of tobacco in the doctor's office or at school may encourage them to urge their parents to quit.

249

Shediac-Rizkallah and Bone (1998) reviewed the determinants of successful community-based programs. They insist that programmatic approaches that favor long-term program maintenance should include: program design and implementation factors (partnership with community members, methods that are perceived to be effective, adequate duration and funding to achieve expected results, and a training component); organizational setting factors (institutional strength, integration with existing services, and a local program champion); and broader community factors (a favorable socioeconomic and political environment and a high level of community participation).

Taken together, social ecological frameworks, which include attention to reciprocal determinism, and community-based planning models, which address sustainability, are conceptual foundations on which our organizational systems approaches have been built. Abrams and colleagues (Abrams, Elder, Carleton, Lasater, & Artz, 1986) have written previously about the reciprocal relationship between the individual and the organization within worksite prevention programs. Here we extend this work to show how these relationships form the basis of interventions in diverse settings, using studies and examples we have conducted in worksites (Abrams, Emmons, Linnan, & Biener, 1994) and primary care offices (Goldstein et al., 1998; Goldstein et al., 1997). Specifically, our research team has explored ways to support individual smoking cessation efforts through organization-level factors such as nonsmoking policies and office system practices that cue providers to assess and treat (if appropriate) all patients who smoke at all visits. Organization-level strategies have been tested at our Brown University Centers for Behavioral and Preventive Medicine with more than 150 New England worksites and over 300 office practice settings in the past 15 years.

This chapter offers organizational principles that have enhanced individual-level cessation efforts. In this chapter, we: (1) briefly describe our conceptual approach to tobacco control; (2) describe steps for implementation of these strategies; and (3) discuss strategies that address macro-social influences on tobacco control efforts, including the role of managed care organizations, health insurers, and other community organizations. These strategies can improve support of providers who deliver tobacco control interventions and ultimately improve support for smokers who are trying to stop. The principles can readily be adapted for application to a variety of community settings or channels of delivery.

WORKSITE "SYSTEMS" FOR TOBACCO CONTROL: MULTILEVEL INTERVENTION STRATEGIES

Overview of Matrix Model for Worksite Approaches

You can think of worksites as "minicommunities," in which individual smoking cessation interventions interact with small-group and organizational change strategies to synergistically accelerate smoking cessation or increase advocacy efforts. Within the larger public health mission of reducing the prevalence of smoking in the United States, worksites are an important channel for reaching people with prevention programs. The majority of U.S. adults are employed, and dependents and retirees may also be included in prevention efforts. Employees embedded within work teams, work units, or job categories are influenced by decisions made across multiple levels of management and exist within a physical work setting that increases or decreases the likelihood of smoking at work.

Applying national estimates, a worksite population will have approximately 25% current smokers, 40–50% ex-smokers, and 25% those who never smoked. Among the smokers at a given worksite, about 80–90% will not be ready to change, and only 10–20% of smokers will be either preparing for or in the process of changing (Biener & Abrams, 1991). It is clear that traditional smoking cessation programs—those aimed at smokers who are ready to quit—are likely to influence only a very small percentage at a given worksite. Our systems approach attempts to target the entire workforce. Both smokers and nonsmokers are involved, and interventions are aimed at (1) cessation promotion (creating the climate to change), (2) action skills (tools to implement change), and (3) cessation maintenance (for those who have already made the change and want to avoid relapse) to sustain and enforce organizational change and policies. We conceptualize this systems approach to tobacco control in the worksite as a matrix of these three intervention targets (cessation promotion, action skills, cessation maintenance) categorized by the level of social complexity at the worksite (individual, group, and organization; see Figure 8.1).

The following section describes intervention strategies that fill each "box" in the matrix model (Figure 8.1). We provide examples and review features of the worksite system ap-

Goals / Levels	Promotion	Action skills	Maintenance
Individual level	Increase awareness and motivation to quit (e.g., screening and tailored motivational feedback).	For smokers: provide coping skills training, access to pharmacological aids, expert consultation and self-help guides, telephone counseling, or Internet-based program access for cessation. For nonsmokers: provide skills training for reducing exposure to secondhand smoke and for supporting smoker efforts to reduce harm or quit smoking.	Provide explicit opportunities for ongoing support and follow-up (e.g., buddy systems) of smokers who are trying to quit or who have recently quit. Sustain messages to motivate smokers to keep trying and to encourage nonsmokers to support efforts to reduce environmental exposures.
Organization/ group level	Build system-wide awareness and support for smoke-free environment (e.g., form a representative workplace task force including occupational health and safety, trade unions, and human resources to build support for policy change).	Provide the policy task force with skills training, sample protocols, and expert consultation on how to achieve a total smoking ban at the workplace. Consider policies that encourage cessation, such as monetary incentives or reimbursement for costs of cessation efforts.	Ensure that smoke-free policies are enforced and that there are systems in place to provide corrective feedback on policy implementation. Provide persistent, novel, repeated messages to smokers and nonsmokers about the importance of sustaining a tobacco-free workplace.

FIGURE 8.1. Matrix conceptual model of intervention goals by levels of social complexity for worksite smoking intervention.

proach that we have found to be particularly helpful and conclude with future directions for worksite-based tobacco control systems.

Individual-Level Interventions

Efforts to increase awareness of the dangers of smoke in the workplace are appropriate for smokers and nonsmokers alike. Environmental tobacco smoke (ETS) has been classified as a Class A carcinogen by the Environmental Protection Agency, and employees should be informed of their rights to clean, smoke-free air at work. Numerous brochures about the harmful effects of secondhand smoke, or ETS, are available from the Office on Smoking and Health of the Centers for Disease Control and Prevention, American Cancer Society, American Lung Association, and others. Excellent videos, news documentaries, and other resources that point out the risk of ETS at work and home are also available to increase awareness among all employees. Although most smokers are aware of the personal increased risk of lung cancer, they are less aware of the negative health effects of ETS on nonsmokers and children. Many smokers do not realize that they are at significantly increased risk of heart attacks, strokes, asthma, and other major chronic illnesses as a result of their smoking. These are compelling awareness-building messages for smokers and nonsmokers that serve as the foundation for other intervention strategies. Modalities used to deliver these messages include a wide range of print (e.g., flyers, posters, brochures), electronic (e.g., e-mail, Internet, intranet, video), or personal (e.g., peer leaders, one-on-one counseling) sources.

Action or skills-based interventions at the individual level differ for smokers and nonsmokers. First, to focus on smokers, we offer a wide menu of options for employees who smoke and who are preparing to quit (or who are in the process of quitting). We have found that providing individualized feedback about changes in personal levels of carbon monoxide before and after smoking is a powerful message that encourages individuals to make a quit attempt. Lung age testing is another powerful way to move smokers into the quit-attempt phase. This process uses handheld spirometry technology to estimate actual versus chronological lung age of smokers. More traditional groups or classes may be offered for those ready to quit, as well as self-help guides, personal counseling to support quit attempts, buddy system strategies, and telephone support services. In all cases, we provide information on the pharmacological aids available to assist smokers in quitting. We recognize that employees making first-time quit attempts have different needs than do those who have tried but failed many times. Smokers who are heavily addicted require additional assistance when quitting than an occasional smoker. Some worksites employ a nurse or case manager who can conduct evaluations and treatments or make appropriate referrals. Third-party payers are beginning to look at treatment as a cost-effective option for helping smokers who are ready to quit (Curry et al., 1998).

Action or skills-based intervention strategies for nonsmokers are aimed at mobilizing employees to advocate for clean air at work, home, and play. Employees who live with smokers are encouraged to reduce their exposure to smoke. Once informed about the health risks of ETS, employees (smokers and nonsmokers) in worksites may band together to advocate for smoke-free policies at work. We have worked with management and employee–management coalitions and trade unions to develop smoke-free policies. There are many guides available about how to design, implement, and enforce a smoke-free policy at work. Two resources we have found helpful are the *Guide to Workplace Tobacco Control* (Li et al., 1993), and *Making Your Workplace Smokefree: A Decision Maker's Guide* from the Centers for Disease Control and Prevention, which is available online at *http://www.cdc.gov/tobacco/research_data/environmental/etsguide.htm*. Our Rhode Island worksite smoking policy tools can be found at *www.rihealth.com/quitsmoke.htm*.

Strategies to sustain and maintain interventions include telephone follow-up support services, support groups for recent quitters, buddy-system check-ins, and reward and recognition programs for employees who have quit. In addition, employees (both smokers and nonsmokers) are encouraged to take personal responsibility for helping to enforce smoke-free policies at work. Timely reports to management are given (e.g., successful case examples, improved employee morale and fewer complaints).

Taken together, these strategies provide individual employees (smokers and nonsmokers alike) with interventions (e.g., awareness, action skills, and maintenance) that appeal to the entire readiness-to-change continuum regarding a personal quit attempt or efforts to advocate for clean, smoke-free air. These individual strategies, however, are not enough to stimulate and sustain long-term changes in smoking prevalence. Multiple levels of intervention are needed, including the development of a parallel set of intervention strategies at the group and organization levels. When we address all three levels (individual, group, and organization), we engage a truly comprehensive approach to tobacco control at the worksite.

Group-Level Interventions

Within worksites, "groups" may be defined by similar interests and/or demographic characteristics (e.g., age, education level, race or ethnicity, gender), work-related characteristics (e.g., job category, work unit, department, union status), or even some type of health-related status (e.g., high claims user, smoker, overweight). Generally, we attempt to intervene with the whole population of employees but then tailor interventions to certain "groups" for special consideration. For each group-level intervention, we devise awareness, action skills, and maintenance strategies. For example, awareness-building messages about the health risks of smoke could be adapted for a department of employees who attend a required safety training program, thereby reaching all smokers and nonsmokers in the unit. The required training program might include a role-play exercise to develop skills on how to secure access to clean air at home and at work. One might organize a departmental challenge to achieve high participation in company-sponsored training programs, with an incentive for the work unit that has the highest percentage of participation. Manager groups are an important target of our intervention efforts. We often present management briefings on the health risks of ETS and strategies for enforcing existing policies about smoking at work. Involving naturally occurring groups (e.g., unions, line supervisors, members of a sports team) in cessation-related messages, programs, or services can provide powerful support for the employee-level interventions at most worksites.

Organization-Level Interventions

At the organization or company level, an important tobacco control intervention strategy is to build awareness for and secure a smoke-free work environment. Restrictive smoking policies have been shown to reduce the number of cigarettes smoked at work and have stimulated quit attempts among smokers. A smoke free policy is a key step toward reducing smoking prevalence at work. It is important to effectively communicate the existence of a policy and to periodically remind all employees (including new hires) about the policy. We have already cited a few of the excellent smoke-free guides available. Although these documents may be circulated or posted, strategically placed signage is also important so that new employees, temporary help, and visitors are aware of the smoke-free policy.

Moving beyond promotion of awareness to skill building, successful implementation of the policy relies on the cooperation of many constituent groups within the organization. The policy implementation plan, including timing of messages, communication, enforcement information, signage, and construction of outside shelters, are all skill-based strategies related to effective policy implementation. Maintenance of a restrictive policy includes clear, consistent enforcement of the policy over time. Other organization-level interventions include: placing dosimeters in various locations throughout the work environment to monitor nicotine exposure levels; serving as a role model or mentor for another company that is interested in going smoke-free; negotiating for discounts on life and/or health insurance for low smoking prevalence rates at the worksite; instituting reward and recognition programs for achieving low smoking rates on a company-wide basis. These organization-level interventions support and may synergistically enhance the individual employee and group-level interventions.

Multiple levels of intervention (individual, group, organization) that respond to all levels of motivational readiness (from not thinking about change to action to maintenance) represent a composite-systems approach to tobacco control. Although this approach includes necessary components of a successful program, it is not sufficient for long-term, sustained change in tobacco prevalence at work. Therefore, in the remaining sections, we address key features of the system that increase the likelihood of success and some thoughts about future directions related to systems change within worksites.

Worksite Features That Enhance Systems Approaches

A comprehensive tobacco control program within a worksite is difficult to achieve without appropriate assessment, monitoring and feedback tools, support from multiple constituent groups within the worksite, and a formal reward and recognition program, all sustained over time. Structural changes within the workplace that support employees and managers in their efforts to reduce smoking are needed. We worked with a company in which a comprehensive program was instituted and commitment from top managers, employee groups, and the union was in place; however, the effort could not be sustained because everyone at the plant knew that a handful of top executives were allowed to smoke cigars in their offices. Because enforcement was not consistent, employees who smoked were angered by the inconsistency. The company failed to institute a smoke-free policy and maintained a much higher than average smoking prevalence rate for many years. The following three "key ingredients" for achieving and sustaining a comprehensive tobacco control program within worksites are important.

Assessment, Monitoring, and Feedback System

Many workplace decision makers are unaware of the smoking prevalence among employees at their companies. An important first step toward developing a successful tobacco control program includes the assessment of smoking status among all employees on a regular basis—annually is a reasonable time frame. Typical assessment tools include: health risk appraisals (HRA) that give self-reported smoking status, along with many other risk factors (available for those who complete the HRA); health care claims data (available for those who use the health care system and file claims); life insurance data (among those who take company-sponsored life insurance and report themselves as smokers); and employee physicals (primarily for new hires). Among all assessment tools mentioned here, health risk appraisals are the most commonly used. Evidence suggests that smokers are less likely to complete an HRA than nonsmokers, so that smokers will be underestimated in smoking prevalence estimates unless they have a very high response rate to the HRA (greater than 80%). Decision makers who monitor the change in smoking prevalence rate over time will be able to determine patterns among those who quit (e.g., males are more likely to quit, shift workers are more likely to smoke). An effective assessment and monitoring system will help select appropriate targets and intervention strategies. These assessment systems also give feedback to decision makers about how successful the interventions have been, including cost-effectiveness estimates.

Assessment tools should also be able to link smoking status to health care claims data, absenteeism, and productivity measures, if available. It may be helpful to aggregate the health care costs for nonsmokers and compare with those for smokers while keeping the identity of individual smokers confidential. Because the costs for smokers tend to be much higher, this information may be used to convince management to offer more organization-level interventions, such as free access to cessation programs or incentives for staying abstinent, that support individual-level change. Monitoring employee complaints and/or violations of the smoking policy may be useful. Enforcement should be consistent with infractions of other personnel policies, and monitoring is likely to point out which aspects of the policy may not be clear to employees. If employees, for example, are not aware that the policy is applicable to company cars, then communication is warranted to clarify the policy. When action is taken to enforce policy, employees realize that violations will not be tolerated in the future.

Multiple Levels of Support

Successful worksite-based tobacco control systems have support from multiple levels within the organization. Support may occur from the top down or from the bottom up. In one worksite, in which we had obvious top management support for a restrictive smoking policy but a very high prevalence of smoking among line supervisors, we found enforcement of the restrictive policy to be very uneven. Our efforts in another worksite resulted in a less than successful outcome: Management at all levels was on board, but the union felt that the new policy was a "smokescreen" to avoid addressing the "real" issues of exposure to other carcinogenic chemicals at the site. All constituent groups within an organization must be convinced that the effort is worthwhile.

Evidence from Witte (1993) found that management style influences the likelihood of adopting health promotion programs. Crump and colleagues (Crump, Earp, Kozma, & Hertz-Picciotto, 1996) suggested that certain subgroups of managers exist who may be more or less likely to encourage employee participation in health promotion programs offered at work. Our own data (Linnan, Graham, Weiner, & Emmons, 2000) found that the predicted quitting probabilities among employees who smoked at baseline nearly doubled when they perceived management support to quit smoking as strong (22% quit rate probability) versus weak (12.5% quit rate probability). Clearly, support is needed when new policies go into effect, when programs are offered, and when enforcement issues arise.

We have utilized employee-driven advisory boards to help plan, deliver, promote, and tailor smoking cessation programs and services to the type of company and employee population. In sites with active employee advisory boards, we have seen very creative, energetic, fun, and successful events take place. Employee-driven boards also may include representation from all levels of management, unions, and smokers to avoid the risk of missing any constituents or their particular concerns. Periodic briefings with management about a tobacco control action plan are recommended. Discussion of the action plan should include goals, objectives, number and timeline of programs and services to be offered, how the objectives will be monitored, and who is responsible for implementing, evaluating, and reporting progress. These meetings ensure that the tobacco control plan remains on the management agenda, along with other business plans. Including cost-effectiveness results of programs and services offered is essential in these reports to management. Obviously, a tobacco control plan could not be developed without having access to effective assessment and monitoring procedures. Integrating the tobacco control plan with other health promotion plans, employee benefits plans, or continuous quality improvement plans represents another useful strategy for incorporating these programs into the overall business plan of the company.

Rewards and Recognition

A third feature of successful worksite-based tobacco control programs is the care and attention given to a comprehensive rewards and recognition system. Companies that are fully committed to a comprehensive tobacco control effort will take the time to recognize employees and managers who contribute to a successful effort. Similar to programs that reward employees who make helpful, cost-effective suggestions or who save the company dollars in other areas of business, recognition programs can make a significant impact on morale and the bottom line. Members of the employee advisory boards at the companies we work with get a certificate T-shirt, giveaways with our logo, and a recognition breakfast or luncheon to which their supervisors are invited and are recognized as well.

Employees who quit smoking should receive certificates and congratulations, have their "stories" placed in the company newsletter (with permission), and be asked to help or talk with other employees who may be interested in trying to quit. We have done "ex-smokers panels" on video so that they can share their success stories about quitting. Employees have told us that this recognition and the knowledge that they may be helping someone quit smoking is enough to keep them involved on a voluntary basis with our programs. Managers are to be congratulated for their involvement or for encouraging the employees they supervise to participate. We offer managers departmental challenges to increase employee participation and to engage them in a spirit of competition among their peers. We also take the time to recognize companies that are (or are going) smoke-free with articles in the local newspaper, the statewide business newspaper, and in the Chamber of Commerce newsletter. We invite successful companies to serve as mentors to other worksites. These efforts serve as both recognition and reward systems at the individual employee and organization levels.

Future Directions in Worksite-Based Systems Approaches

Tobacco control systems within worksites must determine how to best prioritize tobacco control efforts within a comprehensive health promotion program. Our recent research program that focused on smoking, nutrition, physical activity, and sun protection achieved reasonable quit rates but did not outperform the control worksites. As a result, we have begun to question whether we diluted the effects of the tobacco control intervention because we offered too much programming in other topics. Little research is available to understand whether offering multiple-risk-factor programming stimulates increased, synergistic, or decreased effects on single and multiple risk-factor behaviors. This is a question that requires additional research.

Understanding the changing nature of work and its impact on smoking is essential to developing successful tobacco control systems in the future. For example, a recent worksite-based study by investigators in the Netherlands intervened by changing the work design of a manufacturing company to reduce the stress and strain on employees. As a result, employees reported greater control of their work and were successful in significantly reducing smoking rates in sites at which work redesign occurred. The investigators challenged Western and U.S. teams to place more of an emphasis on the structural nature of work and how it affects the health of workers rather than focusing first on lifestyle behavioral choices (Maes, Verhoeven, Kittel, & Scholten, 1998). Future systems that address tobacco control must take into account underinsured employees working multiple shifts, multiple jobs, and in high-demand–low-control working conditions. Changing the way we think of and structure work itself may lead to the development of systems that stand a better chance of long-term success.

A final issue for future directions with worksite-based systems is to better integrate employee, group, and organization-level programs within the larger, macro-level of community and societal influences. Improved linkages with community and society-level interventions will be needed if we are to sustain worksite changes within the health care systems that often drive the delivery and payment of worksite interventions. The final section in this chapter addresses some of these macro-level influences and suggests ways in which providers can make these linkages more effectively.

SYSTEMS SUPPORT FOR TOBACCO TREATMENT IN PRIMARY CARE OFFICES

We focus on the primary care medical office because this is the setting in which the research on office systems has been applied and because it is the setting of our practical experience. We briefly review the history and research basis for this approach. We then present a series of office-system strategies that have been tested and refined during the past 15 years by our team of investigators at Brown Medical School and the Miriam Hospital's Centers for Behavioral and Preventive Medicine. These studies have examined smoking cessation and other lifestyle and screening behaviors in more than 300 medical office settings in New England. Many of the principles could apply to other settings and other intervention targets, such as substance abuse treatment, cardiac rehabilitation, and physical therapy, among others, although the strategies have not been formally tested in other settings. You may wish to substitute your own setting while reading our illustrations and consider whether the principles would apply.

The relationship between patient and physician (or other provider) was the focus of early efforts to help smokers to quit. Interventions addressed barriers to communication—what the smoker heard and was willing to accept and what the provider said and how he/she said it. Recently, intervention efforts have expanded this focus to include the physical space in which the patient–provider exchange occurs, as well as available materials and resources, cues to encourage action, and monitoring and feedback mechanisms. Strategies are incorporated into office routines, with responsibilities shared by all staff.

Rationale for Office-Systems Approach

The doctor's office offers a "unique and powerful" context in which to address smoking (Glynn & Manley, 1989). Patients put a great deal of faith in their doctor's advice, and more than 70% of smokers see a physician and average four visits per year (Davis, 1988). Although the number of smokers quitting in an individual practice may appear to be small, this "small" effect can have a huge public health impact. For example, if 100,000 providers helped just 10% of their smokers quit, we would have 2 million ex-smokers annually (Fiore et al., 1996; see also Tables 1.4 and 1.5).

Surveys of practices indicate that 75–90% of primary care physicians report that they provide cessation advice to all or almost all smoking patients (Ockene et al., 1988; Wechsler, Levine, Idelson, Schor, & Coakley, 1996). Yet only 25–68% report that they go beyond advice to provide assistance to smokers (Goldstein et al., 1998). Population-based surveys of patients have shown that only about half (44–51%) of smokers recall that a physician ever spoke to them about smoking (Goldstein et al., 1997). It is unclear whether physicians overreport their behavior or whether patients do not remember these messages. A number of barriers may explain why it is difficult for physicians to deliver tobacco interventions. These include lack of training in counseling skills, belief that smokers do not want to change, and lack of reimbursement, resources, organizational support, and time (Ockene, 1987). Physicians may not be aware that brief treatments, which are ideal for medical settings (Fiore et al., 2000), are effective. These barriers are reflective of an acute-care culture in today's medicine, in which the priority is treating the presenting problem rather than preventing future conditions.

Research has identified specific office-system strategies to address a variety of barriers and to improve both provider intervention delivery and smokers' cessation rates. Treatments have been most effective when accompanied by training in counseling skills, chart prompts, ancillary staff involvement, and scheduled follow-up visits (Manley, Epps, & Glynn, 1992; Ockene et al., 1991). Successful strategies to improve performance of routine cancer screening tests have included computerized reminder systems, physician audits with feedback, patient education, and use of a flow sheet in the chart (Hahn & Berger, 1990; McPhee & Detmer, 1993). Screening for smoking status has been successfully incorporated as a vital sign in research by Fiore and colleagues (Fiore et al., 1996). They reported that using a preprinted checklist with smoking status during assessment of other vital signs not only increased screening about smoking (from 58% to 81%) but also improved rates of physician advice (from 49% to 70%) and assistance about cessation (from 24% to 43%). Dietrich and colleagues (Dietrich et al., 1992) found that facilitator assistance in implementing an office system increased the provision of smoking cessation counseling. Our own work with community-based primary care practices has incorporated use of prompts to remind staff to address smoking with patients, a flow sheet to monitor counseling progress, patient education materials, and encouragement for ancillary staff to reinforce cessation messages. Our findings (Willey-Lessne et al., 1996) have shown significantly higher quit rates among smokers who reported seeing an intervention physician (25%) versus control physicians (20%). The PHS guideline (Fiore et al., 2000) recommends use of office systems to identify smokers, to treat every smoker at every visit with a cessation or motivational message, to offer nicotine replacement except in special circumstances, and to schedule follow-up.

In this chapter, we advocate specifically for smoking cessation systems. However, we recognize that providers must deal with many patient care concerns, and a comprehensive office system, which includes all clinical preventive services, is more desirable and efficient in the long run. Still, as Solberg and colleagues (Solberg et al., 1997) point out, few comprehensive systems are in use, and where they do exist, they often focus only on a few procedures or preventive services. Although office strategies can address a number of the barriers in tobacco control, there are other, more fundamental impediments, including tradition, economics, lack of time, and difficulty embracing a population (or public health) approach to medical care (rather than an individual, clinical, or acute-care model; Solberg et al., 1997).

The concept of *population medicine*, which is increasingly being demanded by managed care, stands in contrast with traditional medical practice. Population medicine involves orienting medical care to all patients in the practice rather than just those who come in with an acute problem. Fees are generated on a per-patient-per-month basis for all the patients who are enrolled in a health plan (capitated payment plans) rather than a per-visit basis (fee for service). With capitation, there is a greater incentive to keep the whole (or the defined) population well rather than to wait for serious and costly illness to occur. Furthermore, health plans have been reluctant to invest in smoking cessation because any savings generated may not be gained until after the patient has changed health plans, which is typically every 3 to 4 years. If all health plans invested in cessation services, all would benefit.

Few will disagree that we have moved in the right direction by including the broader environment, which provides the context in which providers interact with smokers. Using systems that support smoking cessation and that have broad applicability to other health behaviors can further enhance the promotion and delivery of all preventive health services.

Assessment of Existing Office Systems

It is best to start by reviewing existing office systems to determine what is working well and what might be improved. The overall office system comprises a number of specific subsystems. To be most effective, these routines will be integrated so that they may build on and enhance one another. Efforts for improvement can begin anywhere. We have found that different office teams may choose a different set of strategies to reach the same goal. Although there is some overlap in the functions these systems serve, each office team must tailor these strategies to their setting. We describe each of the following system strategies in more detail: adoption of practice guidelines, screening for tobacco use, monitoring and tracking of interventions, coordination of counseling, maintaining education resources, providing follow-up to smokers, and organizing a team approach to implement and integrate these systems.

Practice Guidelines

Has the practice team formalized what services they will provide to smokers, at what types of visits, and by whom? Do all team members know about and accept this policy? Table 8.1 provides a sample tobacco control practice guideline.

We strongly encourage every practice group to develop its own policy about which tobacco interventions will be provided, by whom in the practice, and at what intervals during ongoing care. This process ensures that team members will be clear about what is expected. Also, when all team members have developed ownership in the process, it is more likely to be implemented and maintained over time. Many professionals resist the use of clinical guidelines out of a belief that all practice should be tailored to the individual. Therefore, it is common for practices to operate without formal guidelines.

Frequently, larger practice groups may require formal written policies and procedures that smaller practices do not. In some practices, policies may be implicit concerning who gets

TABLE 8.1. Sample Tobacco Control Practice Guideline

- The medical assistant or other clinician will ask and record tobacco use status of every patient at every visit while assessing vital signs.
- For tobacco users, at every visit, the primary care provider (PCP) will assess readiness to quit, advise cessation, and offer a motivational message or support in quitting, as appropriate. This advice and disposition will be documented in the medical chart on the preventive care flow sheet.
- Brief counseling for assistance with cessation will be offered in-house by our preventive care coordinator, in concert with the PCP for any necessary medications. He/she will also maintain suitable education resources and provide follow-up support for smokers making a quit attempt. Smokers requiring more intensive treatments will be referred to qualified specialists.

smoking cessation services and when. Although this is not stated as a formal policy, it may be understood by staff. This implicit guideline may work well enough for small offices until new employees are hired who do not carry the history of the practice. Therefore, a written guideline works best to ensure that new employees are appropriately oriented. It also helps to establish a history and record that the practice has suitable standards in case of review or audit by an outside group (e.g., managed care organization or malpractice insurance company). A practice guideline, if it is formally written and posted in the office, can also help communicate to members the value that the practice places on helping them with smoking cessation. Setting a tone geared toward prevention will positively influence future interactions. Therefore, it is useful to write down the guidelines you are using, even if they are still evolving. All guidelines and practice policies should be reviewed and updated periodically.

Screening for Tobacco Use Status

How frequently is tobacco use status assessed by all members of the practice unit? Is this status readily visible in the chart, so that providers are prompted to intervene with all smokers at each visit? Is there a mechanism to assess readiness to quit so that messages can be appropriately tailored?

Proactive screening approaches are critical to ensuring consistency in reaching all tobacco users and maximizing opportunity for interventions. Screening is also a key recommendation from the PHS guideline (Fiore et al., 2000). Many practices use a health history questionnaire or problem list to determine which patients are due for preventive services. This form may be used to assess smoking status, as well as other forms of tobacco use (e.g., cigars, smokeless tobacco). Consider how frequently tobacco use is assessed. Health history forms are sometimes used just for new patients, or they are used periodically at health maintenance visits. It is also important to consider how visible smoking status is in the medical chart in order to prompt providers to perform appropriate services.

The current PHS guideline (Fiore et al., 2000) recommends asking about smoking status at every visit. Because most patients do not come in for a health maintenance checkup, every visit, regardless of its purpose, is an opportunity to intervene in smoking behavior. Providers have a unique advantage if they often have repeated contact with individuals over time and thus have the opportunity to reinforce messages about tobacco. An individual may not be ready to quit on one occasion but may be more ready some months later. Asking about smoking at each visit will provide the entrée to reassess readiness to quit, to continue supporting the smoker to consider quitting, and to offer help as needed.

A specific strategy encouraged as part of the PHS guideline is to include smoking status as a *vital sign*. If smoking status is preprinted on a progress form or encounter form, it is more likely to be asked about and recorded routinely, along with blood pressure, weight, temperature, and any other vital signs at the beginning of the visit (see Table 8.2). The smoking status question may assess whether the patient is a current, former, or never smoked. Readiness to quit may also be asked at this juncture. This strategy improves risk identification and documentation and also acts as a prompt for the provider. The PHS guideline panel reviewed nine studies in which a screening system was used, such as expanding vital signs to include smoking status or use of a smoking status chart sticker. A meta-analysis of these studies found that

TABLE 8.2. Vital Signs

Blood pressure: _____ Temperature: _____	
Pulse: _____ Weight: _____ Respiratory rate: _____	
Tobacco use (circle one): Current Former Never	
Ready to quit (circle one): Not at all Thinking about it Ready now	

such systems markedly increased the rate at which clinicians intervened with their patients who smoke (an estimated rate of 65.6% vs. 38.5% with no screening system; Fiore et al., 2000).

Other screening considerations include assessment of nicotine dependence, more formal questions to assess readiness to change, and questions about mood, psychiatric, or other substance abuse comorbidity (see Chapter 2). The initial vital signs process could prompt an office assistant to distribute other questionnaires specifically for smokers to assess their concerns and further tailor the treatment.

Monitoring and Tracking Intervention Progress

How readily are providers able to find and review a smoker's clinical prevention history to know what the next appropriate action should be? Are there gaps in documentation that may make the practice vulnerable to malpractice litigation or to poor reviews when audited?

Flow sheets, on paper or computer (see Figure 8.2), are increasingly being used by practitioners to ensure documentation of treatment and to allow efficient review of progress from visit to visit. There are a number of reasons that a flow sheet is helpful. In the interest of efficiency, any provider in the office should be able to quickly find and review the status of prior counseling without having to flip through pages of progress notes. The flow sheet may incorporate a number of preventive care issues and list the eligibility and time intervals at which the patient is due for a specific service based on the practice's own policy or adopted guidelines. Another reason is to encourage the documentation needed for legal protection, for quality control audits, or both. Checklists may prompt and simplify necessary documentation. When chart audits are done to evaluate clinician performance, whether they are done by a managed care organization or by internal staff, having a flow sheet in place can streamline the audit. It is desirable to have the system included as part of computerized tracking for key health indicators. The tracking system might include computer-generated provider prompts and internal reports of smoking status and interventions. Although computer systems improve efficiencies, a paper-and-pencil system can accomplish the same tasks and help staff define the procedures.

Smoker Treatment Issues

Who provides treatment to smokers in the office? Does the practice offer only brief interventions to all smokers, or do some providers offer more intensive treatment? Is there a routine for referring those smokers who need additional help to either internal or external providers?

Name: _____

Allergies: _____

Date of Initial Evaluation: _____

	VISIT DATE	PROBLEMS	MEDICATION LIST	START DATE	STOP DATE
1					
2					
3					
4					
5					
6					
7					
8					
9					

Services	Target Group	Interval	Date Performed							
Blood pressure	All	Each visit								
Height	All	Annual								
Weight	All	Annual								
Mammogram	Women age $\geq$ 50	Annual								
Breast exam	Women	Annual								
Pap/pelvic exam	Women	Every 2 yrs								
Influenza vaccine	Age $\geq$ 65	Annual								
Digital rectal exam	Age $\geq$ 40	Annual								
Fecal occult blood	Age $\geq$ 50	Annual								
Sigmoidoscopy	Age $\geq$ 50	Every 10 yrs								
Tobacco counseling	All smokers	Each visit								
Dietary fat and fiber	All	Each visit								
Tetanus	All	Every 10 yrs								
Sun protection	All	Annual								

FIGURE 8.2. Example of preventive care flow sheet.

Treatment techniques are discussed in more detail in Chapters 3–7, but the provision of services within an office practice must be developed as a routine system. The purpose of this system is to assess readiness to quit and to provide personalized advice and assistance to every smoker at every visit. Assistance includes discussing benefits for and barriers to making changes for people who are not ready to quit (see also Chapter 3 on motivational interventions). Assistance also includes providing help with problem solving, behavioral coping skills and support, medications when appropriate, educational materials, and referrals (see also

Chapter 4). The practice team must decide what level of treatment they will provide within the office. According to the PHS guideline (Fiore et al., 2000), a dose–response relationship exists between intensity of counseling and efficacy. Intensive interventions (lasting more than 10 minutes per contact) more than double cessation rates (22.1%) compared with absence of person-to-person contact (10.9%). Brief counseling (> 3 to ≤ 10 minutes) and "minimal counseling" (≤ 3 minutes) both increase cessation rates over no-contact interventions (16% and 13.4% rates, respectively, vs. 10.9% for no contact). All smokers should be offered a minimal or brief intervention whether or not the smoker is referred to a more intensive intervention; intensive interventions should be used when resources permit.

The practice team may consider implementing components of a stepped-care approach, as described in Chapter 1. Stepped care involves varying the intensity of the treatments to meet the needs of smokers who have failed to quit with less intensive intervention. For example, the first step could involve routine minimal counseling of less than 3 minutes. Because the majority of smokers are not ready to quit, the provider may briefly assess readiness to quit, offer advice and motivational messages, and make a point to renew the discussion at the next visit (see Chapters 2–4). Those smokers who are ready to quit would be offered help or referred for treatment. The practice team must decide who will deliver these brief yet critical messages. This person may be the physician or other primary clinician who sees the smoker regularly. Some practices include family planning counselors; women, infants, and children (WIC) counselors; dietitians; psychologists; social workers; nurses; nurse practitioners; and physician assistants who have their own regular caseloads. To maximize opportunity for interventions, all of these professionals should be able to provide the basic smoking cessation messages. Previous research has shown that multiple messages from multiple providers, both physicians and nonphysicians, can have double the effect on cessation outcomes (Fiore et al., 2000).

Having referral opportunities inside the practice, if possible, is advantageous. The benefits include improved integration with other care, greater convenience, and familiarity with clinicians. Nevertheless, the most intensive treatments will usually require outside referrals to specialists or special programs. Referrals to specialists may be needed for those smokers who had great difficulty with prior quit attempts, who have comorbidities, or both. It is critical to identify such referral resources. Obtaining some direct knowledge and familiarity with the specialty program or with the professionals involved is worthwhile to help strengthen your referral recommendation and thus increase the likelihood of its acceptance.

As chronic-disease care management programs are becoming more common for patients with diabetes, asthma, or high blood pressure, they are increasingly incorporating smoking cessation. With these programs, the care manager may provide smoking cessation treatment directly or refer to other cessation services. Alternatively, a more innovative approach would assign each smoker a specialized care manager of his/her own. This provider would proactively follow all smokers in the practice to periodically assess readiness, offer appropriate treatment and support for quit attempts, ensure early recycling or stepped-up treatment following failed attempts, and provide support for relapse prevention and maintenance.

Education Resources

Is there a supply of education resources in the office? How are these obtained and maintained? Who gives these to patients and when is this done in the course of a visit?

Education principles emphasize the value of using multiple modalities (audio and visual) to enhance learning. Many people have difficulty remembering what was said during an office visit. Often the smoker is anxious or preoccupied by the acute condition that precipitated the visit. Therefore, some take-home resources are helpful. These can include simple recommendations written on a prescription pad, printed tip sheets, educational brochures or booklets, or audiotaped or videotaped programs. It takes a serious commitment by the practice team to identify these resources and to keep supplies on hand. Many practices use only what is given to them by pharmaceutical representatives and are left without materials when supplies run out. The lack of a systematic approach to these educational resources limits access to these materials.

To develop a system for managing educational resources, we suggest the following:

1. *Identify an education coordinator* in the office who is responsible for reviewing and selecting education resources, as well as stocking and restocking the materials as needed.

2. *Review the flow* to consider who should distribute materials and when in the course of the visit this should occur. This person also has a valuable opportunity to reinforce educational messages while materials are given out.

3. *Simplify your inventory* by limiting the different selections you keep on hand. Because the inventory across all education topics may be extensive, select a few items you like best on each topic and stick with these. Of course, you should update your choices every year to ensure that information is not outdated and that the educational message is consistent with accepted guidelines for the topic.

4. *Keep a separate file with at least one copy of each item and appropriate ordering information.* It is a problem if the last copy of a special brochure is given out and you do not have the information you need to reorder.

5. *Select materials to suit your audience.* You know who your smokers are. In reviewing materials for them, consider the following features: Will the visuals and language appeal to the predominant age groups? Is the presentation appropriate for the cultural groups you see most often? Are materials available in the languages they most likely read? For printed materials, is the reading level suitable for the most common educational level? For easier reading, look for more pictures, shorter sentences, and words with fewer syllables. Consider in-office video presentations, as many people would rather watch than read.

6. *Select materials to help you match messages with patient's readiness to change.* Tailoring materials to their motivational levels can be helpful in moving smokers along the continuum of readiness to change. For example, smokers who are not ready to change can be asked to review information about the health effects of their smoking and the benefits of quitting. On the other hand, smokers ready to make changes may be given materials on how to quit smoking, including practical and behaviorally specific steps that will help with the gradual process of changing habits over time.

7. *Identify reliable sources of materials, including items you can reproduce on your own copy machine*. There are many excellent sources of good quality, low-cost education materials. Contact government agencies, voluntary agencies, and your own professional organizations (see Table 8.3). Materials from government agencies are often free and usually are not copyrighted, so they can be reproduced without permission.

8. *Take advantage of quality Internet resources*. One example of a useful Web-based resource is QuitNet (*www.quitnet.com*). Chapter 4 provides detailed information about this site.

Follow-Up

Is there a way to contact smokers, either by phone, mail, or a follow-up visit, to reinforce recommendations and support the patient's efforts? Such support is especially critical for smokers making a quit attempt.

Adding even one follow-up contact with smokers making a quit attempt has been shown to significantly increase quit rates, and additional contacts further increase success rates (Fiore et al., 2000). Regardless of whether the smoker is not yet ready to quit, is about to quit, or has just recently quit, follow-up is important to reinforce the provider's recommendations and to provide support for the smoker's efforts. After a quit attempt, a follow-up phone call or visit is especially important and should be made within 1 or 2 days or, at most, a week after a planned quit date. Recall that smoking is a persistent, chronic, relapsing disorder, and thus a quit attempt that does not succeed is an opportunity to learn and acquire new relapse prevention coping skills to help prepare for the next quit attempt.

It is important that the follow-up not be perceived as "checking up" on the smoker, which may come across as negative and may lead to the smoker avoiding further contact. It is a good idea to ask smokers for their permission to contact them and to explain the process

TABLE 8.3. Key Sources for Patient Education Materials on Tobacco Control

Agency address	Notes
National Cancer Institute Building 31, Room 10A24 Bethesda, MD 20892 Phone: 1-800-4-CANCER	The National Cancer Institute (NCI) offers educational materials on all cancers, including information for individuals being treated for cancer. All materials that the NIH produces on smoking are now offered through the NCI.
American Heart Association 1-800-AHA-USA1	Patient materials are available on heart disease risk factors, including smoking, high blood pressure, lack of exercise, and cholesterol, as well as general information on coronary heart disease, cardiovascular disease, and stroke.
American Cancer Society 1-800-ACS-2345	Patient materials are available on cancer prevention, including materials on smoking cessation, diet, sun protection, screening for breast, cervical, colorectal, testicular, prostate, skin, and other cancers. There are also resources for individuals being treated for cancer.
American Lung Association 1-800-LUNG-USA	Patient materials are available on the various lung diseases, their treatment, and prevention. A variety of resources are available on smoking cessation.

and purpose of this contact. For example, the provider might ask, "I would like to give you a call in a couple of weeks to see how this plan is working and see if I can offer any further help. Is this okay?" A follow-up visit is ideal, although we recognize that lack of reimbursement is frequently a barrier for such visits. Often a visit scheduled for follow-up on another problem can be used to review efforts with smoking. Another approach is to use a standard letter that is mailed to smokers who have agreed to make a quit attempt. This letter is an efficient way to express support and to invite those with concerns to call in. The provider can acknowledge that the discussion about smoking can continue at the next regular visit, whenever that will occur.

Use of this continued discussion from visit to visit is a valuable strategy for those smokers who are not ready to quit. For these smokers, the provider should acknowledge that it is the smoker's responsibility to decide when to quit, yet the provider can continue to state concern and offer help when he/she is ready to make a quit attempt (see Chapter 3). Often smokers who have slipped back to smoking have similar beliefs and attitudes as smokers who are not ready to quit. Nonthreatening discussions of reasons for and against quitting may help to motivate the smoker to try again to quit. An especially important strategy may be to explore the smoker's sense of disappointment or "failure" and help him/her reframe these attempts as part of a learning process (see Chapter 3).

Once the office team determines how follow-up will be provided, they will need a mechanism to ensure that these strategies become systematic in the office. For example, many offices have a system by which the receptionist makes another appointment before the patient leaves the office. Adherence with follow-up care is much greater when appointments are made while the smoker is in the office versus when he/she is allowed to make his/her own arrangements (89% vs. 45%; Pinsker, Phillips, Davis, & Iezzoni, 1995). If follow-up care is to be provided by phone, the monitoring system described previously, whether a paper flow sheet or computerized system, may be used to signal a follow-up plan. This form may be linked to a tickler system (such as a log, card file, or computer report), and a designated team member would make follow-up calls or send a standard letter to identified smokers. Although support is most critical in the first few weeks and months after quitting, continued support is also important, because the risk for relapse continues for at least 1 year for many individuals.

A Team Approach

Is the workload for smoking cessation interventions managed by one person in the office, or are different tasks shared across the team? Are there regular team meetings to facilitate communication and problem-solving sessions to continually improve practice routines?

The term "office team" has been used frequently in this chapter. It is intended to include all staff members working in the office, including physicians, other clinicians, medical assistants, receptionists, clerical staff, and the office manager. Most of these individuals have contact with patients and therefore have an opportunity to reinforce messages about smoking and to share in office system tasks. This distribution of office system tasks among clinicians and support staff not only streamlines the process and shares the workload but also produces the best outcomes. Multiple messages from different people, both physicians and nonphysicians, can double the likelihood of successful quitting (Fiore et al., 2000).

An example of such a team process could involve a medical assistant asking about smoking status while assessing vital signs. Then the physician would assess readiness to quit, offer advice to quit, and refer the patient to a nurse or other professional provider. The provider offers more in-depth counseling and checks off recommended self-help materials on the encounter form to alert the receptionist. As the smoker is leaving, the receptionist may distribute the cessation materials and offer his/her own good wishes for the smoker's efforts. Of course, any interaction in more public places in the office must use discretion to protect the patient's confidentiality. The provider may also conduct the follow-up call for further assistance. If a care manager is involved with the practice team, this person may receive referrals and communicate progress to other providers.

Managing this type of team process requires commitment, trust, and good communication. Each person must be clear about what his/her role is and how each step fits into the flow of the practice. They may create message cards with sample scripts for different scenarios or role-play some predictable encounters as part of their training. Periodic staff meetings are valuable to ensure communication opportunities to address problems early on and to find solutions. Unfortunately, busy offices often do not take the time for staff meetings. However, they may find that a staff meeting that devotes time to identifying and solving problems together as a team can save time in the long run. In this fashion, all systems can be periodically reevaluated with necessary changes implemented as soon as possible.

The Importance of Data for Needs Assessment and Feedback to Providers

It is very useful to collect data to better assess areas in which improvement is needed and whether practice changes have improved interventions. For example, a brief chart audit could assess documentation of smoking status. A simple form of chart audit could be conducted by the staff person who pulls charts for the day's appointments (see Table 8.4). He/she might be asked to tally all charts with documentation of smoking status at the last visit (as best

TABLE 8.4. Sample Chart Review Tally Sheet

Record tobacco use status documented at last primary care visit

Tobacco users: _____   Total count: _____

Former users: _____   Total count: _____

Never users: _____   Total count: _____

Status not recorded: _____   Total count: _____

(Total number of charts pulled _____ should equal total of 4 categories above.)

Percent not recorded: # not recorded/total # charts = _____

Among smokers' charts only:

Advice documented at last visit: _____   Total count: _____

Assistance documented at last visit: _____   Total count: _____

Percent advised: # advised/# current smokers = _____

Percent assisted: # assisted/# current smokers = _____

practice) and/or within the last year (as next-best practice). The denominator is the total number of patients seen during the day (to compare with national survey data, you may wish to select only those charts for visits with adult patients). If the smoking status is not easily visible by the chart reviewer, then it is not visible to a busy provider during the visit. A more thorough chart review could check smokers' charts for documentation of advice or assistance. Medical record documentation of smoking interventions may be much lower than either patients or physicians report (McBride, Plane, Underbakke, Brown, & Solberg, 1997). Furthermore, regular documentation is an important standard to uphold to ensure consistency of interventions among all smokers from visit to visit and to facilitate communication between providers who see the patients. Documentation is also important to support claims for reimbursement. The feedback may also help motivate the office team to improve service delivery, and the objective data can help to show progress with improvement efforts.

Implementing and Changing Office Systems

A review of existing systems and/or data collection of office procedures will serve to identify areas in which deficits exist or improvement is desired. It is helpful to review these existing procedures in a group discussion with as many staff members as possible across various job categories. Their participation in problem identification and goal setting is critical for their feeling of ownership in the process. During the assessment of existing systems, it is also necessary to assess the team's readiness to change the office routines. This readiness to change is conceptually similar to an individual's level of readiness to change for smoking cessation or other health behaviors. If one or more influential members of the practice team are not interested in changing office systems, it would be appropriate to provide information for the group to think about. However, if the group is willing and can agree on any focus for change, then that is where team efforts should begin. This specific system becomes their goal for change. Even for office groups who are very motivated to revamp their office structure, it is probably wise to limit the focus to one or two office systems (goals) at a time to ensure success and continued enthusiasm.

With the goal in focus, the team should begin to brainstorm how they will improve their systems (see Table 8.5). The practice team knows best what will work in their setting and what they will implement. Sample tools may also be helpful to review as they relate to the selected goal (e.g., vital signs, flow sheets). In addition to those shown here, samples may be collected from other practices or from commercial vendors. We have found that most practices prefer to adapt and customize the sample forms. The team will also need to consider who will be responsible for choosing and customizing the tool and whose approval is needed for proposed changes. In addition to considering tools, it is important to discuss the context in which the tool will be used. For example, at what point in the flow of patient care will the tool be used and who will use it? Is any training or rehearsal needed to implement the plan? How will this tool or system be communicated to all staff? Then set a start date, and inform staff about this date.

The start date for a new system or office procedure should always be considered the beginning of a pilot test. Everyone should expect that further improvements will be needed. Feedback from staff regarding the ease and usefulness of the selected tools and procedures

TABLE 8.5. Key Steps for Enhancing Office Systems

Goal setting

> What office systems are you looking to improve?
> What outcomes would you like to achieve?

Assessment

> What do you like about your current routine and practices?
> What deficits exist?
> Consider a brief audit or tally of current practices to clarify needs.

Planning

> What are some possible solutions to the deficit areas you identified?
> Does the solution require a new tool and/or procedure?
> Which tool would best fit into your current system?
> Who would be responsible for choosing and/or customizing the tools?
> Where in the flow of patient care will the tool be used and who will use it?
> How will you communicate this new tool or system to all staff?

Start-up/Maintenance

> When will you begin using the tool?
> How will you solicit feedback from staff regarding the ease and usefulness of the tool?
> Who will revise the tool or procedure to address identified problems?
> How and when will you know if the tool or procedure addressed the deficit you identified?
> Who will provide feedback to the staff regarding the implementation of the tool?

Note. From "Changing Office Routines to Enhance Preventive Care," by A. J. Dietrich, C. B. Woodruff, & P. A. Carney, 1994, *Archives of Family Medicine, 3,* 176–183. Copyrighted 1994, American Medical Association.

should be solicited. This can be done through a simple suggestion box, staff opinion polling, or discussions in staff meetings. The recent movement of continuous quality improvement or total quality management incorporates many of the processes described herein for assessing and problem solving to improve organizational function and efficiency (Berwick, 1992; Solberg, Brekke, Kottke, & Steel, 1998). In the philosophy of this movement, staff members on all levels are part of the quality improvement process, and all jobs are interconnected to delivery of care for patients. Each person's job in the office depends on others to work effectively and efficiently. Therefore, all staff members have a critical voice in the ongoing assessment and improvement of quality care.

Adding to the Office System and Maintaining Progress

Once a new system or procedure is operating well, the practice team may choose to focus on another routine in which improvement is needed. As each building block is added, a more comprehensive system can be built and improved over time. In our experience, practice groups are most interested in focusing on systems for screening of smokers, on smoker education, and on monitoring progress. Implementing improvements in one or two of these areas may take several months to a year, given other competing demands in the practice. Referral systems (both in and outside the practice), follow-up systems, and setting practice guidelines have been less often selected as priority issues in the offices we have worked with. As with individuals attempting changes in behavior, practices often start with activities that seem easiest to change, or they select only one or two behaviors to work on at a time. Even after implementing new office systems, maintenance of these systems has been difficult for practices. Having mechanisms in place for ongoing feedback and reviewing key performance indicators may be important for maintenance and improvement of patient care services, although rarely do medical offices devote time and resources to this. As practice-based medical record systems become more computerized, such reviews may be easier to conduct electronically.

The process of changing the behavior of a practice group is similar to that of changing individual health behaviors. The steps described here for assessment of medical office systems, assessment of readiness to change, goal setting, implementing changes in office routines, and maintenance of change parallel the intervention steps with individual smokers described throughout this book. An individual smoker's behavior is influenced by his/her family, friends, and cultural norms, whereas office practice behavior is influenced by group dynamics, practice culture, and health care system norms. Behaviors and habits are difficult to change in either case. Many of the same principles used to guide behavior change for individuals seem to help guide practice group change, such as persistent repeated messages from multiple sources and receiving support for the process of change. Examples of repeated messages to providers include: national guidelines published in medical journals; health plan requests for documentation of smoking status; managed care "report cards" from patient surveys conducted as part of the Health Plan Employer Data and Information Set (HEDIS 3.0) of the National Committee for Quality Assurance (NCQA, 1996); improved benefit plans to stimulate patient demand for cessation services; and availability of clinician skills training at professional meetings. Our staff consultants' visits have often provided the opportunity and guidance to work on office system improvements. However, when our staff involvement ends, there may be little infrastructure or incentive to support these changes, unless the changes have been incorporated into practice policy.

CASE STUDY: COMMUNITY PRACTICE ASSOCIATES

Assessment and Initial Changes in Practice Systems

As a result of a workshop on tobacco control strategies offered at the state nursing association annual meetings, two nurses from Community Practice Associates decided to encourage their colleagues to make some changes in their practice routines. The practice consisted of four family practice physicians, the two nurses, four medical assistants, a receptionist, an office manager, and a billing clerk. While driving home from the conference, the nurses discussed their existing tobacco screening procedure. Their health history form asked about smoking status, but this was seldom updated. They liked the idea of adding smoking status to the vital signs. They knew that counseling of smokers was inconsistent depending on which physician the patient saw, because one physician was very interested in tobacco control, whereas the others were less so. They also realized that their supplies were low on patient education materials about smoking.

Over an impromptu lunchtime meeting, they described the new vital-signs approach they had just learned about. Although not all physicians were on hand at this meeting, the nurses convinced the medical assistants to write a patient's tobacco status in the margin of the progress note when they assessed vital signs at each visit. One of the nurses also decided to update the patient education supplies. This plan was put into action almost immediately, but the tobacco-status notation soon backfired. The physicians who had not been informed of the plan were not sure what to do with this information. They were unclear whether the patient had requested help to quit smoking. They felt awkward about how to broach the issue with their patients. After another impromptu staff meeting, the rationale for the new notation was clarified, and all decided it could be continued. However, over time, its use diminished. Although new smoking cessation materials were now on hand, tobacco screening and counseling continued to be inconsistent in the practice.

Analysis

The nurses in this practice had very good intentions and a realistic plan. However, their plan might have been more successful if they had made a greater effort to win over their less enthusiastic colleagues. Getting agreement from key staff is likely to require a more formal meeting in which the problem—inconsistent screening in this case—is discussed. Without agreement on the problem, commitment to a solution is unlikely. Sometimes data are needed to convince those who feel changes are not needed. A brief chart audit, looking at tobacco screening in the practice, may help to make the case. Agreement to conduct a chart audit might come from this first staff meeting. If the solution decided on is to change the vital-signs procedure, then agreement on a start date is a good idea, allowing all staff to be informed. Further, the prompt is effective only if providers are prepared to give appropriate advice and assistance. The providers may wish to discuss some possible scenarios with patients, as a kind of "rehearsal," in order to be convinced that this new plan will not disrupt other patient care routines. Finally, the use of the margin notation faded with time. Writing a note in the margin can be easy to forget, compared with filling in a preprinted tobacco status line on a progress note page (see Figure 8.2). Periodic review and troubleshooting of new procedures is also helpful.

BEYOND THE ORGANIZATIONAL SETTING: TOWARD MACRO-LEVEL SYSTEMS CHANGES

Up to this point, this chapter has focused on tobacco control systems in two organizational settings: medical offices and worksites. We have explained how they might be developed, implemented, evaluated, and maintained. The remainder of this chapter shares ways in which providers can take action to support these broader systems changes. We challenge readers to look beyond their professional work settings to serve as role models, educators, and advocates for macro-level systems changes in support of tobacco control intervention and its financing and for prevention.

Providers wear many hats. As a result, they are in a position to influence system changes in their office practice settings, the managed care environment in which they may be employed, and in the many other settings in which they work and live. The PHS guideline includes recommendations for systems interventions for administrators, insurers, and purchasers (Fiore et al., 2000). We have summarized their recommendations and added others from our community-based intervention and research experiences.

Formalize Compensation Agreements and Enhance Benefits Packages

Providers often cite lack of reimbursement as a major barrier to the implementation of smoking cessation treatment. Because smoking is the leading cause of preventable death and because evidence now exists that many treatment programs work, providers need to educate contract negotiators about the essential nature of reimbursement agreements for smoking cessation treatment (pharmacological and counseling-based treatment). Getting actively involved in the compensation rate-setting process can be an educational process for contractors and providers alike. This involvement may include volunteering to be on a task force or committee. There are many barriers to inclusion of cessation treatments in health plan benefit packages: (1) the tradition that health insurance has not covered preventive services; (2) the perception that cessation interventions have limited effectiveness; (3) little evidence of cost-effective interventions; and (4) lack of demand from physicians because such services were not part of their medical education and training (Schauffler, 1997). To date, coverage for tobacco cessation treatments is more common in large health maintenance organizations with capitation as the payment system, and it is rare in fee-for-service or discounted fee-for-service systems.

There is increasing evidence to support inclusion of tobacco treatment in benefit plans, as long as the following principles are used in designing such plans: (1) use scientific evidence-based guidelines, such as the clinical practice guideline from PHS (Fiore et al., 2000), as the basis for coverage decisions on effective and cost-effective treatments; (2) reduce barriers to treatment by eliminating copayments that have led to underutilization of tobacco treatments; and (3) define performance measures that will ensure quality (e.g., the Health Plan Employer Data and Information Set, HEDIS 3.0, measures for assessment of smoking status) and advice to quit (Schauffler, 1997). Health plans are likely to share HEDIS (NCQA, 1996) reports with their providers as feedback on performance. When these "report cards" are used in the spirit of quality improvement, patients, providers, and administrators all benefit. Some health plans also incorporate these performance measures to set targets, which in turn are used in provider performance appraisals and become part of the negotiated compensation system for providers. Once benefit coverage for tobacco treatments is secured, it is imperative that health plan administrators inform providers of this coverage. Ensuring that smokers and providers are both aware of the benefits that relate to smoking cessation treatment is likely to increase the utilization of these services.

Influence and Support Policy-Level Changes

Since 1994, every hospital in the United States that is eligible for accreditation by the Joint Commission on Accreditation of Healthcare Organizations (JCAHO) must be smoke free. Clinicians were involved in the development of these requirements for accreditation, and they can continue to be involved in the efforts to successfully work with patients and providers to ensure a smoke-free hospital environment. For example, implementing a system to identify and document the smoking status of all patients on admission, offering appropriate cessation treatment to patients, training providers about how to treat and/or best support patients who smoke, and reimbursing providers who provide treatment and counseling services are all important steps. Performance targets used for quality improvement are also important for JCAHO accreditation (e.g., setting a goal of 100% for recording tobacco status of patients on admission). Progress toward this goal would be monitored over time. The PHS guideline (Fiore et al., 2000) also recommends that hospital formularies include effective pharmacotherapies such as the nicotine patch and gum. Providers are in a unique position to take the lead in developing and supporting these smoking-related policies.

Advocate for Tobacco Control

Health care providers may step out of their traditional work settings to advocate for tobacco control policies in workplaces, playgrounds, schools, and other public places. As members of a community, health professionals are an important source of information and can serve as very credible spokespersons in support of tobacco-related policies (DePue, Miller, & Goldstein, 1995). Macro-level systems change at the local, state, and national levels has been accomplished by such advocacy. If you think back just 30 years, smoking was the norm in hospitals, public places, airplanes, and many other settings. The norms for offices, public transportation, and the health care system have completely shifted, buoyed by the evidence that environmental tobacco smoke is a Class A carcinogen (Jenkins et al., 2000) and the recognition that smoking interventions are cost-effective, as well as lifesaving. Although private practice settings may not be required to be smoke free, providers should serve as role models and advocate for smoke-free practice and office building environments. Being a role model also means that providers who themselves smoke should refrain from smoking in view of their patients and should consider quitting as well. Providers have played an integral role in the advocacy effort to date; for example, Dr. Stanton Glanz conducts research devoted to raising awareness of negative tobacco industry practices and to promoting restrictive policy-level changes (Glantz & Smith, 1997). More work is clearly needed to keep the momentum going.

Develop Partnerships with Community-Based Organizations

Policy interventions have gained momentum in recent years, and many opportunities remain for providers to develop partnerships within and between community-based organizations focused on tobacco prevention, treatment, and control. For example, occupational health nurses play a key role in identifying, treating, and monitoring the smoking status of employed populations. Collaborations between health professionals serving the worksite, such as the occupational health nurses, physicians, health educators, and/or psychologists, can enhance intervention effectiveness by matching treatments to the smoking history and motivational readiness of the smoker. Moreover, organizational changes that create restrictive smoking policies will also support individual employee cessation efforts.

Partnerships among voluntary health organizations, such as that of the Coalition on Smoking or Health with the American Cancer Society, American Lung Association, and American Heart Association, have proven extremely effective in advancing legislative initiatives in some states, as well as in advancing tobacco prevention and control efforts. By collaborating with institutions such as these and state or local health departments, providers reap the following benefits: (1) access to more tobacco control educational materials—especially for diverse audiences; (2) collaborative goal setting that allows organizations to reduce duplicative services and leads to economies of scale for budgeting and intervention delivery; (3) access to additional expertise, as many of these community-based organizations employ tobacco-control specialists with a wealth of knowledge and talent; and (4) opportunities for professional growth and development. Overcoming "turf" issues and enhancing communication among professionals in a variety of settings establishes powerful linkages to increase tobacco control effectiveness. Communities have established state or local coalitions to serve this purpose. Creative work by these coalitions helps to combat the long arms of the tobacco industry.

Develop Collaborations with Researchers

As researchers, we have an inherent bias toward the benefits of collaborations between community-based clinicians and applied researchers. Improvements in treatment options are dependent on these research partnerships. So, too, are advances in systems approaches that assist and support providers in their smoking treatment and prevention efforts. Although participating in research studies involves a time commitment and collection of data, there are many benefits to the professional who forms these partnerships. First, participation usually brings an infusion of assistance and training to staff, as researchers are funded to deliver an intervention and evaluate effectiveness. Second, participation brings with it the opportunity to try out state-of-the-science interventions. Third, research partnerships can bring educational materials and access to current information from federal, state, and local resources. Fourth, collaborations can build bridges to future research partnerships on a wide range of disease and prevention-oriented topics. And fifth, smokers are often pleased to know that their providers are involved with research projects. Being part of a larger effort to improve the health and well-being of the community is usually viewed as worthwhile and appealing.

CONCLUSION

This chapter has reviewed office systems in support of tobacco control and organizational systems in worksites. We assert that these organizational and contextual factors are critical to ensuring that tobacco control interventions are most effective. We have shared specific strategies that have been tested and refined during the past 15 years by our team of investigators at Brown University and the Miriam Hospital Centers for Behavioral and Preventive Medicine. The important role that macro-level systems play in support of smoking control efforts has also been acknowledged. The provider's role in advocating, educating, forming research collaborations, and supporting these macro-level systems changes has been reviewed. We have come a long way in the past three decades toward changing individual, institutional, and community social norms about the dangers of smoking. With careful attention and development of systems that support all the advances in individual treatment, we can expect continued momentum toward a smoke-free society and enhanced continuity of care at every level until the goal is achieved.

9

Ongoing Research and Future Directions

Peter M. Monti
Raymond Niaura
David B. Abrams

This chapter reviews five areas that hold promise for future research to improve interventions for the treatment of nicotine addiction. These areas have evolved, at least in part, from our ongoing work at Brown Medical School. First we present the emergent case for studying adolescent smoking behavior, prevention, and treatment. Increased understanding of the biobehavioral substrates of nicotine addiction with adults has inspired similar questions about etiological mechanisms in adolescents and young adults (Abrams, 1999b). There is a pressing need to develop effective interventions for cessation in youth and young adults. The earlier in the life span the cumulative exposure to the toxic agents in tobacco smoke is stopped, the greater the benefit.

A second area for consideration is the relationship of the neurobiology of nicotine addiction to developing more effective behavioral, pharmacological, and combined treatments for adult smokers. When considered with genetic (Pomerleau & Kardia, 1999) and cellular developments in nicotine research, this line of study illustrates how the neuroscience of nicotine addiction (Dani & Heinemann, 1996; Koob & LeMoal, 2001; Kreek & Koob, 1998) and the study of individual differences (e.g., in nicotine sensitivity) could help isolate new mechanisms to enhance future interventions. The association of comorbidities such as depression, attentional disorders, and substance abuse with nicotine addiction has already prompted new treatments for smoking cessation. Research on nicotine receptors in the mesolimbic areas associated with addiction suggest that designer drugs can be developed that would further improve outcomes.

A third area of emerging research that follows from the study of biobehavioral mechanisms focuses on tailoring treatments to the unique needs and profiles of individual smokers. Perhaps best characterized by the phrase "different strokes for different folks," tailoring implies that no single treatment will prove effective for every smoker, as there are many reasons for people smoking. Nevertheless, smokers who present with certain characteristics may respond to certain treatments more or less favorably. One characteristic common to many smokers is alcohol use. Indeed, because alcohol and nicotine seem to go together and because many heavy smokers are heavy drinkers, a fourth area that we briefly consider is cross-addictions. More specifically, we present some of our ongoing research work with smoking among alcoholics.

The final issue to be considered in this chapter is the potential benefit of using smoking cessation interventions as a template for developing a comprehensive continuum of preventive health care for the future. The elements of such a plan were outlined in Chapter 1 and elaborated on in Chapter 8. In this section we discuss the formidable challenges that remain in evaluating and adopting a comprehensive approach such as a stepped-care treatment plan.

ADOLESCENTS AND TOBACCO ADDICTION

Epidemiology

The rate of smoking among American youth declined during the 1980s but rose sharply by over 32% from 1991 to 1998 (Centers for Disease Control and Prevention, 2000b). Cigarette use increased by 28% on college campuses from 1993 to 1997 (Wechsler, Rigotti, Gledhill-Hoyt, & Lee, 1998). Emmons and colleagues (Emmons et al., 1998) view the rise in college smoking as a consequence of the rise in adolescent smoking that occurred earlier in the 1990s. Unless many smoking teenagers quit during or soon after adolescence, this trend could reverse the 30-year decline in adult smoking prevalence in the United States. A substantial number of youths experiment with smoking (about 70% of all youths will try at least one cigarette) and, of those who try, about 35–40% will progress to regular use and dependence (Centers for Disease Control and Prevention, 2000b).

Smoking among adolescents is a major public health issue and has been receiving increasing attention in the media, among legislators and policy makers, and among behavioral researchers. More than 3 million adolescents in the United States smoke, and 3,000 young people start smoking regularly each day (Pierce, 1991). Two recent review papers (Colby, Tiffany, Shiffman, & Niaura, 2000a, 2000b) note a decline in the age of initiation of smoking behavior, as well as a decline in adolescent perceptions of health risk and peer disapproval related to smoking (Johnston, O'Malley, & Bachman, 1996). Although it is generally known that smoking in early adolescence is a strong predictor of smoking in adulthood (Chassin, Presson, Sherman, & Edwards, 1990), what is remarkable is that smoking during adolescence increases the chances of developing an intractable lifelong dependency (Russell, 1990) and leads to a sixteenfold increase in the risk of adult smoking. Colby and colleagues (Colby et al., 2000a, 2000b) further point out that the earlier a teen starts smoking, the more cigarettes per day he/she will smoke in adulthood and the more severe the tobacco-related health consequences will be. Clearly, although more than a decade's worth of prevention efforts aimed at teens have shown some success (e.g., Flay, Phil, Petraitis, & Hu, 1995), we are most certainly falling short in our efforts at prevention and early cessation with adolescents (Flay, 2000).

Not unlike adult smokers, teens report frequent unsuccessful quit attempts and cite social pressure, urges to smoke, and withdrawal symptoms as reasons for their difficulty quitting (Biglan & Lichtenstein, 1984). Ninety-five percent of high-school-age smokers believe they will quit within 5 years after finishing high school. Of these, in 8 years approximately 53% will try unsuccessfully to quit and about 25% will eventually succeed (Charlton, Melia, & Moyer, 1990). Among college students, survey results (Emmons et al., 1998; Wechsler et al., 1998) suggest that half of college student smokers had quit smoking for at least 24 hours in the past year, including 18% who had made five or more quit attempts. Most adolescent smokers feel they are addicted to nicotine and want to quit but are unable to do so (U.S. Department of Health and Human Services, 1994). Given that many adolescent smokers eventually become addicted to nicotine, more effort needs to be directed toward cessation among youth and young adults.

Another reason to focus on adolescent smoking cessation is that smoking among teens is associated with other dangerous behaviors, such as alcohol and other substance abuse, promiscuity, and reckless driving (Farrell, Danish, & Howard, 1992). Such problem behaviors are positively correlated with each other and negatively correlated with conventional behaviors such as school attendance and grade point average (Farrell et al., 1992). In utero exposure to nicotine (from mothers who smoke during pregnancy) and attentional problems or conduct disorders predict progression to nicotine dependence and criminal or sociopathic behavior in later adolescence and adulthood (Griesler et al., 1998; Levin & Slotkin, 1998). It has been postulated that tobacco is a "gateway" substance in the progression of other drug dependencies, preceding use of other illicit substances (Griesler et al., 1998; Kandel & Yamaguchi, 1993). Some have viewed cigarette smoking as a preventable or interruptable risk factor for abuse of other substances and for other problem behaviors (Henningfield et al., 1993). Interventions to stop smoking before smokers experiment with other substances and negative behaviors could serve to interrupt the progression down the road to severe harm. Although this is an interesting hypothesis, it should be pointed out that a two-way relationship exists. Brown, Lewinsohn, Seeley, and Wagner (1996) recently reported on the reciprocal relationship between major depression and adolescent smoking: Depression at Time 1 predicted smoking at Time 2 and vice versa. There may also be more fundamental mechanisms operating; for example, the cluster of addictive, mood-related, attentional, and other risk-taking behaviors are cofactors of a yet-to-be-discovered set of underlying gene–gene and/or gene–environment interactions (Swan & Carmelli, 1997).

Adolescent Nicotine Dependence

There is increasing evidence that in utero exposure to nicotine may alter the structure of the brain, resulting in greater vulnerability in adolescents to addiction and behavioral problems (Griesler et al., 1998). Understanding how such vulnerability translates into dependence is of paramount importance. Little is known about the critical pathways, transitions, and trajectories, from earliest exposure to nicotine to initial use to experimental use to dependence, among youth (Abrams & Clayton, 2001; Monti, Colby, et al., 2001).

Researchers are calling for a paradigm shift in the focus of research programs toward understanding the etiology and the developmental trajectories of smoking initiation and progression to nicotine dependence in youth (Abrams, 1999a, 1999b). The comprehensive triadic model of social influence advanced by Flay and colleagues (Flay et al., 1995) has mapped how distal (e.g., community, school, neighborhood) and proximal (e.g., peer pressure to conform, social skills, and self-efficacy) levels of social influence are associated with likelihood of smoking. Flay's research demonstrates how social and environmental mediating and moderating variables act through causal pathways to influence smoking. The important ways in which biological, genetic, and gene–environment interactions mediate or moderate the largely sociological and cognitive-behavioral variables in the triadic model have not been fully explored. In order to learn more about how to improve prevention and early cessation treatments for youths and young adults, more basic research studies are needed on the ways in which lifespan developmental factors interact with individual and nested contextual factors along the pathways to initiation, regular tobacco use, and dependence. In particular, research is needed on: parent–offspring and sibling-pair linkage studies to examine gene–environment interactions; longitudinal cohort designs with more than three repeated measures over time; inclusion of high-quality measures from the biological, cognitive, behavioral, and proximal and distal environmental domains; selection of better measures derived from theoretically driven hypotheses; and attending to issues of representative sampling such as subgroups with disproportionate vulnerabilities (Flay, 2000; Flay et al., 1995; Novak & Clayton, 2001).

Our research team at Brown Medical School has begun to tackle the problem of adolescent smoking, both from the perspective of understanding the constructs of nicotine dependence and withdrawal as maintenance factors in adolescent smoking (Colby et al., 2000a, 2000b) and from the perspective of what might constitute effective smoking treatment for teens (Monti, Colby, et al., 2001). Whereas the abstinence syndrome that follows on the abrupt cessation of smoking has been extensively studied among adult smokers (e.g., J. R. Hughes et al., 1990), its study among teens is much less developed and is only recently getting the attention that it deserves (e.g., Colby et al., 2000a, 2000b). A focus on understanding nicotine dependence and withdrawal effects is particularly important because many treatments, such as NRT, are based on this understanding. Such understanding is practically nonexistent in the adolescent literature. Yet, at the same time, many teens are initiating use of NRT. A central question that needs to be addressed is, At what level of smoking does it become safe and effective to consider NRT as part of a cessation treatment plan for teenage or young adult smokers? This issue is addressed in more detail later in this chapter.

In the following sections, we briefly review the results of prevention efforts with adolescents and then review the few intervention studies available, as well as the blueprint of our work in progress.

Prevention

Research has focused on the prevention of smoking initiatives using classroom-based and community approaches (Botvin, Baker, Dusenbury, Botvin, & Diaz, 1995; Pentz, 1999). The more effective prevention approaches have employed psychosocial techniques that address social influences (e.g., peer resistance training). Although social reinforcement–based strategies have been effective in delaying the onset of smoking, with a 30–50% lower rate of smoking onset compared with controls (Flay et al., 1995), the long-term effectiveness of these programs is less impressive, and it is unclear which components of these programs are responsible for significant effects. Indeed, Flay and colleagues (Flay et al., 1995) suggest that the clues to effective prevention programs will be found in the interaction between the intervention program and preexisting macro-socioeconomic, community, neighborhood, school, and other environmental sources of social influence, such as proximal peer and family variables (Flay, 2000; Novak & Clayton, 2001). The largest and most rigorous school-based, social-influences prevention program of its kind, the Hutchinson Smoking Prevention Project, failed to find efficacy both during and after implementation (Peterson, Kealey, Mann, Marek, & Sarason, 2000). Another large and well-controlled cluster-randomized trial, conducted in 52 schools in Great Britain with 8,352 pupils, evaluated the transtheoretical "stages of change" model and, at 1- and 2-year follow-up, reported that the stages of change model was ineffective (Aveyard et al., 2001).

Prevention programs are limited in several respects. First, they are often designed as general substance-use prevention programs. A lack of specificity on smoking behavior may limit their efficacy with respect to smoking outcome. Second, many school-based programs are designed as prevention, not cessation, programs, yet many students are already using—indeed, may already be addicted to—tobacco. Third, prevention programs generally fail to address motivational issues related to use: Most assume that students are motivated to resist use. Motivational enhancement (see Chapter 3) is considered an important element for cessation programs, particularly those targeted to youth (Colby et al., 1998; Monti, Barnett, O'Leary, & Colby, 2001). Fourth, school-based programs fail to reach many high-risk and minority youths. Indeed, one sixth-grade prevention trial found that 68% of subsequent school dropouts were regular smokers at 6-year follow-up compared with 28% of students still in school (Flay et al., 1989). Fifth, the distal macro-socioeconomic, community, and neighborhood sources of influence (including restrictive youth access laws, enforcement, and tax disincentives), as well as prevailing social norms, appear to be strong sources of variability in the success of programs. These factors are rarely targeted for intervention (Chaloupka & Warner, 2000; Forster & Wolfson, 1998; Rigotti et al., 1997).

Youth Cessation Treatment

Although they date back nearly 20 years, documented smoking cessation efforts with adolescents are few and far between. One early study reported that adding a four-session module of prevention and cessation to a regular health education curriculum for tenth graders led to a reduction in the percentage of students who reported smoking compared with controls (Perry, Killen, Telch, Slinkard, & Danaher, 1980). A more recent study using a contingency-based smoking cessation program gave monetary rewards contingent on reductions in carbon monoxide (CO) levels (Weissman, Glasgow, Biglan, & Lichtenstein, 1987). A computer-tailored smoking cessation program for teens recently demonstrated some promise, with short-term quit rates of up to 20% (Pallonen et al., 1998). Tailoring interventions based on an individual assessment of teens' needs is a particularly appealing intervention strategy. The privacy and the confidentiality of computer interactions is another advantage for teens. Those just beginning to contemplate quitting may need more information designed to enhance motivation, whereas those prepared to quit may require more focus on cessation skills and relapse prevention strategies.

Interventions in medical settings are becoming more broadly encouraged as a means to contact and treat smokers who might not otherwise seek help for cessation (Lichtenstein et al., 1996). Our group at Brown Medical School has recently launched a programmatic series of studies that focus on adolescents, using brief interventions in acute-care medical settings. Such approaches with adult smokers resulted in long-term quit rates ranging from 15 to 25% (Glynn, 1988; Orleans et al., 1990). As these brief interventions are most likely to be successful with smokers who have few years of smoking history and are less dependent, they may be particularly suitable for teen or young adult smokers.

One study in this program of research (Colby et al., 1998) tested the feasibility and efficacy of a brief smoking intervention for adolescents being treated for medical problems in an urban children's hospital's emergency department (60%), outpatient clinic (33%), or inpatient unit (7%). All teens received medical care prior to being approached and randomly assigned to receive either brief advice (BA) or motivational enhancement (ME). Forty adolescent smokers, 14 to 17 years old, who had smoked during the past 30 days participated in the research protocol. After completing the baseline assessment, those assigned to BA received advice to stop smoking and an informational handout and were encouraged to stop smoking and to get help if needed. The motivational enhancement intervention was based on the principles of ME first described by W. R. Miller and Rollnick (1991) and described in more detail in Chapter 3. The provider used an empathic style, avoided argumentation and resistance, developed a sense of discrepancy between the teen's goals and behavior, and supported the teen's self-efficacy. Each teen was also given individualized feedback about the negative effects of smoking that emphasized the teen's choice and personal responsibility. To facilitate discussion, each teen watched four videotaped vignettes representing four content areas of smoking: health effects, social consequences, addiction, and financial cost. Each teen was given feedback about his/her level of dependence, as indicated by his/her FTQ (see Chapter 2) responses, and feedback about any smoking-related illness. The teen was given the total cost of his/her smoking during the past year, as well as copies of the feedback sheet and an informational handout. Finally, the provider assisted the teen in identifying goals for change, explored barriers to quitting, and provided advice and strategies.

Results demonstrated the feasibility of the ME intervention in terms of high rates of recruitment, retention, quit attempts, and periods of continuous abstinence. Although the between-group differences in smoking measures were not significant (in part due to the small sample size) at the 3-month follow-up, the effect size was medium, offering support for the potential efficacy of the ME. Furthermore, the sample showed significant decreases in smoking dependence and number of days that the teens smoked. Future research on the mechanisms involved with ME effects with teens is warranted based on these preliminary findings.

Although hospital settings have proven to be good sites for recruitment of teen smokers, young smokers and their families can be reached through a variety of other channels that offer opportunities to conduct prevention and early cessation intervention research. Lichtenstein and colleagues (Lichtenstein et al., 1996) point out that there are many potential channels for delivering smoking cessation and prevention interventions. For example, other studies at Brown Medical School focus on smoking prevention and cessation in pediatric practices, in homes through visiting nurse associations (e.g., families with asthmatic children), in vocational–technical colleges with high-risk young adults, and in low-income populations in public health clinics and state-managed Medicaid programs (Lloyd-Richardson,

Niaura, & Abrams, 2001). Research is needed to address the contextual parameters of the setting, as well as the individuals within the setting, so as to maximize impact.

Little is known regarding the smoking habits of young adults or of the feasibility of implementing intervention strategies. Another study at Brown Medical School is targeting young adults at high risk for smoking and other comorbidities. This research began by investigating smoking rates and characteristics among young adults attending technical school (Lloyd, Niaura, Brown, & Abrams, 2001). A random sample of 784 students attending a large technical school in southern New England was administered an anonymous questionnaire assessing smoking habits, as well as interest and motivation to quit. Questionnaires were administered to one-third of the classrooms, which were randomly selected from a list of all course offerings. The response rate was 82.5%. Respondents were primarily male (70%), and white (85%), with an average age of 26 years. Thirty-three percent were current smokers, smoking an average of 16 cigarettes per day. Ninety-one percent of smokers had tried to quit within the past year, with an average of three 24-hour quit attempts over the past year. Seventy-eight percent of smokers endorsed at least a moderate level of motivation to quit smoking (i.e., "often think of quitting, but no plans yet"), with 50% interested in use of the nicotine patch and 43% interested in use of bupropion hydrochloride (Zyban). These data suggest that the prevalence of smoking among technical school students is higher than among traditional 4-year college students (28%; Wechsler et al., 1998), as well as among the general population of the United States (median 23.2%; Centers for Disease Control and Prevention, 2000a, 2000b).

Given their particular constellation of risk factors, including lower education and socioeconomic status, technical school students may be particularly prone to years of continued smoking, suggesting the need for a powerful early intervention. Therefore, we have opted to investigate the combination of pharmacological (Zyban + nicotine patch) and psychosocial (cognitive-behavioral group therapy) interventions as an effective smoking cessation treatment for this high-risk young adult population. Targeting this group of high-risk adults at a younger age will provide an unexplored window of opportunity for halting the entrenchment of smoking and preventing future detrimental medical, psychological, and economic consequences. Studies of basic mechanisms are needed that can identify leverage points (e.g., different phases of smoking uptake patterns) for prevention, early treatment, or policy formation (Lloyd-Richardson, Papandonatos, Kazura, Stanton, & Niaura, 2002).

Finally, we note that there have been efforts to treat adolescent smokers with NRT. Despite evidence of safety, tolerability, and decreased withdrawal symptoms among adolescents treated with the nicotine patch, efficacy has not been demonstrated (Hurt et al., 2000; Smith et al., 1996). However disappointing, we must recognize that treatment of the adolescent smoker is still in its infancy.

Comorbidity

Another future direction in smoking approaches with adolescents involves comorbidity. The comorbidity between smoking and more general psychopathology among adolescents has been the focus of yet another adolescent initiative by our group at Brown Medical School. Brown and colleagues (Brown et al., 1996) found, in cross-sectional analyses, that a significant association existed between drug abuse and dependence, disruptive behavior disorders, and adolescent smoking, even after controlling for the co-occurrence of other disorders. Major depressive disorder (MDD) and alcohol abuse and dependence were significantly related to smoking before, but not after, controlling for the other disorders. Prospectively, smoking was found to increase the risk of developing an episode of MDD or drug abuse and dependence, and MDD was found to significantly predict smoking onset. Overall, 67% of the teen smokers had a history of psychiatric disorder compared with 33% of the nonsmokers.

In sum, research to date is revealing a complex set of pathways and trajectories that culminate in initiation of smoking, experimental smoking, and progression to regular use and to tobacco dependence (Abrams, 1999b; Abrams & Clayton, 2001). Furthermore, the role of macro-socioeconomic factors and local community, neighborhood, and peer groups, as well as an emerging research literature on genetic and neurobiological mechanisms such as early nicotine exposure in utero, suggest that no one single approach will be sufficient in and of itself to make an impact on reducing population prevalence rates of smoking initiation. Nevertheless, it is expected that early cessation interventions in the adolescent and young adult populations will have to be generalizable to school, community, and health care settings, in which the largest proportion of at-risk teens who smoke may be located. The long-term goal of future research is to translate new discoveries from etiological research on basic mechanisms into promising small-scale clinical treatment efficacy trials and also into larger scale dissemination studies. Interventions will then foster changes in policy and will effect a broad public health impact.

NEUROBIOLOGY, PHARMACOTHERAPY, AND COMBINED TREATMENTS

A common concern of providers who have smokers on various forms of NRT is that these ex-smokers will become dependent on and eventually abuse NRT. This concern is especially true for heavily addicted adults and for adolescent smokers, given the relative lack of scientific evidence for the dependence syndrome in this younger population. However, although there is evidence that NRT with adults can induce phenomena such as tolerance, withdrawal, compulsive use, and misuse, NRT abuse is essentially nonexistent (J. R. Hughes, 1998). Shiffman and colleagues (1998) point out that, despite intensive scrutiny (due to the fact that the FDA prohibits sales of nonprescription NRT to children under age 18), there is no scientific evidence of abuse by minors and that this is probably because NRT products have much lower appeal and abuse potential than cigarettes and because NRT product sales are more restricted than tobacco products. The growing interest in harm minimization strategies for a variety of high-risk behaviors (Marlatt, 1999) is being applied to nicotine addiction and raises new research questions that relate to these exposure reduction strategies (Henningfield, 1997; see later in this section).

Although the major form of NRT misuse is concurrent use of NRT and tobacco in smokers, such use usually results in a decrease in smoking, in carbon monoxide, and in other combustion products, suggesting less exposure to carcinogens and other toxins (J. R. Hughes, 1998). Nevertheless, as concurrent use does result in higher nicotine levels, future research should be focused on studying the potential harmful effects of higher nicotine levels. In addition, Hughes (1998) notes that research is needed to study whether tolerance occurs to the positive effects of NRT and whether withdrawal symptoms occur when nasal spray and inhaler treatments are stopped. In general, Hughes calls for more studies that examine the clinical indices of dependence on NRT, such as difficulty stopping, as well as studies that examine toxin exposure and other potentially harmful effects that might occur from concurrent use of tobacco and NRT.

A recent book on nicotine safety and toxicity concludes that "all of the evidence indicates that nicotine administered as a medication is always safer than that obtained by cigarette smoking" (N. Benowitz, 1998b, p. 183). Clearly, this statement reflects much of the current thinking in the field, but the focus has been on chronic usage by adults rather than adolescents. There are many gaps in our knowledge regarding NRT, and use of NRT indiscriminately can be problematic. Three populations of special concern are pregnant women, children, and those with acute or severe chronic medical illnesses that may be exacerbated by nicotine. Although NRT has been studied in several trials with pregnant women, the safety of patch use during pregnancy has not been established, and it has been recommended that the potential neurotoxicity of continuous nicotine exposure should preclude the use of 24-hour patches with pregnant women (Oncken, Hardardottir, & Smeltzer, 1998). Furthermore, recent findings (Griesler et al., 1998) suggest that in utero exposure results in adolescent addiction among offspring. Given that there is no known safe dose of nicotine that can be taken during pregnancy, NRT should be considered only if it is unlikely that smoking cessation will occur without it (Oncken et al., 1998).

Similarly, the use of NRT with teens and young adults is not adequately studied. Indeed, children are not mentioned by Benowitz (1998b). This clearly reflects the gap in our knowledge base and points to the need for more research. One area about which we are particularly ignorant is at what point in the youth smoking trajectory (from initial use to experimentation to regular use to dependence) it might be helpful to prescribe NRT. Initiation and early smoking among youth is characterized by irregular patterns of use and long periods without exposure to nicotine. Even more regular users typically cannot smoke wherever and whenever they want to. Because upregulation of nicotinic brain receptors occurs (Dani & Heinemann, 1996), a constant infusion of nicotine as delivered by NRT may increase abuse liability and withdrawal sensitivity, especially in irregular smokers. Such potential problems, combined with the ethics involved in possibly exposing naive youth to nicotine for research purposes, are probable reasons that data are not available.

One particularly interesting application of NRT is its use in exposure reduction treatments (ERT) for adults. Shiffman and his colleagues (1998) define ERT as "the systematic application of nicotine-delivering medications and medical and behavioral principles to establish and sustain reduced exposure to tobacco toxins" (p. 350). Although ERT represents a significant modification to smoking treatment policy that has to date focused on cessation, the effectiveness of ERT on the smoking rates of smokers without compensatory behaviors has been well established (Pickworth, Bunker, & Henningfield, 1994) and warrants further attention. Less well studied is the deliberate clinical use of NRT among adult smokers trying to reduce their smoking, and we know of no studies that have used NRT for adolescents trying to reduce. Shiffman and colleagues (1998) point out that the generalizability of findings from adult studies is limited and that more research is needed, with and without NRT, to assess the potential for reduced exposure through reduction in smoking rates.

Nicotine dependence acts as a barrier to cessation, and because smokers with lower dependence can quit more easily, many of the smokers remaining in the population are likely to be more dependent (J. R. Hughes, Goldstein et al., 1999). Hughes and colleagues point out that there are some important differences in the delivery system and in neurobiological mechanisms between nicotine addiction and other drugs of dependence. These differences make even the long-term use of alternative nicotine delivery systems more appealing than the continued use of tobacco products. The delivery device (cigarettes) essentially delivers nicotine in a contaminated form, along with the toxins and carcinogens from the gas phase of burning tobacco, whereas alternative nicotine delivery systems do not. The main toxins are carbon monoxide, carcinogens, and other by-products of smoke rather than nicotine. Zevin and colleagues (1998) evaluated the dose-related cardiovascular and endocrine effects of transdermal nicotine and concluded that high-dose nicotine treatment, even with concomitant smoking, caused no short-term adverse effects on the cardiovascular system.

Nicotine products, both in contaminated forms (cigarettes) and in safer forms (alternative delivery systems—nasal spray, gum, patch, lozenge), are legal and readily available—these already compete on the open market for purchase by consumers, as nicotine gum and patches are over-the-counter products. In general, the dependence liability of most alternative nicotine delivery systems is very low (e.g., gum, patch). There is increasing evidence of their safety, and it may be necessary for some smokers to use NRT over the long term in order to successfully stop smoking (J. R. Hughes, Goldstein, et al., 1999). Recently, new treatments have become available, including the nicotine inhaler and bupropion hydrochloride (Zyban). Hughes and colleagues (J. R. Hughes, Goldstein et al., 1999) conclude that all these new pharmacotherapies should be made available to smokers, as they appear to be equally efficacious and they approximately double the quit rate compared with placebo controls. Behavioral and supportive therapy further increases quit rates and is encouraged in conjunction with all pharmacotherapies.

Advances in biomedical technology, genetics, molecular biology, neuroscience, and pharmacology have dramatically increased our knowledge of the mechanisms involved in nicotine addiction and have resulted in several new and effective intervention options. Among the many questions that remain to be addressed in future research are the following: What is the optimal timing, dose, and duration of NRT, bupropion, and their combinations? What other drugs that are similar in chemical structure to bupropion (e.g., with dopaminergic/noradrenergic properties) should be tested? What is the significance of inhibition of MAO A and B levels in current smokers? How can new pharmacotherapies be best combined with one another and with behavior therapy? Can brief screening tests be developed with sufficient sensitivity and specificity to tailor specific drug therapies to specific biomarkers or behavioral expression of underlying neurobiological individual differences? What implications do all of the above have for adolescent smoking cessation? Because ultimately the neurobiological substrate that underlies addictive processes must be translated into cognitions (e.g., cravings, mood regulation) and expression in behavior (e.g., drug seeking, compulsive use despite harmful consequences), the basic neurobiological disciplines must combine forces with behavioral, social, and population sciences to advance our knowledge of biobehavioral interactions that can inform new treatment and policy (Abrams, 1999a, 1999b).

One technology that has been particularly useful in linking pharmacology and behavioral science is tobacco cue reactivity assessment. This procedure, first developed for research on tobacco addiction (Abrams, 1986) and used extensively by our group at Brown Medical School (Abrams, 1986, 2000; Abrams et al., 1988; Abrams et al., 1987; Niaura et al., 1988; Niaura et al., 1998), enables researchers to study, under controlled laboratory conditions, smokers' physiological and subjective reactions to standardized high-risk-for-relapse situations (Abrams, 2000; Hutchison et al., 1999; Monti, Rohsenow, & Hutchison, 2000). As exposure to smoking cues produces reliable increases in urges to smoke and in negative affect (e.g., Drobes & Tiffany, 1997; Niaura et al., 1988), the cue exposure procedure can and has been used to test the effects of a variety of pharmacological agents that might reduce craving for cigarettes (Abrams, 2000; Hutchison et al., 1999). Thus laboratory studies can bridge the gap between basic human biobehavioral mechanisms, research, and animal studies on the one hand and clinical efficacy trials and larger scale diffusion and dissemination studies of efficiency and cost-effectiveness on the other.

TAILORING TREATMENT TO SMOKER PROFILES

The concept of patient–treatment matching, or tailoring, is not new. There is considerable skepticism concerning the value of patient–treatment matching because studies in the area of alcoholism and mental health have generally failed to produce results that support matching (e.g., Project MATCH Research Group, 1997). The smoking cessation literature contains more evidence in support of specific kinds of tailoring, such as the use of computer-tailored feedback reports (Skinner, Campbell, Rimer, Curry, & Prochaska, 1999) to tailor smoking cessation messages; however, there are insufficient well-controlled studies to draw firm conclusions (Abrams, Mills, & Bulger, 1999). The transtheoretical stages of change model has attracted considerable interest over the past decade, and several studies suggest that matching interventions to stages of change can enhance outcomes (Prochaska et al., 1997). However, the PHS guideline (Fiore et al., 2000) concluded that evidence was insufficient to support the stages of change model. A recent large, well-executed, randomized controlled trial of a stage-based computer expert system was conducted in Great Britain with adolescents ($n = 8,352$). The short- and long-term analysis of outcome efficacy of the stages of change model was reported to be "ineffective" (Aveyard et al., 2001). Because nicotine replacement boosts quit rates across the board, it should be used with all smokers, as recommended in the PHS guideline (Fiore et al., 2000). However, there is also evidence that psychiatric and substance abuse comorbidities result in poorer outcomes and that more dependent smokers may differentially benefit from higher doses of nicotine replacement therapies (Hurt, 1998).

As mentioned previously, Project MATCH (Project MATCH Research Group, 1997), the largest and most rigorous matching trial conducted to date on alcoholics, did not show support for matching. Furthermore, outcomes at 1-year follow-up were similar across the projects' three psychosocial treatments. However, as Marlatt (1999) points out, the negative results of Project MATCH should be interpreted cautiously within the area of alcohol treatment and should not be generalized to other addictive behaviors. The major limitations of Project MATCH have been listed elsewhere (Marlatt, 1999) and include a highly selected sample of motivated alcoholics with limited range in severity of problems, a set of treatments that were exclusively psychosocial and had common and overlapping treatment elements, and the lack of a control group. Most important, Marlatt suggests that in the real world a great deal of "self-matching" occurs as patients seek treatment and as providers decide who they are most qualified to treat. This finer-grained matching is not easily captured in a research protocol. Self-initiated matching results in a strong therapeutic relationship between provider and patient, and the resultant alliance becomes paramount for success (Marlatt, 1999). Thus a true matching study should include self-selection by patients (and/or by the patient and the provider together). Marlatt (1999) believes that matching into self-matched versus randomly assigned conditions may be a better test of the matching hypothesis.

As we have pointed out in earlier chapters, various components of smoking treatment can interact with individual differences to produce tailoring hypotheses. Yet research on tailoring is only just beginning to address the big issues. For example, Abrams and colleagues (Abrams, Clark, & King, 1999) point out that the possibilities for improving smoking outcomes by tailoring smoker characteristics to intervention components is appealing at both macro- and micro-levels. At a macro-level, matching involves a form of stepped care, i.e., the targeting of interventions of varying intensity to community- or group-level characteristics, including the degree of readiness to quit; demographic characteristics such as age, education, and gender; and the needs of special populations such as ethnic minorities. At a micro-level, matching would involve more fine-grained tailoring to biobehavioral factors at the individual level, such as individual motivation, self-efficacy, level of nicotine dependence, and presence of comorbid substance abuse or mood disorders.

A recent study from our Brown Medical School group illustrates one component of smoking treatment that can interact with individual differences. As part of a larger clinical trial (the aim of which was to determine whether fluoxetine would enhance smoking cessation) sponsored by Eli Lilly & Co., Niaura and colleagues (Niaura, Goldstein, Spring, & Keuthen, 1997) conducted a substudy in which they pooled data from 175 smokers on whom they had DSM-III-R SCID diagnostic interviews. They focused specifically on diagnosing lifetime history of major affective disorder. In addition, they administered the Hamilton Depression Scale (HAM-D). Thirty-two percent of the sample met criteria for a diagnosis of lifetime history of major depression. Although outcome results from the substudy showed no overall effect of fluoxetine on smoking cessation, stratifying current symptoms of depression as assessed by the HAM-D interacted with treatment significantly to affect cessation outcomes. Smokers who had two or more signs and symptoms of depression who received a placebo were at significantly greater risk for return to smoking sooner and for treatment failure at follow-up. However, if these high-risk smokers received a high dose (60 mg per day) of fluoxetine, they achieved quit rates similar to those smokers without current symptoms of depression. Subsyndromal signs and symptoms of depression predicted failure to quit smoking in this study. Results further suggest that treatment with an antidepressant will benefit only those smokers who show some, albeit almost any, signs and symptoms of depression prior to quitting.

Future studies must evaluate promising tailoring hypotheses in a scientifically rigorous fashion. Important parameters to be included are (1) smokers with a full range of theory-driven individual difference characteristics (such as various levels of nicotine dependence and nicotine sensitivity), as well as comorbidities and representative populations; (2) assessment tools with reasonable sensitivity and specificity; and (3) experimental designs that include random assignment to both matched and mismatched cohorts or, as Marlatt (1999) suggests, to self-matched and study-matched conditions. Furthermore, given the emergence of innovative and specific pharmacological interventions and a stepped-care approach to smoking treatment, matching studies should include factors at both macro- and micro-levels of social structure. Although numerous empirical studies and reviews (e.g., Abrams, 1993; Abrams et al., 1996; Hughes, 1994a; Orleans & Slade, 1993) suggest the utility of a stepped-care-plus-tailoring approach to smoking cessation, this approach has not been empirically evaluated to date and is clearly a priority area for future research. Lessons learned from Project MATCH and other matching studies can be informative in the design of future research studies on tailoring interventions to smoker characteristics.

SMOKING AND ALCOHOL ABUSE AND DEPENDENCE

Smoking and alcohol go together. Although this notion is not surprising, what is surprising is how little we know about why they go together (Abrams, 1995). Over 85% of adults with a history of alcohol abuse smoke, generally smoke more, and have greater difficulty stopping than smokers without such a history (Burling & Ziff, 1988). Furthermore, drinking alcohol is a significant precipitant of smoking relapse in the general population. Alcohol and tobacco abuse combined is estimated to cost over $150 billion annually (L. T. Kozlowski, Ferrence, & Corbit, 1990). Smoking alcoholics have synergistic health risks for cancer and cardiovascular disease (Zacny, 1990). Hurt and colleagues (1994) reported that more alcoholics die from tobacco use than from their alcoholism. Indeed, Bill W., the cofounder of Alcoholics Anonymous, died of a smoking-related illness. Clearly, reducing smoking prevalence among smoking alcoholics can have a beneficial impact on individuals and society (Bobo, Walker, Lando, McIlvain, & Anderson, 1995). Moreover, there is a need to understand: (1) the mechanisms that regulate alcohol–tobacco interactions; (2) how to reach this alarming majority of smokers; and (3) how to motivate this largely unmotivated group to quit smoking and then help them to stay abstinent (J. R. Hughes, 1995).

Smoking treatments for recovering substance abusers have frequently yielded low cessation rates (Hurt et al., 1994; Joseph, Nichol, & Anderson, 1993), although more recent reports show somewhat more promising results (e.g., Martin et al., 1997). Our group's approach to studying smoking among alcoholics has been first to study alcohol–tobacco interactions in laboratory-based studies, then alcohol–smoking interaction expectancies among alcoholics in treatment; finally we translate the results from basic laboratory research to applications in terms of asking more treatment-outcome-relevant questions.

One early study investigated the relationship between reactions to alcohol cue exposure and urge to smoke among alcoholics in treatment (Abrams et al., 1992). Results showed that urges to smoke at baseline were higher for those with greater alcohol dependence; exposure to alcohol cues significantly increased urges to smoke; and urges to drink correlated positively with urges to smoke (Abrams et al., 1992; Gulliver et al., 1995). A second study (Monti, Rohsenow, Colby, & Abrams, 1995) found that urge to smoke was higher during alcohol cue exposure after negative mood induction than before. Depressed mood affected women's, but not men's, urge to smoke. A third study investigated the effects of exposure to alcohol cues on urge to smoke and smoking topography (Rohsenow et al., 1997). Both urge to drink and urge to smoke were significantly elevated in the alcohol-exposure condition, but no differences in smoking topography were found. From these studies, it can be concluded that urges to smoke are related to drinking variables such as alcohol cues and that smoking cessation may be more difficult in early recovery, when exposure to naturally occurring alcohol cues may increase urges to smoke. However, smoking may not be used as a means of coping with urges to drink (Monti et al., 1995).

An alcohol–smoking interactions questionnaire (Colby et al., 1994) was designed to assess smoking alcoholics' beliefs about the interactions between smoking and drinking during recovery after alcohol treatment. It was administered to 95 alcoholics who were being treated for their alcohol problems. Results from this study showed that: (1) 70% of patients said that it would be harder to stay sober if they quit smoking during alcohol treatment; (2) 60% would try smoking treatment if it were offered; (3) 58% have at times smoked to cope with an urge to drink; and (4) resistance to smoking treatment was greater among alcoholics with higher tobacco dependence or when smoking treatment was mandatory as opposed to voluntary.

Laboratory-based and questionnaire studies have paved the way for two smoking treatment outcome studies with alcoholics that are currently underway at Brown Medical School. One study is designed to evaluate the degree to which a motivational enhancement intervention increases smoking cessation rates compared with a brief intervention in a sample of outpatient alcoholics. All smoking alcoholics are targeted as potential study patients in the context of their outpatient treatments. Following an intake and a baseline assessment, patients are randomly assigned to one of the two treatments, both delivered by a trained health educator/interventionist. Patients assigned to brief advice receive brief counseling (< 5 minutes) and self-help materials (*AHRQ Consumer Guide: You Can Quit Smoking*; see Table 4.8) and a prescription for a nicotine patch. Patients assigned to motivational enhancement receive three 30-minute in-person counseling sessions over a 1-month period, and then two 15-minute telephone counseling sessions over the subsequent 2 months. Nicotine patches and self-help materials are provided to these patients when they become motivated to quit.

A total of 412 patients were approached to take part in this clinical research study (Hitsman et al., 2002) and, of those, 346 (84%) met eligibility criteria. Of these smokers who met eligibility criteria, 298 (86%) were randomized and enrolled in the study. Thus the majority of eligible smokers in busy outpatient alcohol treatment settings agreed to participate in the research, despite the fact that these patients are, on average, only moderately motivated to quit smoking. Adherence to the rigors of the treatment protocol has been remarkable—over 90% of all appointments with enrolled patients have been kept. Patients in the study are heavy smokers (smoking an average of 27.5 cigarettes per day), 22% had comorbid psychiatric illnesses, and only 28% wanted to set a quit date. Moreover, the follow-up rate through 3 months has been over 90%, and at 12 months, it has been over 80%. Clearly, this experience suggests that the majority of alcoholics receiving outpatient treatment are willing to at least talk about their smoking, even if they are not quite ready to quit yet, which may be in contrast to traditional clinical lore that most alcoholics do not want to discuss concurrent smoking for fear that it will undermine their sobriety. The results of this study promise to provide key insights into the most effective ways to help alcoholics quit smoking.

A second study is designed to test the effects of enhancing motivation among smoking alcoholics who may or may not be interested in smoking cessation by offering them the opportunity to receive information about the effects of their smoking on their lives. The important issue of timing of smoking treatment for alcoholics is addressed in this study. Similar to the previous study, this study evaluates the effectiveness of motivational interviewing as an intervention for tobacco use among alcoholics, as compared with a widely recommended intervention that involves brief advice and assistance. In addition, the study evaluates the effectiveness of adding booster sessions of the same intervention about 1 and 4 weeks later, when patients may be more receptive, and examines individual differences in motivationally relevant variables that may effect responsiveness.

Thus, with both alcoholic outpatients and residential treatment patients, we have demonstrated the feasibility and transportability of these brief interventions and the ability to target a unique subset of particularly high-risk smokers. Given that such individuals are otherwise unlikely to receive smoking treatment, the potential for a clinically meaningful application of this treatment is promising.

CHALLENGES IN FORMULATING THE STEPPED-CARE PLAN OF THE FUTURE

This book has focused primarily on the assessment and treatment elements needed for development of an individual treatment plan for a single provider treating a smoker. Although we recommend in Chapters 1 and 8 that the provider role can be broadened from simply delivering a one-shot intervention, the reality is that many providers will neither have the time, resources, reimbursement incentives, nor access to a team of specialists needed to fully manage the more complicated comorbidities found among many smokers. Thus the providers of today will fall short of being able to implement a comprehensive and more idealistic version of what we envision as a broader care management plan (i.e., to treat smoking cessation as a chronic illness, like diabetes or schizophrenia, and provide continuity of care, persistent positive support, and offer options for different levels of treatment [stepped care] for as long as it takes to achieve at least 12 months of continuous cessation).

In the future, the contextual and organizational support for a more comprehensive care management plan (CMP) at the level of policy and delivery systems (rather than at the level of individual providers and smokers) must be considered and evaluated for cost-effectiveness. Within an organizational infrastructure, the task of identifying all who smoke, reaching them proactively, assessing their specific profiles of risk, and then enrolling them in a CMP requires considerable planning, infrastructure, investment of resources, and top-down support from the leadership of health care organizations and government. The sometimes lengthy process of coordinating care across multiple providers and settings suggests that a special unit staffed by full-time care managers may be needed. The care manager is someone who does not deliver direct care at all but who assures that appropriate care will be delivered by a qualified specialist.

As outlined in Chapters 1 and 8, a good CMP is designed to overcome systemic barriers to continuity of care and to ensure that appropriate levels of care are delivered at the right place and time. Ideally, health care delivery systems and communities should have adequate capacity to support service providers in delivering coordinated individual care management. In reality, the infrastructure and capacity do not exist in most health care or public health delivery systems in the United States today. Current barriers include competition, small profit margins, and turf battles among health care entities. Lack of infrastructure and support for a CMP perpetuates the present delivery system (one we call the "spray and pray," or uncoordinated, approach), in which inefficient care, inequitable care, no care, and sometimes even inappropriate care are being delivered. Smokers in the lowest socioeconomic groups and the uninsured are most affected by the current status quo and likely will continue to have little access to, or opportunity for obtaining, the more specialized, intensive, effective, and expensive levels of care. The provider who is developing a CMP may want to consider these contextual factors and even become an advocate for social action and policy change within his/ her own organization, community, state, or nation.

A crucial issue is where to place the locus of responsibility for developing the infrastructure to permit a comprehensive approach to treatment. How should the entire model be centrally managed within the health care system? An integrated medical record that is agreed on as a standard by all providers would help to manage such a CMP approach with the capability of tracking patients over time and across delivery systems. Computer management information systems make it possible to create an integrated medical record. An ongoing tracking system could be developed for individuals and could be tailored to their high-risk conditions, ranging from nicotine addiction to diabetes to heart failure.

Consumers and developers of clinical guidelines will also need to be educated about what constitutes a high-quality and comprehensive nicotine addiction treatment program and the benefits it can provide to individuals and to society at large. As time goes on, the mature managed care markets may eventually see the wisdom of prevention as a longer term return on investment. Once the more obvious short-term demand-reduction strategies are in place (to ensure efficient acute and emergency care) and these reengineered systems have reached the upper limit of their cost-saving potential, then primary care and primary prevention will have more value and will become the only other source of possible improvement of care and of return on investment.

Cost-Effectiveness and Cost per Quality Adjusted Life Years Saved

Although improving quality of life for the entire society is the ultimate goal of health care, comparative cost factors cannot be ignored. Table 9.1 provides some indicators of cost, such as cost per quality adjusted life years saved by smoking cessation treatment programs. The most expensive treatment programs for smoking cessation only begin to approach the cost of other well-accepted medical practices, such as management of hypertension or hypercholes-

TABLE 9.1. Cost Savings in Dollars ($) per Quality Adjusted Life Year Saved for Smoking Cessation and Other Medical Strategies

Smoking cessation: self-help (Step 1)	$100–500
Smoking cessation: brief physician counseling (Step 2)	$1,000–3,000
Smoking cessation: behavioral specialty clinic (Step 3)	$3,000–6,000
Common disease prevention	$7,500–15,000
Hypertension management	$11,000–23,000
Hyperlipidemia treatment	$20,000–100,000
Palliative medicine: tertiary care/rehab	$20,000–150,000+

Samples of smoker's excess cost to health care system

14% higher for health care utilization
$650–1,200 more per year to worksites
Pregnant smokers—if quit in first trimester would save $22–56 million (due to prevention of low birth weight)

Note. Sources referenced in table: "The Cost-Effectiveness of Three Smoking Cessation Programs," by D. G. Altman, J. A. Flora, S. P. Fortmann, & J. W. Farquhar, 1987, *American Journal of Public Health, 77*(2), 162–165; "The Cost-Effectiveness of Counseling Smokers to Quit," by S. R. Cummings, S. M. Rubin, & G. Oster, 1989, *Journal of the American Medical Association, 276,* 75–79; "Pregnancy and Medical Cost Outcomes of a Self-Help Prenatal Smoking Cessation Program in an HMO," by D. H. Ershoff, V. P. Quinn, P. D. Mullen, & D. R. Lairson, 1990, *Public Health Reports, 105,* 340–347; "Effect of Cost on the Self-Administration and Efficacy of Nicotine Gum: A Preliminary Study," by J. Hughes, W. Wadland, J. Fenwick, J. Lewis, & W. K. Bickel, 1991, *Preventive Medicine, 20,* 486–496; "A Cost-Benefit/Cost-Effectiveness Analysis of Smoking Cessation for Pregnant Women," by J. S. Marks, J. P. Koplan, C. J. Hogue, & M. E. Dalmat, 1990, *American Journal of Preventive Medicine, 6*(5), 282–289; "The Economic Costs of Smoking and the Benefits of Quitting," by G. Oster, G. A. Colditz, & N. L. Kelly, 1984, *Preventive Medicine, 13,* 377–389; "Cost-Effectiveness of Nicotine Gum as an Adjunct to Physician's Advice Against Cigarette Smoking," by G. Oster, D. M. Huse, T. E. Delea, & G. A. Colditz, 1986, *Journal of the American Medical Association, 256*(10), 1315–1318; "Report of the Tobacco Policy Research Study Group on Reimbursement and Insurance in the United States," by M. D. Parkinson, H. H. Schauffler, T. E. Kottke, S. J. Curry, L. I. Solberg, C. B. Arnold, R. H. Butz, R. Taylor, J. B. Holloway, & C. Meltzer, 1992, *Tobacco Control, S1,* S52–S56; "Health Insurance Coverage for Smoking Cessation Services," by H. H. Schauffler & M. D. Parkinson, 1993, *Health Education Quarterly, 20,* 185–206; "Multivariate Cost-Effectiveness Analysis: An Application to Optimizing Ambulatory Care for Hypertension," by D. S. Shepard, W. B. Stason, H. M. Perry, B. A. Carmen, & J. T. Nagurney, 1995, *Inquiry, 32*(3), 320–331; "Dose and Nicotine Dependence as Determinants of Nicotine Gum Efficacy," by P. Tonnesen, in *Nicotine Replacement: A Critical Evaluation,* O. F. Pomerleau & C. S. Pomerleau, Eds., 1988, New York: Alan R. Liss; and "Where Now for Saving Lives?," by R. J. Zeckhauser & D. S. Shepard, 1976, *Law and Contemporary Problems, 40*(4), 5–45.

terolemia. Smoking cessation interventions are orders of magnitude more valuable than typical palliative treatments, such as coronary artery bypass surgery. It should also be noted (see Chapter 1) that lung cancer is virtually untreatable—the 5-year survival rate is under 15% for both men and women. Indeed, for most of the serious chronic diseases caused by use of tobacco products, prevention or cessation is the best "treatment." Once symptoms of serious illness develop (e.g., cancers, cardiovascular diseases, pulmonary diseases), the medical treatments are palliative and in many instances can be viewed as "too little, too late."

There are formidable challenges to adoption of a comprehensive CMP model across the continuum of care. As Abrams and colleagues state (1996), at least six areas need to be addressed: (1) providing evidence for return on investment, both long and short term; (2) providing incentives to health care providers for support of high-quality delivery of brief treatment programs; (3) creating the infrastructure within current practice guidelines to mainstream delivery of preventive services; (4) educating providers, consumers, and payers; (5) coordinating and integrating community-wide services beyond medical care and across the continuum of care; and (6) a renewed emphasis on youth and prevention or early cessation across the developmental life span.

Several methods could help improve access and accelerate the adoption of comprehensive stepped-care models, including:

1. Establishing a central, standardized core medical information system.
2. Approving federal and state legislation to create policies for the mandatory adoption of prevention services that must be covered by all health services suppliers.
3. Educating consumers.
4. Providing reimbursement for assessment and triage into all levels of stepped care.
5. Developing standards, guidelines, and report cards for both adults and adolescents, with meaningful enforceable consequences for nonadherence.
6. Implementing legislative policies and financial incentives for health care delivery systems to focus on primary prevention and on care management for chronic disease states.

The financial barriers for the uninsured and lower-SES consumers should not be permitted to drive treatment decisions about level of care needed, especially concerning the more costly treatment options.

There are also at least five key elements that managed health care systems are likely to share in the not-too-distant future that may facilitate adoption of an infrastructure for CMPs for nicotine addiction. These include:

1. Primary care as the "gatekeeper" to specialist health care. This means that patients are likely to have more frequent contact with their primary care provider, as she/he will be harder to bypass to get to other medical providers.
2. Some preventive services will be covered (e.g., immunizations, mammograms, well-adult check-ups).
3. Automated data systems to track utilization of services (clinic visits, laboratory tests, X rays, etc.).
4. Clinical information systems to prompt providers to deliver preventive services and track management of chronic diseases.
5. Clinical practice guidelines to promote standardization of health care services across multiple providers.

It is these (and other) characteristics of managed care services and the informatics revolution that afford some optimism for adoption of a CMP.

There are many other factors outside of health care delivery that can powerfully influence our society toward improving smoking cessation treatments. Environmental and public health strategies, such as earmarked tobacco taxes and smoking bans in offices, hospitals, airlines, and public places, are all crucial to help move the vast majority of adult smokers into quitting (Abrams, Emmons, Niaura, Goldstein, & Sherman, 1991). Other strategies that can help accelerate prevalence reduction include better primary prevention among youth, education, community activation, advocacy, mass media, and other incentives to quit and disincentives to smoke. Taxation of tobacco products and public health messages about the dangers of environmental tobacco exposure can be very powerful, as they influence the whole of society.

The results of all this concerted effort can be supported by the health care system in a three-way reciprocal partnership of medical, preventive, and public health disciplines.

If society truly values prevention, then the current practice of holding preventive medicine to a higher standard than palliative and curative medicine needs to be challenged. For example, the benefits of coronary bypass surgery or cholesterol management are not questioned in the funding process the way those of smoking cessation are. Diabetes is treated as a chronic disease and is fully integrated into the health care delivery system. Medical care is not based only on costs and profits but also on the value of improved quality for the whole of society. Of greatest concern is how to ensure a safety net of appropriate levels of quality and quantity of preventive services for younger, less educated, lower income, and uninsured citizens. These fellow members of our society are in reality denied access to even brief or moderate types of interventions. Poverty itself is a major risk factor, and it clusters with other poor lifestyle habits, breeding drug abuse, violence, and unrest. Smoking is increasingly a problem of the lower socioeconomic status members of society, and smokers are increasingly challenging: hard to reach, hard to motivate, and hard to treat. There is now considerable evidence that smoking is a serious addictive behavior with enormous human and financial costs to society.

This chapter raises many questions for future researchers and practitioners to consider. Greater collaboration between researchers and practitioners will be needed to advance the field and improve our treatments for nicotine addiction. At the present time, we do have many safe, effective, and cost-effective treatments available, as reviewed in the evidence-based clinical practice guidelines of the PHS (Fiore et al., 2000). It is challenging to put what is known into practice and to disseminate interventions widely enough to make a measurable impact on population and societal statistics of smoking prevalence, of health-damaging consequences, and of personal and societal burdens on quality of life and on our economic well-being. A partnership between basic, clinical, dissemination, and policy researchers and practitioners will help define the challenges and address them in the most parsimonious manner as we traverse the 21st century.

Appendix

Reproducible Handouts

READINESS TO QUIT LADDER

INSTRUCTIONS: Below are some thoughts that smokers have about quitting. On this ladder, circle the one number that shows what you think about quitting. Please read each sentence carefully before deciding.

10	I have quit smoking and I will never smoke again.
9	I have quit smoking, but I still worry about slipping back, so I need to keep working on living smoke free.
8	I still smoke, but I have begun to change, like cutting back on the number of cigarettes I smoke. I am ready to set a quit date.
7	I definitely plan to quit smoking within the next 30 days.
6	I definitely plan to quit smoking in the next 6 months.
5	I often think about quitting smoking, but I have no plans to quit.
4	I sometimes think about quitting smoking, but I have no plans to quit.
3	I rarely think about quitting smoking, and I have no plans to quit.
2	I never think about quitting smoking, and I have no plans to quit.
1	I enjoy smoking and have decided not to quit smoking for my lifetime. I have no interest in quitting.

BARRIERS TO SMOKING CESSATION CHECKLIST

INSTRUCTIONS: Please indicate the extent to which each of the following factors influences your thoughts about quitting smoking.

	Not at all	Some-what	A lot
There are too many difficult things going on in my life right now.	1	2	3
Without cigarettes, I would feel too anxious or worried about things.	1	2	3
Without cigarettes, I would feel too down or sad.	1	2	3
Without cigarettes, I would feel too irritable to be around.	1	2	3
I enjoy smoking too much to give it up.	1	2	3
It would be too hard to control my weight without smoking.	1	2	3
Smoking helps me control other behaviors that I have already changed.	1	2	3
My family and friends don't think it is important to quit smoking.	1	2	3
I don't know how to go about quitting smoking.	1	2	3
I have tried to quit smoking in the past so many times, I've given up.	1	2	3
I can't afford or find a smoking cessation program.	1	2	3

IMPACT OF ENVIRONMENTAL TOBACCO SMOKE

Environmental tobacco smoke exposure:

1. Is a group A carcinogen
2. Increases risk for lung cancer
3. Increases risk for coronary heart disease
4. Increases children's risk of
    - developing coughs, colds
    - tonsillectomy and adenoidectomy
    - otitis media
    - sudden infant death syndrome
    - developing and exacerbating asthma
    - lower respiratory infections
    - hospitalization during first 3 years of life due to respiratory illness
    - having reduced lung function

CONSTITUENTS OF ENVIRONMENTAL TOBACCO SMOKE

Compared with cigarette (mainstream) smoke, environmental tobacco smoke contains
- 2 to 3 times the amount of nicotine
- 3 to 5 times the amount of carbon monoxide
- 8 to 11 times the amount of carbon dioxide
- 5 to 10 times the amount of benzene[a]
- 13 to 30 times the amount of nickel[a]
- 30 times the amount of 2-naphthylamine[a]
- 31 times the amount of 4-aminobiphenyl[a]

[a]Known animal or human carcinogen.

BENEFITS OF SMOKING CESSATION FOR ALL SMOKERS

Short-term benefits

- Improved circulation
- Improved sleep, taste, and smell
- Less shortness of breath
- Reduced risk of home fires
- Improved effectiveness of medications that are affected by smoking (e.g., propranolol, theophylline, insulin, phenylbutazone, as well as medications for pain, depression, anxiety, and insomnia)
- Availability of money that was previously spent on cigarettes

Longer-term benefits

- Risk of dying from a heart attack is cut by half within 1 year of quitting
- Risk of developing emphysema and bronchitis is greatly reduced
- Improved memory, compared with those who continue to smoke
- Reduced risk of osteoporosis and cervical cancer
- Increased life expectancy and quality of life

THE HEALTH AND SOCIAL CONSEQUENCES OF SMOKING

Acute risks

Health risks
- Shortness of breath
- Exacerbation of asthma
- Impotence
- Infertility
- Increased levels of carbon monoxide, carbon dioxide, benzene,[a] nickel,[a] 2-naphthylamine,[a] and 4-aminobiphenyl[a]

Social risks
- Expensive
- Bad breath
- Less accepted socially
- Family's exposure to environmental tobacco smoke

Long-term risks

Health risks
- Myocardial infarction
- Stroke
- Chronic obstructive pulmonary disease
- Emphysema
- Cancer, including cancer of the
  - lung
  - cervix
  - bladder
  - oral cavity
  - pharynx
  - esophagus
  - pancreas
  - colon

Social risks
- Wrinkles
- Children are more likely to smoke
- Some employers may not hire smokers

---

[a]Known animal or human carcinogen.

THE POSITIVE IMPACT OF SMOKING CESSATION ON HEALTH

Within 20 minutes of quitting smoking, a quitter's body begins a series of long-term changes, including:

20 minutes:	Blood pressure drops to normal.
	Pulse rate drops to normal.
	Body temperature of hands and feet increases to normal.
8 hours:	Carbon monoxide level in blood drops to normal.
	Oxygen level in blood increases to normal.
24 hours:	Chance of heart attack decreases.
48 hours:	Nerve endings start regrowing.
	Ability to smell and taste is enhanced.
2 weeks to 3 months:	Circulation improves.
	Walking becomes easier.
	Lung function increases as much as 30%.
1 to 9 months:	Coughing, sinus congestion, fatigue, shortness of breath decrease.
	Cilia regrow in lungs, increasing ability to handle mucus, clean the lungs, reduce infection.
	Energy level increases.
1 year:	Excess risk of coronary heart disease is half that of a smoker.
5 years:	Stroke risk is reduced to that of a nonsmoker within 5–15 years after quitting.
	Risk of cancer of the mouth, throat, and esophagus is half that of a smoker.
10 years:	Precancerous cells are replaced.
	Risk of cancer of the mouth, throat, esophagus, bladder, kidney, and pancreas decreases.
15 years:	Risk of coronary heart disease is equal to that of a nonsmoker.

Source. American Cancer Society, Centers for Disease Control and Prevention.

DECISIONAL WORKSHEET

THINGS I LIKE ABOUT SMOKING	THINGS I DON'T LIKE ABOUT SMOKING

THINGS I WOULD DISLIKE ABOUT QUITTING	THINGS I WOULD LIKE ABOUT QUITTING

REASONS TO STAY THE SAME	REASONS FOR MAKING A CHANGE

GOALS WORKSHEET

The changes I want to make are:

GOAL #1:	GOAL #2:

The steps I plan to take in meeting my goals are:

To smoke less at work . . .	To stop smoking in my house . . .

Other people can help me by:

Person who can help:	Possible ways to help:

Some things that I could do if problems get in the way of my plan are:

Problems:	Things I can do:

MY BUDDY CONTRACT

My goal(s) are to:

1. _____
2. _____

My buddy _____ has agreed to help me meet these goals in the following ways:

1. _____
2. _____

If I need additional help, I can call on my buddy at any time!

_____   _____

My Signature   Buddy's Signature

SAMPLE RELAXATION EXERCISE

The goal of this relaxation exercise is to learn the difference between muscle tension and relaxation. Once that distinction is mastered, it's much easier to evoke a feeling of relaxation, even in stressful settings!

Here's how to get started:

1. Find a quiet, darkened room. Lie on your back or sit in a comfortable, straight-backed chair.
2. Slowly draw as much air as you can into your chest and release it. Do this three or four times. Then let your breathing go back to its normal rhythm. Listen to it.
3. Starting with your face, you are going to tighten and relax groups of muscles as you move down the body. Scrunch your face up tightly for 5 seconds, then relax it. Do this for each of these muscle groups: the neck and shoulders, the arms, the stomach and chest, the legs, and the feet. As each part of your body relaxes, let it go limp. Feel the tension leave your body. You should feel like you are floating in space.

SAMPLE SMOKING INTERVENTION FORM

Client Name: _____   Chart ID#: _____

Visit Date: _____   Type of Visit: _____

Nurse Name: _____

Currently smoking?   ☐ Yes   ☐ No

  If yes, # cigarettes/day: _____

  If no, quit date: _____

Decisional worksheet completed/reviewed?   ☐ Yes   ☐ No

Health-related feedback given?   ☐ Yes   ☐ No

Motivational readiness for *Cutting Back* (circle one):

1	2	3
Not thinking about it	Thinking about it	Ready for change

Motivational readiness for *Quitting* (circle one):

1	2	3
Not thinking about it	Thinking about it	Ready for change

Goal Setting and Plans to Achieve Goal(s):

  Goal #1: _____   Goal #2: _____

  Plan #1: _____   Plan #2: _____

Materials given: _____

Comments: _____

BRIEF COPING SKILLS TRAINING

Smoking doesn't just happen automatically, though it might seem like it sometimes. There are usually triggers or events that cause you to have an urge and then to smoke. These triggers can be feelings, thoughts, or situations. There are three types of *behavioral* or habit changing strategies you can use to cope with these triggers, to break up the chain of events that lead to smoking:

1. *Avoid the trigger.* Avoiding the trigger obviously can be the most powerful strategy. If you are not around the trigger, you will not have an urge and you will not smoke. For example, if you know that having a cup of coffee is a big trigger for you, then not having a cup of coffee will decrease your desire for a cigarette. However, sometimes avoiding a trigger is not always the most practical strategy; if waking up in the morning is a trigger, you can't simply avoid waking up, as much as you might like to sometimes. That's why there are two additional types of strategies to help you manage your smoking triggers.

2. *Alter the trigger situation.* Think of your triggers to smoke as very fixed parts of your daily routine—anything that you can do to alter that routine can help you to manage your smoking urges. What you're doing is essentially taking control of your environment so that you can control your smoking. For example, let's take that cup of coffee as a trigger. If you always drink that cup of coffee in the same place using the same cup at the same time of the day, change any one or all of those parts of the routine: change the cup you use, drink your coffee in a different chair or part of the house. The key with altering a trigger is to be creative. Use it as an opportunity to challenge yourself to outsmart the environment to give you control of your smoking.

3. *Substitute* something else for the cigarette when you encounter the trigger. This can be as simple as putting a piece of gum or hard candy in your mouth when you want a cigarette. Again, think of this as an opportunity to be creative.

Another type of coping strategy is a *cognitive* strategy that involves changing your thoughts or telling yourself things so that you will not want to smoke. These self-statements can include:

    a. Reasons you want to quit
    b. Benefits of quitting
    c. Statements of determination (e.g., "I can do it")
    d. Delay statements (e.g., "only five more minutes").

(continued)

Other types of self-statements include getting a new perspective on the situation. Take a step back when you feel the urge to smoke and ask yourself a simple question: "Do I really want to smoke here?" Then redefine the situation and your reaction (e.g., "I don't really want to smoke, I really just want to relax here"), and use other coping strategies (e.g., substitute a piece of gum for the cigarette).

Practice these strategies before you quit. Imagine yourself successfully coping with these trigger situations. Think of this as your road map to becoming a successful nonsmoker.

You may have to try different types of strategies to cope with your triggers. It can be discouraging if you try things, but they just do not work, and you still feel the need for a cigarette. Don't give up! Have fun with it! It just means you haven't found the right strategy or combinations of strategies to use yet. Although it is important to get advice on some possible strategies, it is equally important to remember that what works for someone else may not necessarily work for you.

A SAMPLE RELAPSE PREVENTION HANDOUT

A. *Withdrawal symptoms.* Common withdrawal symptoms include: irritability, increased tension and frustration, trouble concentrating, cravings, trouble sleeping, and increased hunger.

B. *Withdrawal symptom duration.* Not everybody will have the same withdrawal symptoms for the same amount of time. Generally speaking, though, your symptoms will gradually decrease over the 2 to 3 weeks after you've quit. Many people feel better within 2 to 3 days. You may find that you hit some peaks and valleys along the way. Many people report their withdrawal symptoms get worse during the evening hours. In any case, you may not feel like yourself for a few days and that's okay. This will not be a permanent change.

C. *High-risk situations.* The situations that triggered a cigarette before you quit are your high-risk situations now. These are times that you are at most risk for going back to smoking. Understanding these connections gives you the ability to develop a coping plan for those high-risk times.

D. *Abstinence violation effect* (AVE). How do you think you would feel if you did smoke a cigarette? It would be perfectly natural for you to feel guilty, frustrated, or angry, like you've failed. Recognize that these feelings are natural and do not use them as an excuse to start smoking again. Are you really a failure? A failure might be someone who gives up and never thinks of quitting again. If you slip and have a cigarette, use it as a source of information; take a step back and analyze the situation that just occurred. Use it as a learning experience. Find out what happened by asking yourself the following questions: What did you feel like when you smoked? Where were you? Who were you with? Use this information to plan coping strategies for the next time this set of circumstances presents itself so that you can decrease the chances that you'll smoke the next time around.

WRAP SHEET

CIGARETTES	TIME	HOW DO YOU FEEL?								WHAT ARE YOU DOING?
		Happy	Sad or depressed	Relaxed	Bored	Anxious	Angry	Tired	Frustrated	
1										
2										
3										
4										
5										
6										
7										
8										
9										
10										
11										
12										
13										
14										

TRIGGERS FOR SMOKING

Think about the different times or situations in which you usually smoke. These situations may trigger your smoking in different ways. For example, you may automatically light up a cigarette whenever you get in the car. The trigger here is "getting in the car." We call such situations "Triggers for Smoking."

You can begin to understand your own triggers for smoking by looking over the Wrap Sheets you keep this week. After keeping Wrap Sheets for 3 days, list below as many of your own triggers as possible. In addition to the event or what you were doing when smoking, also list how you are feeling (your mood) and what you might be thinking at the time.

Learning about your own triggers can help you quit and quit for keeps. Read the example below before beginning to list your own trigger situations.

	Event or What You're Doing	Feeling	Thinking
EX:	Driving to work	Tense, frustrated	How will I ever get anything done today!

1.
2.
3.
4.
5.
6.
7.
8.

MANAGING TRIGGERS
FOR SMOKING WORKSHEET

How did you manage your triggers for smoking this week?

Continue to keep a record of your triggers for smoking and the strategies you used to deal with them. This week, reduce the number of cigarettes you smoked last week by 10% and smoke only your newly assigned lower-nicotine brand.

Trigger	Strategy
Example: Driving to work	*Chew gum, listen to relaxing music, keep cigarettes in trunk*

NICOTINE FADING WORKSHEET

Week 1 – Regular brand: _____

Average number smoked per day:		Mg. nicotine per cigarette		Average nicotine per day
_____	×	_____	=	_____

Week 2 – 30% Reduction of nicotine   Brand: _____

Average number smoked per day:		Mg. nicotine per cigarette		Average nicotine per day
_____	×	_____	=	_____

Week 3 – 60% Reduction of nicotine   Brand: _____

Average number smoked per day:		Mg. nicotine per cigarette		Average nicotine per day
_____	×	_____	=	_____

Week 4 – 90% Reduction of nicotine   Brand: _____

Average number smoked per day:		Mg. nicotine per cigarette		Average nicotine per day
_____	×	_____	=	_____

NONSMOKING GAME PLAN: LIFESTYLE CHANGE WORKSHEET

As part of your Nonsmoking Game Plan, you can plan to make changes in your daily behaviors that can help you remain a nonsmoker. Below, list specific answers to some general lifestyle questions important to quitting smoking and remaining a nonsmoker.

1. What will you do to make cigarettes unavailable to you?

    _____

    _____

    _____

2. What will you do to increase time spent in nonsmoking places or time spent doing nonsmoking activities?

    _____

    _____

    _____

3. How can you develop a "buddy system" or get support from others when quitting?

    _____

    _____

    _____

4. What will you do to manage stress successfully?

    _____

    _____

    _____

5. What will you do to keep from gaining weight?

    _____

    _____

    _____

6. What will you do to become more physically active?

    _____

    _____

    _____

NONSMOKING GAME PLAN: COPING WITH HIGH-RISK SITUATIONS WORKSHEET

High-Risk Situations Week of _____

For each specific high-risk situation, describe the event, persons you might be with, what you might be doing, thinking, or feeling at the time. List the specific coping strategies you will use to avoid smoking in each case. Remember: Avoid, Alter, use Alternatives.

High-Risk Situations   Specific Coping Strategies

1. _____
2. _____
3. _____
4. _____
5. _____
6. _____
7. _____
8. _____
9. _____
10. _____

SOCIAL SUPPORT
FOR NONSMOKING WORKSHEET

Getting support and encouragement from others while you quit and work at being a nonsmoker can be very helpful. Complete this handout to help you determine what other people do that is helpful or not helpful to you and what you can do to ask them to be more helpful.

Supportive Behaviors for Nonsmoking:
List behaviors from others that you consider to be helpful or supportive to your nonsmoking efforts:

1. _____
2. _____
3. _____
4. _____

Nonsupportive Behaviors for Nonsmoking:
List behaviors from others that you consider to be not helpful or that interfere with your efforts to quit smoking:

1. _____
2. _____
3. _____
4. _____

Requesting Behavior Changes from Others:
What can you ask or request of others to have them engage in more actions or behaviors that you find supportive of nonsmoking?

1. _____
2. _____
3. _____
4. _____

What can you ask or request of others to have them engage in fewer (or eliminate completely) behaviors that you find not helpful or interfere with your efforts to quit smoking?

1. _____
2. _____
3. _____
4. _____

STRATEGIES FOR IDENTIFYING AND COUNTERACTING RESUMPTION THOUGHTS

Types of Smoking Resumption Thoughts:

1. Nostalgia–longing for the times when one could smoke; "It sure was fun to smoke while sitting around the campfire drinking a beer."

2. Testing control–due to overconfidence or curiosity, testing out one's control by smoking one or more cigarettes; "I bet I could smoke just one cigarette and then put them down."

3. Crisis–telling oneself that it is okay to smoke under "exceptional" circumstances, such as in a crisis; "Ordinarily I wouldn't smoke, but I'm under so much pressure right now, I need a cigarette."

4. Unwanted changes–worrying that changes (such as weight gain, irritability, inability to concentrate, withdrawal symptoms) one feels may be associated with nonsmoking; "I'm not willing to regain the weight I lost this summer, even if I have to start smoking again."

5. Self-doubts–self-doubts can undermine efforts to remain abstinent; "This is so hard for me—maybe I'm just meant to be a smoker."

Strategies to Counteract the Effects of These Thoughts:

1. Challenging–the most straightforward way to counteract thoughts about smoking is to directly confront or challenge them; "I cannot have one cigarette without smoking more."

2. Benefits of nonsmoking–another useful strategy is to think about the personal benefits of not smoking; "The best feeling in the world will be breathing freely again and not being congested once I've quit smoking."

3. Remembering unpleasant smoking experiences–another strategy is to recall specific unpleasant aspects of smoking; "I won't have to worry about my wife feeling like she's kissing an ashtray when she kisses me."

4. Distractions–another effective means of coping is for smokers to simply divert their attention from any aspect of smoking; "I'm going to ignore this urge and imagine, in vivid detail, that I'm skiing down my favorite slope in Colorado."

5. Self-rewarding thoughts–another strategy involves thinking about one's successes and strengths; "Good job! It wasn't easy but I didn't smoke in that tempting situation."

DAILY MOOD RATING FORM

INSTRUCTIONS: At the end of each day, about an hour before going to bed, rate your mood on three dimensions for that day. If your mood was *negative* (depressed, angry/irritable, or anxious), mark a *lower* number on the chart for that day for each mood. If your mood was *positive* (happy, calm, or relaxed), mark a *higher* number for each mood. Write down events or situations that might have contributed to your mood, either positively or negatively over the past week.

Events or situations that resulted in *positive* moods:

_____

_____

_____

_____

Events or situations that resulted in *negative* moods:

_____

_____

_____

_____

Date: _____

Happy								Depressed
9	8	7	6	5	4	3	2	1

Calm								Angry/irritable
9	8	7	6	5	4	3	2	1

Relaxed								Anxious
9	8	7	6	5	4	3	2	1

Date: _____

Happy								Depressed
9	8	7	6	5	4	3	2	1

Calm								Angry/irritable
9	8	7	6	5	4	3	2	1

Relaxed								Anxious
9	8	7	6	5	4	3	2	1

Date: _____

Happy								Depressed
9	8	7	6	5	4	3	2	1

Calm								Angry/irritable
9	8	7	6	5	4	3	2	1

Relaxed								Anxious
9	8	7	6	5	4	3	2	1

Date: _____

Happy								Depressed
9	8	7	6	5	4	3	2	1

Calm								Angry/irritable
9	8	7	6	5	4	3	2	1

Relaxed								Anxious
9	8	7	6	5	4	3	2	1

Date: _____

Happy								Depressed
9	8	7	6	5	4	3	2	1

Calm								Angry/irritable
9	8	7	6	5	4	3	2	1

Relaxed								Anxious
9	8	7	6	5	4	3	2	1

Date: _____

Happy								Depressed
9	8	7	6	5	4	3	2	1

Calm								Angry/irritable
9	8	7	6	5	4	3	2	1

Relaxed								Anxious
9	8	7	6	5	4	3	2	1

Date: _____

Happy								Depressed
9	8	7	6	5	4	3	2	1

Calm								Angry/irritable
9	8	7	6	5	4	3	2	1

Relaxed								Anxious
9	8	7	6	5	4	3	2	1

Date: _____

Happy								Depressed
9	8	7	6	5	4	3	2	1

Calm								Angry/irritable
9	8	7	6	5	4	3	2	1

Relaxed								Anxious
9	8	7	6	5	4	3	2	1

ABC OVERVIEW

In managing negative mood, it is helpful to take a look at your thinking patterns. A method developed by a well-known psychologist, Dr. Albert Ellis, can help you understand the connection between what you think and how you feel. This method is called the ABC technique.

The <u>A</u> stands for <u>A</u>ctivating event, the event you feel upset about.

The <u>B</u> stands for <u>B</u>eliefs about the activating event, or what you tell yourself about the event.

The <u>C</u> stands for the emotional <u>C</u>onsequences, or reaction to the event.

The ABC technique is not intended to help you avoid <u>reasonable</u> emotional reactions to events but rather to avoid <u>emotional overreactions</u>. To best describe the ABC technique, look at the following example:

> Jack reports that he is angry and sad (emotional consequence: <u>C</u>) because he did not get a raise in pay at work (activating event: <u>A</u>). He is so upset that he does not go to work for the next two days.

In this example, Jack might conclude that <u>A</u> (the activating event) caused <u>C</u> (the emotional consequence). This is not surprising, because people commonly believe that events cause their emotional reactions:

$$\underline{A} \quad \rightarrow ? \rightarrow \quad \underline{C}$$
<u>A</u>ctivating Event   <u>C</u>onsequence

However, this is not accurate. When Jack felt angry and sad, it was not <u>A</u> (the activating event) that <u>caused</u> his emotional reaction; rather it was <u>B</u> (his beliefs or what he said to himself) that resulted in <u>C</u> (his emotional reaction).

$$\underline{A} \quad \rightarrow \quad \underline{B} \quad \rightarrow \quad \underline{C}$$
<u>A</u>ctivating   <u>B</u>eliefs   <u>C</u>onsequence
Event

In the example, Jack's beliefs or self-talk included statements such as:
"I should have gotten a raise."
"Since I didn't, I must be a total failure."
"I didn't get it because the boss hates me."

(continued)

The ABC technique correctly identifies Jack's beliefs or self-talk statements as leading to his emotional overreaction. Jack's beliefs or self-talk about why he didn't get a raise are directly related to his feelings of anger and sadness.

<u>A</u>	→	<u>B</u>	→	<u>C</u>
<u>A</u>ctivating Event		<u>B</u>eliefs		<u>C</u>onsequence
Not getting a raise		*"I must be a total failure."*		*Angry and sad*

> Many times it is not what happens that makes us upset; rather, it is what we tell ourselves about the situation. If, at times, your thinking patterns cause you to overreact, as in this example, the ABC technique can help you.

In future sessions, we will discuss how you can change your emotional overreactions (<u>C</u>) by learning to evaluate and change what you say or believe (<u>B</u>) about upsetting events (<u>A</u>).

ABC METHOD:
CHANGING FAULTY THINKING

In previous exercises using the ABC technique, you learned to identify beliefs and self-talk statements that can result in emotional overreactions. The next step is to change these beliefs or self-talk in order to reduce or avoid emotional overreactions.

To change your emotional Consequences (C), you need to Dispute (D) your Beliefs (B) about Activating events (A). If any beliefs are irrational or not constructive, then you can dispute and change them.

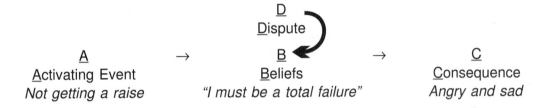

You can Dispute or challenge beliefs that are not constructive by *arguing against the beliefs*. Ask yourself the following questions to help you Dispute irrational or nonconstructive beliefs or self-talk:

1. What is the evidence for my belief?
2. What are the alternative views?
3. What's the worst that could happen now? What could I do if it did happen?
4. Is it helpful in some way for me to believe what I do?
5. What would I say to a friend in the same situation (or who had experienced the same Activating event)?

Challenging your irrational or nonconstructive beliefs in this way can lead to new, more constructive beliefs (counterthoughts) that will better fit the situation. By changing your beliefs, emotional overreactions will be replaced by new, more positive feelings.

ABC METHOD WORKSHEET: IDENTIFYING FAULTY THINKING

The ABC technique can help you identify faulty thinking patterns. To understand C (your feelings or emotional overreactions), you can first learn how to evaluate B (your beliefs, or self-talk) about A (activating events).

INSTRUCTIONS: Step 1: Complete Box C; Step 2: Complete Box A; Step 3: Complete Box B

Step 2, Box A
A = Activating Event

Describe Event:

_____
_____
_____
_____
_____
_____
_____

Step 3, Box B
B = Beliefs or Self-Talk

List each of the things you said to yourself about A that resulted in C:

_____
_____
_____
_____
_____
_____

Step 1, Box C
C = Emotional Consequence

Describe how you felt when A happened:

I felt:

_____
_____
_____
_____
_____
_____

Step 4: Place a check mark beside each statement in Box B that is nonconstructive or "irrational."

INVENTORY OF THOUGHTS

INVENTORY OF POSITIVE AND NEGATIVE THOUGHTS

INSTRUCTIONS: For the next week, keep track of your positive and negative thoughts. Write down the positive and negative thoughts that are the most powerful or that tend to occur over and over again. You don't need to write down every thought you have, just the ones important to this exercise—those thoughts that send you clear positive or negative messages.

Positive Thoughts   Negative Thoughts

_____

_____

_____

_____

_____

_____

_____

_____

_____

_____

_____

ABC(D) WORKSHEET: CHANGING FAULTY THINKING

The ABC technique can help you change faulty thinking patterns by Disputing your Beliefs about an Activating event.

Instructions

1. Complete box C.
2. Complete box A.
3. Complete box B.
4. Place an X by each statement in box B that is irrational or not constructive.
5. Complete box D. Use questions from ABC(D) overview to help you Dispute beliefs.
6. Complete "New Feelings" box.

Step 2, Box A
Activating Event
(Describe Event)

Step 3, Box B
Beliefs or Self Talk
(List each of the things you said to yourself about A that resulted in C.)

Step 1, Box C
Emotional Consequence
(Describe how you felt when A happened)

I felt:

Step 5, Box D
D Counterthoughts
(After disputing statements in Box B, list your counterthoughts.)

Step 6
New Feelings
(After reading your statement in Box D, describe how you feel about A.)

I feel:

328

POSITIVE AND NEGATIVE THOUGHTS WORKSHEET

INSTRUCTIONS: For the next week, continue to keep track of your positive and negative thoughts. Remember, you don't need to write down every thought, just the ones that send you clear positive or negative messages.

Positive Thoughts	Negative Thoughts

Write down one technique that you used to increase positive thoughts:	Write down one technique that you used to decrease negative thoughts:

How effective was it for you?

1	2	3	4	5
Not Effective			Very Effective	

How effective was it for you?

1	2	3	4	5
Not Effective			Very Effective	

TOP 20 PLEASANT EVENTS

INSTRUCTIONS: List 20 events that you enjoy and find pleasant. Choose events that you can do frequently, that you have control over, and that are affordable.

Examples: Have coffee, tea, Coke with a friend.
Watch favorite TV show.
Take a ride in the country.
Help another person.

1. _____
2. _____
3. _____
4. _____
5. _____
6. _____
7. _____
8. _____
9. _____
10. _____
11. _____
12. _____
13. _____
14. _____
15. _____
16. _____
17. _____
18. _____
19. _____
20. _____

CONTRACT FOR INCREASING PLEASANT ACTIVITIES

My goal for the next week is to bring my total pleasant activity count up to ____.

This means that I will try to engage in ____ pleasant activities each day.

I will also try to keep my pleasant activities level from falling below ____ on any given day.

If my daily total is ____, I will reward myself by ____.

If my total for the week is ____, I will reward myself by ____.

Signed: _____   Date: _____

Weekly Plan for Pleasant Activities

Time	Monday	Tuesday	Wednesday	Thursday	Friday	Saturday	Sunday
8:00 a.m.							
9:00							
10:00							
11:00							
12:00							
1:00							
2:00							
3:00							
4:00							
5:00							
6:00							
7:00							
8:00							
9:00							
10:00 p.m.							

A PLAN FOR ASSERTIVENESS

Think of situations in which you would like to be more assertive. You probably don't feel very positive about these situations and would like to change your feelings in the future. The first step in acting more assertively is to identify situations that fit the following pattern:

1. You have not been assertive in the past.
2. The situation occurs regularly in your life (at least once a month).
3. The situation is troubling you.
4. The situation is not too specific or too general.

Once you have identified these situations, work on developing assertive responses one situation at a time. Use the following steps to help you.

Step 1: Describe the other person's behavior *accurately in neutral terms* so that they (or anyone else) cannot argue.

> Example: "When you asked me a question while I was talking to your sister on the telephone . . . "

Step 2: Use "I feel" statements to describe your feeling about what has happened. These statements will let the other person know you are responsible for your *own* feelings and that you are not blaming him/her. Avoid *"you" statements* that are hostile or blaming.

> Example: "I felt angry . . . "

Step 3: Let the person know what you want. Request a specific behavior change on his or her part.

> Example: "In the future, I'd appreciate it if you would wait until I'm off the phone before asking me questions."

Using these steps can help you to be assertive in specific situations and to improve communication with others. Recognize that a person may not change his or her behavior because of your request. By being assertive, you have the best chance of getting what you want, and you will feel better about yourself for stating your request assertively.

(continued)

Other Helpful Tips When Using Assertiveness

1. Before approaching a person, *practice* what you will say. Use assertive imagery. Imagine the following:
    a. The entire scene
    b. Your assertive statement
    c. How the other person responds
    You can change the details of the scene and practice again. Imagine the person responding positively. After several practices, imagine the person responding more negatively.

2. *Listen* to the other person's answer. Acknowledge and accept his or her feelings.

3. *Avoid "you" statements* that are hostile or judgmental (such as "When you acted like a jerk . . . ").

4. End the conversation on a *positive note* . . . even if it means you agree to disagree.

5. Praise and *reward yourself* for practicing assertiveness.

ASSERTIVENESS WORKSHEET

1. Situation you want to respond to (what happened):

    _____

2. Developing the assertive response:
    Step 1: "WHEN YOU _____
               (Describe his or her behavior in neutral terms.)
    Step 2: "I FELT _____
                (Describe your emotional reaction.)
    Step 3: "I WOULD LIKE YOU _____
                (Request specific behavior change.)

3. Assertive imagery practice:

    Before practicing, rate your comfort with assertiveness and your level of
    assertiveness skill on a scale of 0–10, where 0 = very low and 10 = very high.

    Level of Comfort: _____ Level of Skill: _____

    NOW PRACTICE:

    Step 1: Imagine the scene.
    Step 2: Practice your assertive statement. Say it out loud.
    Step 3: Imagine how the other person will respond.

    After practicing, rate your comfort with assertiveness and your level of assertiveness
    skill on a scale of 0–10, where 0 = very low and 10 = very high.

    Level of Comfort: _____ Level of Skill: _____

4. Using assertiveness skills in actual situations.

    Try out the assertiveness technique in a real situation. After practicing, rate your comfort
    with assertiveness and your level of assertiveness skill on a scale of 0–10 points, where 0 =
    very low and 10 = very high.

    Level of Comfort: _____ Level of Skill: _____

334

VITAL SIGNS

Blood pressure: _____   Temperature: _____

Pulse: _____   Weight: _____   Respiratory rate: _____

Tobacco use (circle one):   Current   Former   Never

Ready to quit (circle one):   Not at all   Thinking about it   Ready now

SAMPLE CHART REVIEW TALLY SHEET

Record tobacco use status documented at last primary care visit

Tobacco users: _____ Total count: _____

Former users: _____ Total count: _____

Never users: _____ Total count: _____

Status not recorded _____ Total count: _____

(Total number of charts pulled _____ should equal total of 4 categories above.)

Percent not recorded: # not recorded/total # charts = _____

Among smokers' charts only:

Advice documented at last visit: _____ Total count: _____

Assistance documented at last visit: _____ Total count: _____

Percent advised: # advised/# current smokers = _____

Percent assisted: # assisted/# current smokers = _____

PATIENT PREVENTIVE CARE FLOWSHEET

Name: _____

Allergies: _____

Date of Initial Evaluation: _____

	VISIT DATE	PROBLEMS	MEDICATION LIST	START DATE	STOP DATE
1					
2					
3					
4					
5					
6					
7					
8					
9					

Services	Target Group	Interval	Date Performed						
Blood pressure	All	Each visit							
Height	All	Annual							
Weight	All	Annual							
Mammogram	Women age ≥ 50	Annual							
Breast exam	Women	Annual							
Pap/pelvic exam	Women	Every 2 yrs							
Influenza vaccine	Age ≥ 65	Annual							
Digital rectal exam	Age ≥ 40	Annual							
Fecal occult blood	Age ≥ 50	Annual							
Sigmoidoscopy	Age ≥ 50	Every 10 yrs							
Tobacco counseling	All smokers	Each visit							
Dietary fat and fiber	All	Each visit							
Tetanus	All	Every 10 yrs							
Sun protection	All	Annual							

337

References

Abrams, D. B. (1986). Roles of psychosocial stress, smoking cues, and coping in smoking-relapse prevention. *Health Psychology, 5*, 91–92.

Abrams, D. B. (1993). Treatment issues: Towards a stepped care model. *Tobacco Control, 2*(Suppl.), S17–S37.

Abrams, D. B. (1995). Integrating basic, clinical and public health research for alcohol–tobacco interactions. In J. B. Fertig & J. P. Allen (Eds.), *Alcohol and tobacco: From basic science to policy* (National Institute on Alcohol Abuse and Alcoholism Research Monograph No. 30, NIH Publication No. 95-3931, pp. 3–16). Bethesda, MD: U.S. Department of Health and Human Services, National Institutes of Health, National Institute on Alcohol Abuse and Alcoholism.

Abrams, D. B. (1999a). Nicotine addiction: Paradigms for research in the 21st century. *Nicotine and Tobacco Research, 1*(Suppl. 2), S211–S215.

Abrams, D. B. (1999b). Transdisciplinary paradigms for tobacco prevention research. *Nicotine and Tobacco Research, 1*(Suppl. 1), S15–S23.

Abrams, D. B. (2000). Transdisciplinary concepts and measures of craving: Commentary and future directions. *Addiction, 95*(Suppl. 2), S237–S246.

Abrams, D. B., & Biener, L. (1992). Motivational characteristics of smokers at the workplace: A public health challenge. *Preventive Medicine, 21*, 679–687.

Abrams, D. B., Borrelli, B., Shadel, W. G., King, T., Bock, B., & Niaura, R. (1998). Adherence to treatment for nicotine dependence. In S. Shumaker, E. Schron, J. Ockene, & W. McBee (Eds.), *Handbook of health behavior change* (2nd ed., pp. 137–165). New York: Springer.

Abrams, D. B., Boutwell, W. B., Grizzle, J., Heimendinger, J., Sorensen, G., & Varnes, J. (1994). Cancer control at the workplace: The working well trial. *Preventive Medicine, 23*, 15–27.

Abrams, D. B., Clark, M. M., & King, T. K. (1999). Increasing the impact of nicotine dependence treatment: Conceptual and practical considerations in a stepped-care plus treatment-matching approach. In J. A. Tucker, D. M. Donovan, & G. A. Marlatt (Eds.), *Changing addictive behavior: Bridging clinical and public health strategies* (pp. 307–330). New York: Guilford Press.

Abrams, D. B., & Clayton, R. R. (2001). Transdisciplinary research to improve brief interventions for addictive behaviors. In P. M. Monti, S. M. Colby, & T. A. O'Leary (Eds.), *Adolescents, alcohol, and substance abuse: Reaching teens through brief interventions* (pp. 321–341). New York: Guilford Press.

Abrams, D. B., Elder, J. P., Carleton, R. A., Lasater, T. M., & Artz, L. M. (1986). Social learning principles for organizational health promotion: An integrated approach. In M. F. Cataldo & T. J. Coates (Eds.), *Health and industry: A behavioral medicine perspective* (pp. 28–51). New York: Wiley.

Abrams, D. B., Emmons, K. M., Linnan, L., & Biener, L. (1994). Smoking cessation at the workplace: Conceptual and practical issues. In R. Richmond (Ed.), *Interventions for smokers: An international perspective* (pp. 137–169). Baltimore: Williams & Wilkins.

Abrams, D. B., Emmons, K. M., Niaura, R. S., Goldstein, M. G., & Sherman, C. B. (1991). Tobacco dependence: An integration of individual and public health perspectives. In P. E. Nathan, J. W. Langenbucher, B. S. McCrady, & W. Frankenstein (Eds.), *Annual review of addiction research and treatment* (Vol. 1, pp. 331–396). New York: Pergamon Press.

Abrams, D. B., Marlatt, G. A., & Sobell, M. B. (1995). Overview of Section II: Treatment, early intervention, and policy. In J. Fertig & J. P. Allen (Eds.), *Alcohol and tobacco: From basic science to policy* (National Institute of Alcohol Abuse and Alcoholism Research Monograph No. 30, NIH Publication No. 95-3931, pp. 307–323). Bethesda, MD: U.S. Department of Health and Human Services, National Institutes of Health, National Institute on Alcohol Abuse and Alcoholism.

Abrams, D. B., Mills, S., & Bulger, D. (1999). Challenges and future directions for tailored communication research. *Annals of Behavioral Medicine, 21*(4), 299–306.

Abrams, D. B., Monti, P. M., Carey, K. B., Pinto, R. P., & Jacobus, S. I. (1988). Reactivity to smoking cues and relapse: Two studies of discriminant validity. *Behaviour Research and Therapy, 26*(3), 225–233.

Abrams, D. B., Monti, P. M., Pinto, R., Elder, J. P., Brown, R. A., & Jacobus, S. I. (1987). Psychosocial stress and coping in smokers who relapse or quit. *Health Psychology, 6*, 289–304.

Abrams, D. B., Orleans, C. T., Niaura, R. S., Goldstein, M. G., Prochaska, J. O., & Velicer, W. (1996). Integrating individual and public health perspectives for treatment of tobacco dependence under managed health care: A combined stepped care and matching model. *Annals of Behavioral Medicine, 18*(4), 290–304.

Abrams, D. B., Rohsenow, D., Niaura, R., Pedraza, M., Longabaugh, R., Beattie, M., Binkoff, J., Noel, N., & Monti, P. (1992). Smoking and treatment outcome for alcoholics: Effects on coping skills, urge to drink and drinking rates. *Behavior Therapy, 23*(2), 283–297.

Abrams, D. B., & Wilson, G. T. (1979a). Effects of alcohol on social anxiety in women: Cognitive versus physiological processes. *Journal of Abnormal Psychology, 88*, 161–173.

Abrams, D. B., & Wilson, G. T. (1979b). Self-monitoring and reactivity in the modification of cigarette smoking. *Journal of Consulting and Clinical Psychology, 47*(2), 243–251.

Abrams, D. B., & Wilson, G. T. (1986). Clinical advances in treatment of smoking and alcohol addiction. In A. J. Frances & R. E. Hales (Eds.), *The American Psychiatric Association annual review: Psychiatric update* (Vol. 5, pp. 606–626). Washington, DC: American Psychiatric Association Press.

American Cancer Society. (1999). *Cancer facts and figures—1999.* Atlanta, GA: Author.

American Cancer Society. (2000). *Cancer facts and figures.* Atlanta, GA: Author.

American Psychiatric Association. (1994). *Diagnostic and statistical manual of mental disorders* (4th ed.). Washington, DC: Author.

American Psychiatric Association Work Group on Nicotine Dependence. (1996). Practice guideline for the treatment of patients with nicotine dependence. *American Journal of Psychiatry, 153*(Suppl. 10), 1–31.

Anda, R. F., Williamson, D. F., Escobedo, L. G., Mast, E. E., Giovino, G. A., & Remington, P. L. (1990). Depression and the dynamics of smoking. *Journal of the American Medical Association, 264*(12), 1541–1545.

Ascher, J. A., Cole, J. O., Colin, J. N., Feighner, J. P., Ferris, R. M., Fibiger, H. C., Golden, R. N., Martin, P., Potter, W. Z., Richelson, E., & Sulser, F. (1995). Bupropion: A review of its mechanism of antidepressant activity. *Journal of Clinical Psychiatry, 56*(9), 395–401.

Aveyard, P., Sherratt, E., Almond, J., Lawrence, T., Lancashire, R., Griffin, C., & Cheng, K. K. (2001). Change-in-stage and updated smoking status results from a cluster-randomized trial of smoking prevention and cessation using the transtheoretical model among British adolescents. *Preventive Medicine, 33*(4), 313–324.

Baer, J., & Lichtenstein, E. (1988). Classification and prediction of smoking relapse episodes: An exploration of individual differences. *Journal of Consulting and Clinical Psychology, 56*(1), 104–110.

Baer, J. S., Marlatt, G. A., & McMahon, R. J. (1993). *Addictive behaviors across the life span: Prevention, treatment, and policy issues.* Newbury Park, CA: Sage.

Bandura, A. (1997). *Self-efficacy: The exercise of control.* New York: Freeman.

Baranowski, T., Lin, L., Wetter, D., Resnicow, K., & Hearn, M. D. (2001). Theory as mediating variables: Why aren't community interventions working as desired? *Annals of Epidemiology, S7*(1), S89–S95.

Battjes, R. J. (1988). Smoking as an issue in alcohol and drug abuse treatment. *Addictive Behaviors, 13,* 225–230.

Bayer, D. (1995). Results: A comparison of chemical dependency treatment outcomes when clients are given full choice. *Employee Assistance Quarterly, 10*(4), 53–65.

Benowitz, N. (1998a). Nicotine pharmacology and addiction. In N. Benowitz (Ed.), *Nicotine safety and toxicity* (pp. 3–16). New York: Oxford University Press.

Benowitz, N. (1998b). *Nicotine safety and toxicity.* New York: Oxford University Press.

Benowitz, N. L. (1988). Pharmacologic aspects of cigarette smoking and nicotine addiction. *New England Journal of Medicine, 319,* 1318–1330.

Benowitz, N. L. (1993). Nicotine replacement therapy: What has been accomplished—can we do better? *Drugs, 45,* 157–170.

Benowitz, N. L. (1996). Pharmacology of nicotine: Addiction and therapeutics. *Annual Review of Pharmacology and Toxicology, 36,* 597–613.

Benson, H. (1975). *The relaxation response.* New York: Avon Books.

Berwick, D. M. (1992). The clinical process and the quality process. *Quality Management in Health Care, 1,* 1–8.

Biener, L., & Abrams, D. B. (1991). The contemplation ladder: Validation of a measure of readiness to consider smoking cessation. *Health Psychology, 10*(5), 360–365.

Biglan, A., & Lichtenstein, E. (1984). A behavior-analytic approach to smoking acquisition: Some recent findings. *Journal of Applied Social Psychology, 14,* 207–223.

Blair, S. N., Dunn, A. L., Marcus, B. H., Carpenter, R. A., & Jaret, P. (2001). *Active living every day: 20 weeks to lifelong vitality.* Champaign, IL: Human Kinetics.

Bobo, J. K., Anderson, J. R., & Bowman, A. (1997). Training chemical dependency counselors to treat nicotine dependence. *Addictive Behaviors, 22*(1), 23–30.

Bobo, J. K., McIlvain, H. E., Lando, H. A., Walker, R. D., & Leed-Kelly, A. (1998). Effect of smoking cessation counseling on recovery from alcoholism: Findings from a randomized community intervention trial. *Addiction, 93*(6), 877–887.

Bobo, J. K., Walker, R. D., Lando, H. A., McIlvain, H. E., & Anderson, J. R. (1995). Enhancing alcohol control with counseling on nicotine dependence: Pilot study findings and treatment recommendations. In J. B. Fertig & J. P. Allen (Eds.), *Alcohol and tobacco: From basic science to policy* (National Institute of Alcohol Abuse and Alcoholism Research Monograph No. 30, NIH Publication No. 95-3931, pp. 225–238). Bethesda, MD: U.S. Department of Health and Human Services, National Institutes of Health, National Institute on Alcohol Abuse and Alcoholism.

Borrelli, B., Marcus, B. H., Clark, M. M., Bock, B. C., King, T. K., & Roberts, M. (1999). History of major depression and subsyndromal depression in women smokers. *Addictive Behaviors, 24*(3), 781–794.

Borrelli, B., & Mermelstein, R. (1994). Goal setting and behavior change in a smoking cessation program. *Cognitive Therapy and Research, 18*(1), 69–83.

Borrelli, B., & Mermelstein, R. M. (1998). The role of weight concern and self-efficacy in smoking cessation and weight gain among smokers in a clinic-based cessation program. *Addictive Behaviors, 23*(5), 609–622.

Botvin, G. J., Baker, E., Dusenbury, L., Botvin, E. M., & Diaz, T. (1995). Long-term follow-up results of a randomized drug abuse prevention trial in a white middle-class population. *Journal of the American Medical Association, 273,* 1106–1112.

Brandon, T., & Baker, T. (1991). The smoking consequences questionnaire: The subjective expected utility of smoking in college students. *Psychological Assessment, 3*(3), 484–491.

Brennan, P. A., Grekin, E. R., & Mednick, S. A. (1999). Maternal smoking during pregnancy and adult male criminal outcomes. *Archives of General Psychiatry, 56,* 215–219.

Brown, R. A., Herman, K. C., Ramsey, S. E., & Stout, R. L. (1999, October). *Characteristics of smoking cessation participants who lapse on quit date.* Paper presented at the international meeting of the Society for Research on Nicotine and Tobacco, Copenhagen, Denmark.

Brown, R. A., Kahler, C. W., Niaura, R., Abrams, D. B., Sales, S. D., Ramsey, S. E., Goldstein, M. G., Burgess, E. S., & Miller, I. W. (2001). Cognitive-behavioral treatment for depression in smoking cessation. *Journal of Consulting and Clinical Psychology, 69*(3), 471–480.

Brown, R. A., Lewinsohn, P. M., Seeley, J. R., & Wagner, E. F. (1996). Cigarette smoking, major depression and other psychiatric disorders among adolescents. *Journal of the American Academy of Child and Adolescent Psychiatry, 35*(12), 1602–1610.

Brownell, K., Marlatt, G. A., Lichtenstein, E., & Wilson, G. T. (1986). Understanding and preventing relapse. *American Psychologist, 41,* 765–782.

Burling, T. A., & Ziff, D. C. (1988). Tobacco smoking: A comparison between alcohol and drug abuse inpatients. *Addictive Behavior, 13,* 185–190.

Burton, D., Graham, M., Flay, B. R., Hahn, G., Craig, S., Sussman, S., Dent, C., & Stacy, A. (1989, November). *Motivating tobacco cessation among high school students.* Paper presented at the annual meeting of the Society for Public Health Educators, Chicago, IL.

Centers for Disease Control. (1994a). Cigarette smoking among adults—United States, 1993. *Morbidity and Mortality Weekly Report, 43,* 925–930.

Centers for Disease Control. (1994b). Medical care expenditures attributable to cigarette smoking—United States, 1993. *Morbidity and Mortality Weekly Report, 43,* 469–472.

Centers for Disease Control. (1998). Tobacco use among high school students—United States, 1997. *Morbidity and Mortality Weekly Report, 47*(12), 229–233.

Centers for Disease Control and Prevention. (2000a). Cigarette smoking among adults—United States, 1998. *Morbidity and Mortality Weekly Report, 49*(39), 881–884.

Centers for Disease Control and Prevention. (2000b). Tobacco use among middle and high school students—United States, 1999. *Morbidity and Mortality Weekly Report, 49*(3), 49–53.

Cervone, D., & Scott, W. (1995). Self-efficacy theory of behavioral change: Foundations, conceptual issues, and therapeutic implications. In W. O'Donohue & L. Krasner (Eds.), *Theories of behavior therapy: Exploring behavior change* (pp. 349–384). Washington, DC: American Psychological Association Books.

Chaloupka, F. J., & Warner, K. E. (2000). The economics of smoking. In A. J. Cuyler & J. P. Newhouse (Eds.), *The handbook of health economics* (pp. 1539–1627). Amsterdam: Elsevier.

Charlton, A., Melia, P., & Moyer, C. (1990). *A manual on tobacco and young people for the industrialized world.* Toronto, Ontario, Canada: Canadian Cancer Society.

Chassin, L., Presson, C. C., Sherman, S. J., & Edwards, D. A. (1990). The natural history of cigarette smoking: Predicting young-adult outcomes from adolescent smoking. *Health Psychology, 9,* 701–716.

Cheng, L. S., Swan, G. E., & Carmelli, D. (2000). A genetic analysis of smoking behavior in family members of older adult males. *Addiction, 95,* 426–436.

Cochrane Collaboration Library. (1998). *The Cochrane library* (issue 2). Retrieved 6/23/02 from *www.cochranelibrary.com/cochrane.*

Cohen, S., Kamark, T., & Mermelstein, R. (1983). A global measure of perceived stress. *Journal of Health and Behavior, 24,* 385–396.

Cohen, S., & Lichtenstein, E. (1990). Perceived stress, quitting smoking, and smoking relapse. *Health Psychology, 9*(4), 466–478.

Cohen, S., Lichtenstein, E., Prochaska, J. O., Rossi, J. S., Gritz, E. R., Carr, C. R., Orleans, C. T., Schoenbach, V. J., Biener, L., Abrams, D., DiClemente, C., Curry, S., Marlatt, G. A., Cummings, K. M., Emont, S. L., Giovino, G., & Ossip-Klein, D. (1989). Debunking myths about self-quitting: Evidence from 10 prospective studies of persons who attempt to quit smoking by themselves. *American Psychologist, 44*, 1355–1365.

Colby, S., Monti, P., Barnett, N., Weissman, K., Rohsenow, D., Spirito, A., Woolard, R., & Lewander, W. (1998). Brief motivational interviewing in a hospital setting for adolescent smoking: A preliminary study. *Journal of Consulting and Clinical Psychology, 66*(3), 574–578.

Colby, S. M., Monti, P. M., Rohsenow, D. J., Sirota, A. D., Abrams, D. B., & Niaura, R. S. (1994). *Alcoholics' beliefs about quitting smoking during alcohol treatment: Do they make a difference?* Paper presented at the annual meeting of the Research Society on Alcoholism, Maui, HI.

Colby, S. M., Tiffany, S. T., Shiffman, S., & Niaura, R. S. (2000a). Are adolescent smokers dependent on nicotine? A review of the evidence. *Drug and Alcohol Dependence, 59*(Suppl. 1), S83–S95.

Colby, S. M., Tiffany, S. T., Shiffman, S., & Niaura, R. S. (2000b). Measuring nicotine dependence among youth: A review of available approaches and instruments. *Drug and Alcohol Dependence, 59*(Suppl. 1), S23–S39.

Cole, P., & Rodu, B. (1996). Declining cancer mortality in the United States. *Cancer, 78*(10), 2045–2048.

Cooper, T. M., & Clayton, R. R. (1993). *How heavy smokers can become nonsmokers using a comprehensive behavioral smoking-cessation program with Nicoderm (nicotine transdermal system): The Cooper/Clayton method.* Lexington, KY: SBC/SBC.

Copeland, A. L., Brandon, T. H., & Quinn, E. P. (1995). The Smoking Consequences Questionnaire—Adult: Measurement of smoking outcome expectancies of experienced smokers. *Psychological Assessment, 7*(4), 484–494.

Covey, L. S., Glassman, A. H., & Stetner, F. (1997). Major depression following smoking cessation. *American Journal of Psychiatry, 154*, 263–265.

Cromwell, J., Bartosch, W. J., Fiore, M. C., Hasselblad, V., & Baker, T. (1997). Cost-effectiveness of the clinical practice recommendations in the AHCPR guideline for smoking cessation. *Journal of the American Medical Association, 278*(21), 1759–1766.

Crump, C. E., Earp, J. L., Kozma, C. M., & Hertz-Picciotto, I. (1996). Effect of organization-level variables on differential employee participation in 10 federal worksite health promotion programs. *Health Education Quarterly, 23*(2), 204–223.

Curry, S. J., & Emmons, K. M. (1994). Theoretical models for predicting and improving compliance with breast cancer screening. *Annals of Behavioral Medicine, 16*(4), 302–316.

Curry, S. J., Grothaus, L., & McBride, C. (1997). Reasons for quitting: Intrinsic and extrinsic motivation for smoking cessation in a population-based sample of smokers. *Addictive Behaviors, 22*(6), 727–739.

Curry, S. J., Grothaus, L. C., McAfee, T., & Pabiniak, M. S. (1998). Use and cost-effectiveness of smoking cessation services under four insurance plans in a health maintenance organization. *New England Journal of Medicine, 339*(10), 673–679.

Curry, S. J., Wagner, E. H., & Grothaus, L. C. (1990). Intrinsic and extrinsic motivation for smoking cessation. *Journal of Consulting and Clinical Psychology, 58*(3), 310–316.

Curry, S. J., Wagner, E. H., & Grothaus, L. C. (1991). Evaluation of intrinsic and extrinsic motivation interventions with a self-help smoking cessation program. *Journal of Consulting and Clinical Psychology, 59*(2), 318–324.

Dalack, G. W., Glassman, A. H., Rivelli, S., Covey, L., & Stetner, F. (1995). Mood, major depression, and fluoxetine response in cigarette smokers. *American Journal of Psychiatry, 152*(3), 398–403.

Dani, J. A., & Heinemann, S. (1996). Molecular and cellular aspects of nicotine abuse. *Neuron, 16*, 905–908.

Davis, R. M. (1988). Uniting physicians against smoking: The need for a coordinated national strategy. *Journal of the American Medical Association, 259*, 2900–2901.

DePue, J., Miller, J., & Goldstein, M. (1995). The physicians' challenge in tobacco control. *Rhode Island Medicine, 78,* 82–85.

Dietrich, A. J., O'Connor, G. T., Keller, A., Carney, P. A., Levy, D., & Whaley, F. S. (1992). Cancer: Improving early detection and prevention. A community practice randomized trial. *British Medical Journal, 304,* 687–691.

Dietrich, A. J., Woodruff, C. B., & Carney, P. A. (1994). Changing office routines to enhance preventive care. *Archives of Family Medicine, 3,* 176–183.

DiFranza, J. R., & Guerrera, M. P. (1990). Alcoholism and smoking. *Journal of Studies on Alcohol, 51,* 130–135.

Drobes, D., & Tiffany, S. (1997). Induction of smoking urge through imaginal and in vivo procedures: Psychological and self-report manifestations. *Journal of Abnormal Psychology, 106,* 15–25.

Durbren, R. (1977). Self-reinforcement by recorded telephone messages to maintain nonsmoking behavior. *Journal of Consulting and Clinical Psychology, 45,* 358–360.

Elash, C. A., Tiffany, S. T., & Vrana, S. R. (1995). Manipulation of smoking urges and affect through a brief imagery procedure: Self-report, physiological, and startle probe responses. *Experimental and Clinical Psychopharmacology, 3*(2), 156–162.

Elford, R. W., Jennett, P., Bell, N., Szafran, O., & Meadows, L. (1994). Putting prevention into practice. *Health Reports, 6,* 142–153.

Emmons, K. M. (1994). *Evaluation of a motivational intervention for hospitalized smokers.* Unpublished manuscript.

Emmons, K. M., Goldstein, M. G., Roberts, M., Cargill, B., Sherman, C. B., Millman, R., Brown, R., & Abrams, D. B. (2000). The use of nicotine replacement therapy during hospitalization. *Annals of Behavioral Medicine, 22*(4), 325–329.

Emmons, K. M., Hammond, S. K., & Abrams, D. B. (1995). Smoking at home: The impact of smoking cessation on nonsmokers' exposure to environmental tobacco smoke. *Health Psychology, 13,* 516–520.

Emmons, K. M., Hammond, S. K., Fava, J. L., Velicer, W. F., Evans, J. L., & Monroe, A. D. (2001). A randomized trial to reduce passive smoke exposure in low-income households with young children. *Pediatrics, 108*(1), 18–24.

Emmons, K. M., Marcus, B. H., Linnan, L., Rossi, J. S., & Abrams, D. B. (1994). Mechanisms in multiple risk factor interventions: Smoking, physical activity, and dietary fat intake among manufacturing workers. *Preventive Medicine, 23,* 481–489.

Emmons, K. M., & Wall, M. (1999). Environmental tobacco smoke and smoking cessation. In R. A. Etzel & S. J. Balk (Eds.), *Handbook of pediatric environmental health* (pp. 97–106). Elk Grove Village, IL: American Academy of Pediatrics.

Emmons, K. M., Wechsler, H., Dowdall, G., & Abraham, M. (1998). Predictors of smoking among U.S. college students. *American Journal of Public Health, 88,* 104–107.

Emmons, K. M., Weidner, G., Foster, W. M., & Collins, R. L. (1992). Improvement in pulmonary function following smoking cessation. *Addictive Behaviors, 17,* 301–306.

Environmental Protection Agency. (1992). *Respiratory health effects of passive smoking: Lung cancer and other disorders.* Washington, DC: Author.

Epstein, L., & Perkins, K. (1988). Smoking, stress, and coronary heart disease. *Journal of Consulting and Clinical Psychology, 56*(3), 342–349.

Ershoff, D. H., Quinn, V. P., Boyd, N. R., Stern, J., Gregory, M., & Wirtschafter, D. (1999). The Kaiser Permanente Prenatal Smoking-Cessation Trial: When more isn't better: What is enough? *American Journal of Preventive Medicine, 17*(3), 161–168.

Ershoff, D. H., Quinn, V. P., Mullen, P. D., & Lairson, D. R. (1990). Pregnancy and medical cost outcomes of a self-help prenatal smoking cessation program in an HMO. *Public Health Reports, 105,* 340–347.

Fagerstrom, K. (1978). Measuring degree of physical dependence to tobacco smoking with reference to individuation of treatment. *Addictive Behaviors, 3,* 235–241.

Fagerstrom, K., & Schneider, N. G. (1989). Measuring nicotine dependence: A review of the Fagerstrom Tolerance Questionnaire. *Journal of Behavioral Medicine, 12,* 159–182.

Farkas, A., Pierce, J., Gilpin, E., Zhu, S., Rosbrook, B., Berry, C., & Kaplan, R. (1996). Is stage of change a useful measure of the likelihood of smoking cessation? *Annals of Behavioral Medicine, 18*(2), 79–86.

Farkas, A. J., Pierce, J. P., Zhu, S. H., Rosbrook, B., Gilpin, E. A., Berry, C., & Kaplan, R. M. (1996). Addiction versus stages of change models in predicting smoking cessation in California. *Addiction, 91*(9), 1271–1280.

Farrell, A., Danish, S., & Howard, C. (1992). Relationship between drug use and other problem behaviors in urban adolescents. *Journal of Consulting and Clinical Psychology, 60,* 705–712.

Federal Trade Commission. (1997). *Tar, nicotine, and carbon monoxide of the smoke of 1206 varieties of domestic cigarettes for the year 1994.* Washington, DC: Author.

Fertig, J., & Allen, J. P. (Eds.). (1995). *Alcohol and tobacco: From basic science to policy* (National Institute on Alcohol Abuse and Alcoholism Research Monograph No. 30, NIH Publication No. 95-3931). Bethesda, MD: U.S. Department of Health and Human Services, National Institutes of Health, National Institute on Alcohol Abuse and Alcoholism.

Fichtenberg, C. M., & Glantz, S. A. (2000). Association of the California Tobacco Control Program with declines in cigarette consumption and mortality from heart disease. *New England Journal of Medicine, 343*(24), 1772–1777.

Fiore, M. C., Bailey, W. C., Cohen, S. J., Dorfman, S. F., Goldstein, M. G., Gritz, E. R., Heyman, R. B., Holbrook, J., Jaen, C. R., Kottke, T. E., Lando, H. A., Mecklenberg, R., Mullen, P. D., Nett, L. M., Robinson, L., Stitzer, M. L., Tommasello, A., Villejo, L., & Wewers, M. E. (1996). *Smoking cessation* (Clinical practice guideline no 18, AHCPR Publication No. 96–0692). Rockville, MD: U.S. Department of Health and Human Services, Public Health Service, Agency for Health Care Policy and Research.

Fiore, M. C., Bailey, W. C., Cohen, S. J., Dorfman, S. F., Goldstein, M. G., Gritz, E. R., Heyman, R. B., Jaen, C. R., Kottke, T. E., Lando, H. A., Mecklenburg, R. E., Mullen, P. D., Nett, L. M., Robinson, L., Stitzer, M. L., Tommasello, A. C., Villejo, L., & Wewers, M. E. (2000, June 20). *Treating tobacco use and dependence. Clinical practice guideline.* Rockville, MD: U.S. Department of Health and Human Services, Public Health Service.

Fiore, M. C., Jorenby, D. E., Baker, T. B., & Kenford, S. L. (1992). Tobacco dependence and the nicotine patch: Clinical guidelines on effective use. *Journal of the American Medical Association, 26,* 2687–2694.

Fisher, E. B., Haire-Joshu, D., Morgan, G. D., Rehberg, H., & Rost, K. (1990). Smoking and smoking cessation. *American Review of Respiratory Disease, 143,* 702–720.

Fisher, E. B., Jr. (1997). Two approaches to social support in smoking cessation: Commodity model and nondirective support. *Addictive Behaviors, 22*(6), 819–833.

Flay, B. R. (2000). Approaches to substance use prevention utilizing school curriculum plus social environment change. *Addictive Behaviors, 25*(6), 861–885.

Flay, B. R., Koepke, D., Thomson, S. J., Santi, S., Best, J. A., & Brown, K. S. (1989). Six-year follow-up of the first Waterloo School smoking prevention trial. *American Journal of Public Health, 79,* 1371–1376.

Flay, B. R., Phil, D., Petraitis, J., & Hu, F. B. (1995). The theory of triadic influence: Preliminary evidence related to alcohol and tobacco use. In J. Fertig & R. Allen (Eds.), *Alcohol and tobacco: From basic science to policy* (National Institute on Alcohol Abuse and Alcoholism Research Monograph No. 30, NIH Publication No. 95-3931, pp. 37–57). Bethesda, MD: U.S. Department of Health and Human Services, National Institutes of Health, National Institute on Alcohol Abuse and Alcoholism.

Forster, J. L., & Wolfson, M. (1998). Youth access to tobacco: Policies and politics. *Annual Review of Public Health, 19,* 203–235.

Foxx, R. M., & Brown, R. A. (1979). Nicotine fading and self-monitoring for cigarette abstinence or controlled smoking. *Journal of Applied Behavior Analysis, 12,* 111–125.

Garvey, A. J., Bliss, R. E., Hitchcock, J. L., Heinold, J. W., & Rosner, B. (1992). Predictors of smoking relapse among self-quitters: A report from the Normative Aging Study. *Addictive Behaviors, 17,* 367–377.

Gibbons, F. X., & Gerrard, M. (1996). Smoker networks and the typical smoker: A prospective analysis of smoking cessation. *Health Psychology, 15,* 469–477.

Glantz, S. A., & Smith, L. R. (1997). The effect of ordinances requiring smoke-free restaurants and bars on revenues: A follow-up. *American Journal of Public Health, 10,* 1687–1693.

Glanz, K., Lewis, F., & Rimer, B. (1997). Linking theory, research, and practice. In K. Glanz, F. Lewis, & B. Rimer (Eds.), *Health behavior and health education: Theory, research and practice* (pp. 19–40). San Francisco, CA: Jossey-Bass.

Glassman, A. H. (1993). Cigarette smoking: Implications for psychiatric illness. *American Journal of Psychiatry, 150*(4), 546–553.

Glassman, A. H. (1997). *Cigarette smoking and its comorbidity* (NIDA Research Monograph No. 172, pp. 52–60). Rockville, MD: National Institute on Drug Abuse.

Glassman, A. H., Stetner, F., Walsh, B. T., Raizman, P. S., Fleiss, J. L., Cooper, T. B., & Covey, L. S. (1988). Heavy smokers, smoking cessation, and clonidine: Results of a double-blind, randomized trial. *Journal of the American Medical Association, 259*(19), 2863–2866.

Glynn, T. J. (1988). Relative effectiveness of physician-initiated smoking cessation programs. *Cancer Bulletin, 40*(6), 359–364.

Glynn, T. J., & Manley, M. W. (1989). *How to help your patients stop smoking: A National Cancer Institute manual for physicians* (NIH Publication No. 89-3064). Bethesda, MD: Smoking, Tobacco and Cancer Program, Division of Cancer Prevention and Control, National Cancer Institute.

Goldstein, M., DePue, J., Monroe, A., Willey-Lessne, C., Rakowski, W., Prokhorov, A., Niaura, R., & Dubé, C. (1998). A population-based survey of physician smoking cessation counseling practices. *Preventive Medicine, 27,* 720–729.

Goldstein, M. G., & Niaura, R. S. (1991). Nicotine gum: Pharmacological and clinical aspects. In J. A. Cocores (Ed.), *Clinical management of nicotine dependence* (pp. 181–195). New York: Springer-Verlag.

Goldstein, M. G., & Niaura, R. (1998). Smoking. In E. J. Topol, M. Bristow, R. M. Califf, J. Isner, E. N. Prsytowsky, P. Serruys, J. Swain, J. Thomas, & P. Thompson (Eds.), *Textbook of cardiovascular medicine* (pp. 145–169). Philadelphia: Lippincott-Raven.

Goldstein, M. G., Niaura, R., Follick, M. J., & Abrams, D. B. (1989). Effects of behavioral skills training and schedule of nicotine gum administration on smoking cessation. *American Journal of Psychiatry, 146*(1), 56–60.

Goldstein, M. G., Niaura, R., Willey-Lessne, C., DePue, J., Eaton, C., Rakowski, W., & Dubé, C. (1997). Physicians counseling smokers: A population-based survey of patients' perceptions of health care provider-delivered smoking cessation interventions. *Archives of Internal Medicine, 157,* 1313–1319.

Gourlay, S., & Benowitz, N. (1995). Is clonidine an effective smoking cessation therapy? *Drugs, 50,* 197–207.

Griesler, P. C., Kandel, D. B., & Davies, M. (1998). Maternal smoking in pregnancy, child behavior problems, and adolescent smoking. *Journal of Research on Adolescence, 8*(2), 159–189.

Gritz, E. R., Klesges, R. C., & Meyers, A. W. (1989). The smoking and body weight relationship: Implications for intervention and postcessation weight control. *Annals of Behavioral Medicine, 11,* 144–153.

Gritz, E. R., Kristeller, J., & Burns, D. M. (1993). High-risk groups and patients with medical co-morbidity. In C. T. Orleans, & J. Slade (Eds.), *Nicotine addiction: Principles and management* (pp. 279–309). New York: Oxford University Press.

Gross, J., Stitzer, M., & Maldonadok, J. (1989). Nicotine replacement: Effects on postcessation weight gain. *Journal of Consulting and Clinical Psychology, 37*, 87–92.

Gulliver, S. B., Rohsenow, D. J., Colby, S. M., Dey, A. N., Abrams, D. B., Niaura, R. S., & Monti, P. M. (1995). Interrelationship of smoking and alcohol dependence, use and urges to use. *Journal of Studies on Alcohol, 56*, 202–206.

Haaga, D. A. F., & Stewart, B. L. (1992). Self-efficacy for recovery from a lapse after smoking cessation. *Journal of Consulting and Clinical Psychology, 60*(1), 24–28.

Hahn, D. L., & Berger, M. G. (1990). Implementation of a systematic health maintenance protocol in a private practice. *Journal of Family Practice, 31*, 492–504.

Hajek, P., West, R., Foulds, J., Nilsson, F., Burrows, S., & Meadow, A. (1999). Randomized comparative trial of nicotine polacrilex, a transdermal patch, nasal spray, and an inhaler. *Archives of Internal Medicine, 159*, 2033–2038.

Hale, K., Hughes, J., Oliverto, A., Helzar, J. E., Higgins, S. T., Bickel, W. K., & Cottler, L. B. (1993). *Nicotine dependence in a population-based sample: Problems of drug dependence, 1992* (NIDA Research Monograph No. 132). Rockville, MD: National Institute on Drug Abuse.

Hall, S. M., Reus, V. I., Munoz, R. F., Sees, K. L., Humfleet, G., Hartz, D. T., Frederick, S., & Triffleman, E. (1998). Nortriptyline and cognitive-behavioral therapy in the treatment of cigarette smoking [Comments]. *Archives of General Psychiatry, 55*(8), 683–690.

Hall, S. M., Tunstall, C. D., Vila, K. L., & Duffy, J. (1992). Weight gain prevention and smoking cessation: Cautionary findings. *American Journal of Public Health, 82*(6), 799–803.

Hanrahan, J., Sherman, C., & Emmons, K. M. (1996). Cigarette smoking and health: Official statement of the American Thoracic Society. *American Journal of Respiratory and Critical Care Medicine, 153*, 861–865.

Hatsukami, D. K., & Boyle, R. G. (1997). Prevention and treatment of smokeless tobacco use. *Advances in Dental Research, 11*(3), 342–349.

Hayford, K., Patten, C., Rummans, T., Schroider, D., Offord, K., Croghan, I., Glover, E., Sachs, D., & Hurt, R. (1999). Efficacy of bupropion for smoking cessation in smokers with a former history of major depression or alcoholism. *British Journal of Psychiatry, 174*, 173–178.

Heatherton, T. F., Kozlowski, L. T., Frecker, R. C., & Fagerstrom, K. O. (1991). The Fagerstrom Test for Nicotine Dependence: A revision of the Fagerstrom Tolerance Questionnaire. *British Journal of Addiction, 86*, 1119–1127.

Heatherton, T., Kozlowski, L., Frecker, R., Rickert, W., & Robinson, J. (1989). Measuring the heaviness of smoking: Using self-reported time to the first cigarette of the day and number of cigarettes smoked per day. *British Journal of Addiction, 84*(7), 791–799.

Henningfield, J. E. (1997). *Comparing the abuse potential of nicotine delivery systems.* Paper presented at the Alternative Nicotine Delivery System Harm Reduction Public Health Conference, Toronto, Canada.

Henningfield, J. E., Cohen, C., & Pickworth, W. B. (1993). Psychopharmacology of nicotine. In C. T. Orleans & J. Slade (Eds.), *Nicotine addictions: Principles and management* (pp. 24–45). New York: Oxford University Press.

Henschke, C. I., McCauley, D. I., Yankelevitz, D. F., Naidich, D. P., McGuiness, G., Miettinen, O. S., Libby, D. M., Pasmantier, M. W., Koizumi, J., Altorki, N. K., & Smith, J. P. (1999). Early Lung Cancer Action Project: Overall design and findings from baseline screening. *Lancet, 354*, 99–105.

Henschke, C. I., Naidich, D. P., Yankelevitz, D. F., McGuiness, G., McCauley, D. I., Smith, J. P., Libby, D., Pasmantier, M., Vazquez, M., Koizumi, J., Flieder, D., Altorki, N., & Miettinen, O. S. (2001). Early Lung Cancer Action Project: Initial findings on repeat screenings. *Cancer, 92*(1), 153–159.

Herzog, T. A., Abrams, D. B., Emmons, K. M., Linnan, L., & Shadel, W. G. (1999). Do processes of change predict smoking stage movements?: A prospective analysis of the transtheoretical model. *Health Psychology, 18*(4), 369–375.

Hitsman, B., Abrams, D. B., Shadel, W. G., Niaura, R., Borrelli, B., Emmons, K. M., Brown, R. A., Swift, R. M., Monti, P. M., Rohsenow, D. J., & Colby, S. M. (2002, April). *Motivating alcoholics to quit smoking: Baseline data from a novel motivational intervention.* Paper presented at the annual meeting of the Society of Behavioral Medicine, Washington, DC.

Hollis, J. F., Lichtenstein, E., Vogt, T. M., Stevens, V. J., & Biglan, A. (1993). Nurse-assisted counseling for smokers in primary care. *Annals of Internal Medicine, 118,* 521–525.

Hovell, M., Meltzer, S., Zakarian, J., Wahlgren, D., Emerson, J., Hofsetter, C., Leaderer, B., Meltzer, E., Zeiger, R., & O'Connor, R. (1994). Reduction of environmental tobacco smoke exposure among asthmatic children: A controlled trial. *Chest, 106*(2), 440–446.

Hovell, M. F., Zakarian, J. M., Matt, G. E., Hofstetter, C. R., Bernert, J. T., & Pirkle, J. (2000). Effect of counseling mothers on their children's exposure to environmental tobacco smoke: Randomised controlled trial. *British Medical Journal, 321*(7257), 337–342.

Hughes, J., & Hatsukami, D. (1992). The nicotine withdrawal syndrome: A brief review and update. *International Journal of Smoking Cessation, 1,* 22–26.

Hughes, J. R. (1992). Tobacco withdrawal in self-quitters. *Journal of Consulting and Clinical Psychology, 60*(5), 689–697.

Hughes, J. R. (1993). Treatment of smoking cessation in smokers with a past history of alcohol/drug problems. *Journal of Substance Abuse Treatment, 10,* 181–187.

Hughes, J. R. (1994a). An algorithm for smoking cessation. *Archives of Family Medicine, 3,* 280–285.

Hughes, J. R. (1994b). Smoking and alcoholism. In J. Cox & D. Hatsukami (Eds.), *Behavioral approaches to addiction* (pp. 1–3). Belle Mead, NJ: Calmers Heathcare Communications.

Hughes, J. R. (1995). Clinical implications of the association between smoking and alcoholism. In J. Fertig & R. Fuller (Eds.), *Alcohol and tobacco: From basic science to policy* (National Institute of Alcohol Abuse and Alcoholism Research Monograph No. 30, NIH Publication No. 95-3931, pp. 171–181). Bethesda, MD: U.S. Department of Health and Human Services, National Institutes of Health, National Institute on Alcohol Abuse and Alcoholism.

Hughes, J. R. (1996). Pharmacotherapy of nicotine dependence. In C. R. Schuster & M. J. Kuhar (Eds.), *Pharmacological aspects of drug dependence: Toward an integrative neurobehavioral approach* (pp. 599–626). New York: Springer-Verlag.

Hughes, J. R. (1998). Dependence on the abuse of nicotine replacement medications: An update. In N. L. Benowitz (Ed.), *Nicotine safety and toxicity* (pp. 147–157). New York: Oxford University Press.

Hughes, J. R., Cummings, K. M., & Hyland, A. (1999). Ability of smokers to reduce their smoking and its association with future smoking cessation. *Addiction, 94*(1), 109–114.

Hughes, J. R., Fiester, S., Goldstein, M., Resnick, M., Rock, N., & Ziedonis, D. (1996). Practice guideline for the treatment of patients with nicotine dependence. *American Journal of Psychiatry, 153*(Suppl. 10), 1–31.

Hughes, J. R., Goldstein, M. G., Hurt, R. D., & Shiffman, S. (1999). Recent advances in the pharmacotherapy of smoking cessation. *Journal of the American Medical Association, 281*(1), 72–76.

Hughes, J. R., & Hatsukami, D. (1986). Signs and symptoms of tobacco withdrawal. *Archives of General Psychiatry, 43,* 289–294.

Hughes, J. R., Hatsukami, D. K., Mitchell, J. E., & Dahlgren, L. A. (1986). Prevalence of smoking among psychiatric outpatients. *American Journal of Psychiatry, 143*(8), 993–997.

Hughes, J. R., Higgins, S. T., & Hatsukami, D. K. (1990). Effects of abstinence from tobacco: A critical review. In L. T. Kozlowski, H. M. Annis, & H. D. Capell (Eds.), *Recent advances in alcohol and drug problems* (Vol. 10, pp. 317–397). New York: Plenum Press.

Hughes, J. R., & Liguori, A. (1997). Bibliographical analysis of research on smoking cessation therapy. *Tobacco Control, 6,* 111–114.

Hughes, J. R., Stead, L. F., & Lancaster, T. R. (2002). Anxiolytics for smoking cessation. Cochrane Review. Retrieved 6/23/02 from Cochrane Library, *www.cochranelibrary.com/cochrane.*

Hunt, W. A., & Bespalec, D. A. (1974). An evaluation of current methods of modifying smoking behavior. *Journal of Clinical Psychology, 30,* 431–438.

Hurt, R. D. (1998, July). *New medications for nicotine dependence treatment.* Paper presented at the

National Research Forum: Addicted to Nicotine, National Institutes of Health, Bethesda, Maryland.

Hurt, R. D., Croghan, G. A., Beede, S., Wolter, T. D., Croghan, I. T., & Patten, C. A. (2000). Nicotine patch therapy in 101 adolescent smokers: Efficacy, withdrawal symptom relief, and carbon monoxide and plasma cotinine levels. *Archives of Pediatric and Adolescent Medicine, 154,* 31–37.

Hurt, R. D., Dale, L. C., Croghan, G. A., Croghan, I. T., Gomez-Dahl, L. C., & Offord, K. P. (1998). Nicotine nasal spray for smoking cessation: Pattern of use, side effects, relief of withdrawal symptoms, and cotinine levels. *Mayo Clinic Proceedings, 73*(2), 118–125.

Hurt, R. D., Dale, L. C., McClain, F. L., Eberman, K. M., Offord, K. P., Bruce, B. K., & Lauger, G. G. (1992). A comprehensive model for the treatment of nicotine dependence in a medical setting. *Medical Clinics of North America, 76*(2), 495–514.

Hurt, R. D., Eberman, K. M., Croghan, I. T., Offord, K. P., Davis, L. J., Jr., Morse, R. M., Palmen, M. A., & Bruce, B. K. (1994). Nicotine dependence treatment during inpatient treatment for other addictions: A prospective intervention trial. *Alcoholism: Clinical and Experimental Research, 18*(4), 867–872.

Hurt, R. D., Sachs, D. P. L., Glover, E. D., Offord, K. P., Johnston, J. A., Dale, L. C., Khayrallah, M. A., Schroeder, D. R., Glover, P. N., Sullivan, C. R., Croghan, I. T., & Sullivan, P. M. (1997). A comparison of sustained-release bupropion and placebo for smoking cessation. *New England Journal of Medicine, 337*(17), 1195–1202.

Hutchison, K. E., Monti, P. M., Rohsenow, D. J., Swift, R. M., Colby, S. M., Gnys, M., Niaura, R. S., & Sirota, A. D. (1999). Effects of naltrexone with nicotine replacement on smoking cue reactivity: Preliminary results. *Psychopharmacology, 142*(2), 139–143.

Jack, B. W., Campanile, C., McQuade, W., & Kogan, M. D. (1995). The Negative Pregnancy Test: An opportunity for preconception care. *Archives of Family Medicine, 4,* 340–345.

Jacobson, E. (1938). *Progressive relaxation* (2nd ed.). Chicago: University of Chicago Press.

Jaen, C., Cummings, K., Emont, S., Sciandra, R., Feldman, R., & Humphrey, J. (1991). Promotion of a stop smoking telephone information and referral service. In R. Feldman & J. Humphrey (Eds.), *Advances in health education: Current research* (pp. 27–36). New York: AMS Press.

Jaen, C., Cummings, K., Zielenzy, M., & O'Shea, R. (1993). Patterns and predictors of smoking cessation among users of a telephone hotline. *Public Health Reports, 108,* 772–778.

Janis, I. L., & Mann, L. (1977). *Decision making: A psychological analysis of conflict, choice, and commitment.* New York: Free Press.

Janz, N. K., & Becker, M. H. (1984). The health belief model: A decade later. *Health Education Quarterly, 11,* 1–47.

Jarvik, M., & Henningfield, J. (1988). Pharmacologic treatment of tobacco dependence. *Pharmacology, Biochemistry, and Behavior, 30,* 279–284.

Jenkins, R. A., Guerin, M. R., & Tomkins, B. A. (2000). Mainstream and sidestream cigarette smoke. In R. A. Jenkins, M. R. Guerin, & B. A. Tomkins (Eds.), *The chemistry of environmental tobacco smoke: Composition and measurement* (pp. 49–75). Boca Raton, FL: Lewis.

Johnston, L. D., O'Malley, P. M., & Bachman, J. G. (1996). *National survey results on drug use from the Monitoring the Future Study, 1975–1995: Vol. 1. Secondary School Students* (NIH Publication No. 96-4139). Rockville, MD: National Institute on Drug Abuse.

Jorenby, D. E., Hatsukami, D. K., Smith, S. S., Fiore, M. C., Allen, S., Jensen, J., & Baker, T. B. (1996). Characterization of tobacco withdrawal symptoms: Transdermal nicotine reduces hunger and weight gain. *Psychopharmacology (Berlin), 128*(2), 130–138.

Jorenby, D. E., Leischow, S. J., Nides, M. A., Rennard, S. I., Johnston, J. A., Hughes, A. R., Smith, S. S., Muramoto, M. L., Daughton, D. M., Doan, K., Fiore, M. C., & Baker, T. B. (1999). A controlled trial of sustained-release bupropion, a nicotine patch, or both for smoking cessation. *New England Journal of Medicine, 340*(9), 685–691.

Joseph, A. M., Nichol, K. L., & Anderson, H. (1993). Effect of treatment for nicotine dependence on alcohol and drug treatment outcomes. *Addictive Behavior, 18,* 635–644.

Joseph, A. M., Norman, S. M., Ferry, L. H., Prochazka, A. V., Westman, E. C., Steele, B. G., Sherman, S. E., Cleveland, M., Antonnucio, D. O., Hartman, N., & McGovern, P. G. (1996). The safety of transdermal nicotine as an aid to smoking cessation in patients with cardiac disease. *New England Journal of Medicine, 335,* 1792–1798.

Kandel, D. B., & Yamaguchi, K. (1993). From beer to crack: Developmental patterns of drug involvement. *American Journal of Public Health, 83,* 851–855.

Kawachi, I., Troisi, R. J., Rotnitzky, A. G., Coakely, E. H., & Colditz, G. A. (1996). Can physical activity minimize weight gain in women after smoking cessation? *American Journal of Public Health, 86,* 999–1004.

Killen, J., & Fortman, S. (1997). Craving is associated with smoking relapse: Evidence from three prospective studies. *Experimental and Clinical Psychopharmacology, 5*(2), 137–142.

King, T. K., Matacin, M., Bock, B. C., & Marcus, B. H. (1997, November). *Body image evaluations in women smokers.* Paper presented at the annual meeting of the Association for the Advancement of Behavior Therapy, Miami, FL.

King, T. K., Matacin, M., Marcus, B. H., Bock, B. C., & Tripolone, J. (2000). Body image evaluations in women smokers. *Addictive Behaviors, 25*(4), 613–618.

Kinne, S., Thompson, B., & Wooldridge, J. (1991). Response to a telephone smoking information line. *American Journal of Health Promotion, 5,* 410–413.

Klesges, R. C., Benowitz, N. L., & Meyers, A. W. (1991). Behavioral and biobehavioral aspects of smoking and smoking cessation: The problem of postcessation weight gain. *Behavior Therapy, 22,* 179–199.

Koob, G. F., & LeMoal, M. (2001). Drug addiction, dysregulation of reward, and allostasis. *Neuropsychopharmacology, 24*(2), 97–129.

Kottke, T. E., Battista, R. N., DeFriese, G. H., & Brekke, M. L. (1988). Attributes of successful smoking cessation interventions in medical practice: A meta-analysis of 39 controlled trials. *Journal of the American Medical Association, 259,* 2883–2889.

Kozlowski, L., & Ferrence, R. G. (1990). Statistical control in research on alcohol and tobacco mortality. *British Journal of Addiction, 85,* 271–278.

Kozlowski, L., & Herlig, S. (1988). Objective measures. In D. M. Donovan & G. A. Marlatt (Eds.), *Assessment of addictive behaviors* (pp. 214–238). New York: Guilford Press.

Kozlowski, L., Pillitteri, J., Sweeney, C., Whitfield, K., & Graham, J. (1996). Asking about urges or cravings for cigarettes. *Psychology of Addictive Behaviors, 10*(4), 248–260.

Kozlowski, L. T., Ferrence, R. G., & Corbit, T. (1990). Tobacco use: A perspective for alcohol and drug researchers. *British Journal of Addiction, 85,* 245.

Kozlowski, L. T., Pope, M. A., & Lux, J. E. (1988). Prevalence of the misuse of ultra-low tar cigarettes by blocking filter vents. *American Journal of Public Health, 78,* 694–695.

Kreek, M. J., & Koob, G. F. (1998). Drug dependence: Stress and dysregulation of brain reward pathways. *Drug and Alcohol Dependence, 51,* 23–47.

Lawson, G. M., Hurt, R. D., Dale, L. C., Offord, K. P., Croghan, I. T., Schroeder, D. R., & Jiang, N. S. (1998). Application of serum nicotine and plasma cotinine concentrations to assessment of nicotine replacement in light, moderate and heavy smokers undergoing transdermal therapy. *Journal of Clinical Pharmacology, 38*(6), 502–509.

Leischow, S. J., Valente, S. N., Hill, A. L., Otte, P. S., Aickin, M., Holden, T., Kligman, E., & Cook, G. (1997). Effects of nicotine dose and administration method on withdrawal symptoms and side effects during short-term smoking abstinence. *Experimental and Clinical Psychopharmacology, 5*(1), 54–64.

Lerman, C., Caporaso, N. E., Audrain, J., Main, D., Bowman, E. D., Lockshin, B., Boyd, N. R., & Shields, P. G. (1999). Evidence suggesting the role of specific genetic factors in cigarette smoking. *Health Psychology, 18,* 14–20.

Levin, E. D., & Slotkin, T. A. (1998). Developmental neurotoxicity of nicotine. In W. Slikker & L. W. Chang (Eds.), *Handbook of developmental neurotoxicology* (pp. 587–615). San Diego, CA: Academic Press.

Levinson, B. L., Shapiro, D., Schwartz, G. E., & Tursky, B. (1971). Smoking elimination by gradual reduction. *Behavior Therapy, 2,* 477–487.

Lewinsohn, P. M., Munoz, R. F., Youngren, M. A., & Zeiss, A. M. (1986). *Control your depression.* New York: Prentice-Hall.

Li, F. P., Sorensen, G., Hunt, M. K., Pucci, L., Thompson, J. E., Harden, E., Graham-Meho, L., Youngstrom, R., Burak, L., McGill, K., Rosenblum, L. B., Farr, E., Burke, C., Eskow, R., Benjamin, G., Adams, L. A., Pinney, J., & Linnan, L. (1993). *Guide to workplace tobacco control: Tobacco free worksite training and technical assistance initiative.* Boston, MA: Dana–Farber Cancer Institute.

Lichtenstein, E. (1999). Nicotine anonymous: Community resource and research implications. *Psychology of Addictive Behaviors, 13*(1), 60–68.

Lichtenstein, E., Antonnuccio, D. O., & Rainwater, G. (1977, April). *Unkicking the habit: The resumption of cigarette smoking.* Paper presented at the annual meeting of the Western Psychological Association, Seattle, WA.

Lichtenstein, E., & Glasgow, R. E. (1992). Smoking cessation: What have we learned over the past decade? *Journal of Consulting and Clinical Psychology, 60*(4), 518–527.

Lichtenstein, E., Glasgow, R. E., & Abrams, D. B. (1986). Social support in smoking cessation: In search of effective interventions. *Behavior Therapy, 17,* 607–619.

Lichtenstein, E., & Hollis, J. (1992). Patient referral to a smoking cessation program: Who follows through? *Journal of Family Practice, 34,* 739–744.

Lichtenstein, E., Hollis, J. F., Severson, H. H., Stevens, V. J., Vogt, T. M., Glasgow, R. E., & Andrews, J. A. (1996). Tobacco cessation interventions in health care settings: Rationale, model, outcomes. *Addictive Behaviors, 21*(6), 709–720.

Lindsay, M. E., Wilson, D., Best, J. A., Gilbert, J. R., Taylor, W., Willms, D., & Singer, J. (1987). The impact of a continuing education package for smoking cessation on physicians' clinical behavior and patient smoking. *Proceedings of the Annual Conference of Research and Medical Education, 26*(14), 14–19.

Linnan, L., Graham, A., Weiner, B., & Emmons, K. (2000, November). *Managers' knowledge, attitudes, and beliefs about worksite health promotion.* Paper presented at the annual meeting of the American Public Health Association, Boston, MA.

Lloyd, E. E., Niaura, R., Brown, R., & Abrams, D. (2001). [A survey of smoking among young adults in technical school]. Unpublished raw data.

Lloyd-Richardson, E. E., Niaura, R., & Abrams, D. (2001, June). *Informed development of smoking cessation interventions: Addressing the needs of college and technical school students.* Symposium conducted at the Society for Prevention Research, Developing Effective Tobacco Interventions: Transdisciplinary Research Informing Target, Policy, and Content Decisions, L. Dierker, chairperson, Washington, DC.

Lloyd-Richardson, E. E., Papandonatos, G., Kazura, A., Stanton, C., & Niaura, R. (2002). Differentiating stages of smoking intensity among adolescents: Stage-specific psychological, and social influences. *Journal of Consulting and Clinical Psychology, 70,* 998–1009.

MacGregor, I. (1996). Efficacy of dental health advice as an aid to reducing cigarette smoking. *British Dental Journal, 180,* 292–296.

MacPhillamy, D. J., & Lewinsohn, P. M. (1982). The Pleasant Events Schedule: Studies on reliability, validity, and scale intercorrelation. *Journal of Consulting and Clinical Psychology, 50*(3), 363–380.

Maes, S., Verhoeven, C., Kittel, F., & Scholten, H. (1998). Effects of a Dutch worksite wellness-health program: The Brabantia Project. *American Journal of Public Health, 88*(7), 1037–1041.

Manley, M. W., Epps, R. P., & Glynn, T. J. (1992). The clinician's role in promoting smoking cessation among clinic patients. *Medical Clinics of North America, 76,* 477–494.

Mannuzza, S., Fryer, A., Klein, D., & Endicott, J. (1986). Schedule for Affective Disorders and Schizophrenia—Lifetime Version modified for the study of anxiety disorders (SADS-LA): Rationale and conceptual development. *Journal of Psychiatric Research, 20*(4), 317–325.

Marcus, B. H., Albrecht, A. E., King, T. K., Parisi, A. F., Pinto, B. M., Roberts, M., Niaura, R. S., & Abrams, D. B. (1999). The efficacy of exercise as an aid for smoking cessation in women: A randomized controlled trial. *Archives of Internal Medicine, 159,* 1229–1234.

Marcus, B. H., Emmons, K. M., Abrams, D. B., Marshall, R. J., Novotny, T. E., & Etzel, R. A. (1992). Restrictive smoking policies: Impact on nonsmokers' tobacco exposure. *Journal of Public Health Policy, 13*(1), 42–51.

Marks, J. S., Koplan, J. P., Hogue, C. J., & Dalmat, M. E. (1990). A cost-benefit/cost-effectiveness analysis of smoking cessation for pregnant women. *American Journal of Preventive Medicine, 6*(5), 282–289.

Marlatt, G. A. (Ed.). (1998). *Harm reduction: Pragmatic strategies for managing high-risk behaviors.* New York: Guilford Press.

Marlatt, G. A. (1999). From hindsight to foresight: A commentary on Project MATCH. In J. A. Tucker, D. M. Donovan, & G. A. Marlatt (Eds.), *Changing addictive behavior: Bridging clinical and public health strategies* (pp. 45–66). New York: Guilford Press.

Marlatt, G. A., & Gordon, J. R. (Eds.). (1985). *Relapse prevention: Maintenance strategies in the treatment of addictive behaviors.* New York: Guilford Press.

Martin, J. E., Calfas, K. J., Patten, C. A., Polarek, M., Hofstetter, C. R., Noto, J., & Beach, D. (1997). Prospective evaluation of three smoking interventions in 205 recovering alcoholics: One-year results of project SCRAP—tobacco. *Journal of Consulting and Clinical Psychology, 65*(1), 190–194.

Martinez, M. E., McPherson, R. S., Annegers, J. F., & Levin, B. (1995). Cigarette smoking and alcohol consumption as risk factors for colorectal adenomatous polyps. *Journal of the National Cancer Institute, 87*(4), 274–279.

McBride, P. E., Plane, M. B., Underbakke, G., Brown, R. L., & Solberg, L. I. (1997). Smoking screening and management in primary care practices. *Archives of Family Medicine, 6,* 165–172.

McGinnis, J. M., & Foege, W. H. (1993). Actual causes of death in the United States. *Journal of the American Medical Association, 270,* 2207–2212.

McLellan, A. T., Hagan, T. A., Levine, M., Gould, F., Meyers, K., Bencivengo, M., & Durell, J. (1998). Supplemental social services improve outcomes in public addiction treatment. *Addiction, 93*(10), 1489–1499.

McPhee, S. J., & Detmer, W. M. (1993). Office-based interventions to improve delivery of cancer prevention services by primary care physicians. *Cancer, 72,* 1100–1112.

Mermelstein, R., Lichtenstein, E., & McIntyre, K. (1983). Partner support and relapse in smoking cessation programs. *Journal of Consulting and Clinical Psychology, 51,* 465–466.

Mermelstein, R. J., Cohen, S., Lichtenstein, E., Baer, J. S., & Kamarck, T. (1986). Social support and smoking cessation and maintenance. *Journal of Consulting and Clinical Psychology, 54,* 447–453.

Miller, S. M. (1995). Monitoring versus blunting styles of coping with cancer influence the information patients want and need about their disease. *Cancer, 76*(2), 167–177.

Miller, W. (1985). Motivation for treatment: A review with special emphasis on alcoholism. *Psychological Bulletin, 98,* 84–107.

Miller, W. R., & Rollnick, S. (1991). *Motivational interviewing: Preparing people to change addictive behavior.* New York: Guilford Press.

Miller, W. R., & Rollnick, S. (2002). *Motivational interviewing* (2nd ed.): *Preparing people for change.* New York: Guilford Press.

Monti, P., Rohsenow, D., Colby, S., & Abrams, D. (1995). Smoking among alcoholics during and after treatment: Implications for models, treatment strategies, and policy. In J. Fertig & J. Allen (Eds.), *Alcohol and tobacco: From basic science to policy* (National Institute on Alcohol Abuse and Alcoholism Research Monograph No. 30, NIH Publication No. 95-3931, pp. 187–206). Bethesda, MD: U.S. Department of Health and Human Services, National Institutes of Health, National Institute on Alcohol Abuse and Alcoholism.

Monti, P., Rohsenow, D., & Hutchison, K. (2000). Toward bridging the gap between biological, psychobiological and psychosocial models of alcohol craving. *Addiction, 95*(Suppl. 2), S229–S236.

Monti, P. M., Barnett, N. P., O'Leary, T. A., & Colby, S. M. (2001). Motivational enhancement for alcohol-involved adolescents. In P. M. Monti, S. M. Colby, & T. A. O'Leary (Eds.), *Adolescents, alcohol, and substance abuse: Reaching teens through brief interventions* (pp. 145–182). New York: Guilford Press.

Monti, P. M., Colby, S. M., Barnett, N. P., Spirito, A., Rohsenow, D. J., Myers, M., Woolard, R., & Lewander, W. (1999). Brief intervention for harm reduction with alcohol-positive older adolescents in a hospital emergency department. *Journal of Consulting and Clinical Psychology, 67*(6), 989–994.

Monti, P. M., Colby, S. M., & O'Leary, T. A. (Eds.). (2001). *Adolescents, alcohol, and substance abuse: Reaching teens through brief interventions.* New York: Guilford Press.

Murray, C. J. L., & Lopez, A. D. (Eds.). (1996). *The global burden of disease: A comprehensive assessment of mortality and disability from diseases, injuries, and risk factors in 1990 and projected to 2020.* Boston, MA: Harvard School of Public Health.

Murray, R., Johnston, J., Dolce, J., Lee, W., & O'Hara, P. (1995). Social support for smoking cessation and abstinence: The Lung Health Study. *Addictive Behaviors, 20*(2), 159–170.

Murray, R. P., Bailey, W. C., Daniels, K., Bjornson, W. M., Kurnow, K., Connett, J. E., Nides, M. A., & Kiley, J. P. (1996). Safety of nicotine polacrilex gum used by 3,094 participants in the Lung Health Study. *Chest, 109*(2), 438–445.

National Committee for Quality Assurance. (1996). *HEDIS 3.0 Health Plan Employer Data and Information Set.* Washington, DC: National Committee for Quality Assurance.

Niaura, R., Abrams, D., Shadel, W. G., Rohsenow, D., Monti, P., & Sirota, A. (1999). Cue exposure treatment for smoking relapse prevention: A controlled clinical trial. *Addiction, 94*(5), 685–695.

Niaura, R., & Abrams, D. B. (2002). Smoking cessation: Progress, priorities, and prospectus. *Journal of Consulting and Clinical Psychology, 70*(3), 494–509.

Niaura, R., Goldstein, M., DePue, J., Keuthen, N., Kristeler, J., & Abrams, D. B. (1995). Fluoxetine, symptoms of depression, and smoking cessation. *Annals of Behavioral Medicine, 17*(Suppl.), S061.

Niaura, R., Goldstein, M., Spring, B., & Keuthen, N. (1997). Fluoxetine for smoking cessation: A multicenter randomized double blind dose response study. *Annals of Behavioral Medicine, 19,* S042.

Niaura, R. S., Brown, R., Goldstein, M., Murphy, J., & Abrams, D. B. (1996). Transdermal clonidine for smoking cessation: A double-blind randomized dose-response study. *Experimental and Clinical Psychopharmacology, 4,* 285–291.

Niaura, R. S., Rohsenow, D. J., Binkoff, J. A., Monti, P. M., Pedraza, M., & Abrams, D. B. (1988). Relevance of cue reactivity to understanding alcohol and smoking relapse. *Journal of Abnormal Psychology, 97*(2), 133–152.

Niaura, R. S., Shadel, W. G., Abrams, D. B., Monti, P. M., Rohsenow, D. J., & Sirota, A. (1998). Individual differences in cue reactivity among smokers trying to quit: Effects of gender and cue type. *Addictive Behaviors, 23,* 209–224.

Novak, S. P., & Clayton, R. R. (2001). The influence of school environment and self-regulation on transitions between stages of cigarette smoking: A multilevel analysis. *Health Psychology, 20*(3), 196–207.

Ockene, J., Kristeller, J., Goldberg, R., Ockene, I., Merriam, P., Barrett, S., Pekow, P., Hosmer, D., & Gianelli, R. (1992). Smoking cessation and severity of disease: The coronary artery smoking intervention study. *Health Psychology, 11,* 119–126.

Ockene, J. K. (1987). Physician-delivered interventions for smoking cessation: Strategies for increasing effectiveness. *Preventive Medicine, 16,* 723–737.

Ockene, J. K., Kristeller, J., Goldberg, R., Amick, T. L., Pekow, P. S., Hosmer, D., Quirk, M., & Kalan, K. (1991). Increasing the efficacy of physician-delivered smoking interventions: A randomized clinical trial. *Journal of General Internal Medicine, 6,* 1–8.

Ockene, J. K., Kristeller, J., Pbert, L., Hebert, J. R., Luippold, R., Goldberg, R. J., Landon, J., & Kalan,

K. (1994). The physician-delivered smoking intervention projects: Can short-term interventions produce long-term effects for a general outpatient population? *Health Psychology, 13*(3), 278–281.

Ockene, J. K., Quirk, M. E., Goldberg, R. J., Kristeller, J. L., Donnelly, G., Kalan, K. L., Gould, B., Greene, H. L., Harrison-Atlas, R., Pease, J., Pickens, S., & Williams, J. W. (1988). A residents' training program for the development of smoking intervention skills. *Archives of Internal Medicine, 148*(5), 1039–1045.

O'Leary, K. D., & Wilson, G. T. (1987). *Behavior therapy: Application and outcome* (2nd ed.). Englewood Cliffs, NJ: Prentice-Hall.

Oncken, C., Hardardottir, H., & Smeltzer, J. (1998). Human studies of nicotine replacement during pregnancy. In N. Benowitz (Ed.), *Nicotine safety and toxicity* (pp. 107–116). New York: Oxford University Press.

Orleans, C., Rimer, B., Cristinzio, S., Keintz, M., & Fleisher, L. (1991). A national survey of older smokers: Treatment needs of a growing population. *Health Psychology, 110*, 343–351.

Orleans, C. T., Boyd, N. R., Bingler, R., Sutton, C., Fairclough, D., Heller, D., McClatchey, M., Ward, J., Graves, C., Fleisher, L., & Baum, S. (1998). A self-help intervention for African American smokers: Tailoring cancer information service counseling for a special population. *Preventive Medicine, 27*, S61–S70.

Orleans, C. T., Rimer, B., Telepchak, J., Fleisher, L., Keintz, M. K., Boyd, N. R., Noll, E. L., & Robinson, R. (1997). *Clear horizons*. Philadelphia: Fox Chase Cancer Center.

Orleans, C. T., Rotberg, H., Quade, D., & Lees, P. (1990). A hospital quit-smoking consult service: Clinical report and intervention guidelines. *Preventive Medicine, 19*, 198–212.

Orleans, C. T., & Slade, J. E. (1993). *Nicotine addiction: Principles and management*. New York: Oxford University Press.

Pallonen, U. E., Velicer, W. F., Prochaska, J., Rossi, J. S., Bellis, J. M., Tsoh, J. Y., Migneault, J. P., Smith, N. F., & Prokhorov, A. V. (1998). Computer-based smoking cessation interventions in adolescents: Description, feasibility, and six-month follow-up findings. *Substance Use and Misuse, 33*, 935–965.

Parrott, S., Godfrey, C., Raw, M., West, R., & McNeill, A. (1998). Guidance for commissioners on the cost effectiveness of smoking cessation interventions. *Thorax, 53*(Suppl. 5, Pt. 2), S1–S38.

Patten, C. A., Martin, J. E., Myers, M. G., Calfas, K. J., & Williams, C. D. (1998). Effectiveness of cognitive-behavioral therapy for smokers with histories of alcohol dependence and depression. *Journal of Studies on Alcohol, 59*, 327–335.

Pentz, M. A. (1999). Prevention. In M. Galanter & H. D. Kleber (Eds.), *American Psychiatric Press textbook of substance abuse treatment* (2nd ed., pp. 535–544). Washington, DC: American Psychiatric Press.

Perkins, K. A., Donny, E., & Caggiula, A. R. (1999). Sex differences in nicotine effects and self-administration: Review of human and animal evidence. *Nicotine and Tobacco Research, 1*, 301–315.

Perkins, K. A., Marcus, M. D., Levine, M. D., D'Amico, D., Miller, A., Broge, M., Ashcom, J., & Shiffman, S. (2001). Cognitive-behavioral therapy to reduce weight concerns improves smoking cessation outcome in weight-concerned women. *Journal of Consulting and Clinical Psychology, 69*(4), 604–613.

Perry, C., Killen, J., Telch, M., Slinkard, L., & Danaher, B. (1980). Modifying smoking behavior of teenagers: A school-based intervention. *American Journal of Public Health, 70*, 722–725.

Peterson, A. V., Kealey, K. A., Mann, S. L., Marek, P. M., & Sarason, I. G. (2000). Hutchinson Smoking Prevention Project: Long-term randomized trial in school-based tobacco use prevention—results on smoking. *Journal of the National Cancer Institute, 92*, 1979–1991.

Peto, R., Lopez, A. D., Boreham, J., Thun, M., & Heath, C., Jr. (1994). *Mortality from smoking in developed countries 1950–2000*. Oxford, England: Oxford University Press.

Piasecki, T., Fiore, M., & Baker, T. (1997). Profiles in discouragement: Two studies of variability in the timecourse of smoking withdrawal symptoms. *Journal of Abnormal Psychology, 107*, 238–251.

Piasecki, T. M., Niaura, R., Shadel, W. G., Goldstein, M. G., Abrams, D. B., Fiore, M. C., & Baker, T. B. (2000). Withdrawal dynamics predict smoking relapse: Tracing an affective path to relapse? *Journal of Abnormal Psychology, 109*(1), 74–86.

Pickworth, W., Bunker, E., & Henningfield, J. (1994). Transdermal nicotine: Reduction of smoking with minimal abuse liability. *Psychopharmacology, 115*, 9–14.

Pierce, T. (1991). Dual-disordered adolescents: A special population. *Journal of Adolescent Chemical Dependence, 1*, 11–28.

Pinsker, J., Phillips, R. S., Davis, R. B., & Iezzoni, I. (1995). Use of follow-up services by patients referred from a walk-in unit: How can patient compliance be improved? *American Journal of Medical Quality, 19*, 81–87.

Pirie, P. L., McBride, C., Hellerstedt, W., Jeffery, R. W., Hatsukami, D., Allen, S., & Lando, H. (1992). Smoking cessation in women concerned about weight. *American Journal of Public Health, 82*(9), 799–803.

Pirie, P. L., Murray, D. M., & Luepker, R. V. (1991). Gender differences in cigarette smoking and quitting in a cohort of young adults. *American Journal of Public Health, 81*(3), 324–327.

Pomerleau, C., Aubin, H., & Pomerleau, O. (1997). Self-reported alcohol use patterns in a sample of male and female heavy smokers. *Journal of Addictive Diseases, 16*(3), 19–24.

Pomerleau, C., & Kurth, C. (1996). Willingness of female smokers to tolerate postcessation weight gain. *Journal of Substance Abuse, 8*, 371–378.

Pomerleau, O. F., Collins, A. C., Shiffman, S., & Pomerleau, C. S. (1993). Why some people smoke and others do not: New perspectives. *Journal of Consulting and Clinical Psychology, 61*, 723–731.

Pomerleau, O. F., & Kardia, S. L. R. (1999). Introduction to the featured section: Genetic research on smoking. *Health Psychology, 18*, 3–6.

Prochaska, J. O., & DiClemente, C. C. (1983). Stages and processes of self-change of smoking: Toward an integrative model of change. *Journal of Consulting and Clinical Psychology, 51*(3), 390–395.

Prochaska, J. O., & Goldstein, M. G. (1991). Process of smoking cessation: Implications for clinicians. *Clinics in Chest Medicine, 12*, 727–735.

Prochaska, J. O., Redding, C. A., & Evers, K. E. (1997). The transtheoretical model and stages of change. In K. Glanz, F. M. Lewis, & B. K. Rimer (Eds.), *Health behavior and health education* (2nd ed., pp. 60–84). San Francisco: Jossey-Bass.

Prochazka, A. V., Weaver, M. J., Keller, R. T., Fryer, G. E., Licari, P. A., & Lofaso, D. (1998). A randomized trial of nortriptyline for smoking cessation. *Archives of Internal Medicine, 158*, 2035–2039.

Project MATCH Research Group. (1997). Matching alcoholism treatments to client heterogeneity: Project MATCH posttreatment drinking outcomes. *Journal of Studies on Alcohol, 58*, 7–29.

Radloff, L. S. (1977). The CES-D: A self-report depression scale for research in the general population. *Applied Psychological Measurement, 1*, 385–401.

Raw, M., McNeill, A., & West, R. (1998). Smoking cessation guidelines for health professionals: A guide to effective smoking cessation interventions for the health care system. *Thorax, 53*(Suppl. 5, Pt. 1), S1–S19.

Rigotti, N. A., DiFranza, J. R., Chang, Y. C., Tisdale, T., Kemp, B., & Singer, D. E. (1997). The effect of enforcing tobacco sales laws on adolescents' access to tobacco and smoking behavior. *New England Journal of Medicine, 337*, 1044–1051.

Rigotti, N. A., Lee, J. E., & Wechsler, H. (2000). U.S. college students' use of tobacco products: Results of a national survey. *Journal of the American Medical Association, 284*, 699–705.

Rimer, B. K., Orleans, C. T., Fleisher, L., Cristinzio, S., Resch, N., Telepchak, J., & Keintz, M. K. (1994). Does tailoring matter? The impact of a tailored guide on ratings and short-term smoking-related outcomes for older smokers. *Health Education Research, 2*, 69–84.

Risser, N. L., & Belcher, D. W. (1990). Adding spirometry, carbon monoxide, and pulmonary symptom results to smoking cessation counseling. *Journal of General Internal Medicine, 5*, 16–22.

Rohsenow, D. J., Monti, P. M., Colby, S. M., Gulliver, S. B., Sirota, A. D., Niaura, R. S., & Abrams, D. B.

(1997). Effects of alcohol cues on smoking urges and topography among alcoholic men. *Alcoholism: Clinical and Experimental Research, 21*(1), 101–107.

Rounsaville, B. J., Kosten, T. R., Weissman, M. M., & Kleber, H. D. (Eds.). (1985). Evaluating and treating depressive disorders in opiate addicts. *National Institute on Drug Abuse Treatment Research Monograph Series* (DHHS Publication No. [ADM] 85-1406). Washington, DC: U.S. Government Printing Office.

Russell, M. (1990). The nicotine addiction trap: A 40–year sentence for four cigarettes. *British Journal of Addiction, 85,* 293–300.

Schachter, S. (1982). Recidivism and self-cure of smoking and obesity. *American Psychologist, 37*(4), 436–444.

Schauffler, H. H. (1997). Defining benefits and payment for smoking cessation treatment. *Tobacco Control, 6*(Suppl. 1), S81–S85.

Schwartz, J. L. (1987). *Review and evaluation of smoking control methods: United States and Canada 1978–1985* (NIH Publication No. 87-2940). Bethesda, MD: U.S. Department of Health and Human Services, Public Health Service, National Institutes of Health.

Shadel, W., Niaura, R., & Abrams, D. (2000). An idiographic approach to understanding personality structure and individual differences among smokers. *Cognitive Therapy and Research, 24,* 345–359.

Shadel, W. G., & Mermelstein, R. (1993a, March). *Characteristics of smokers who frequently relapse and recycle.* Paper presented at the Society of Behavioral Medicine, San Francisco, CA.

Shadel, W. G., & Mermelstein, R. J. (1993b). Cigarette smoking under stress: The role of coping expectancies among smokers in a clinic-based smoking cessation program. *Health Psychology, 12,* 443–450.

Shadel, W. G., & Mermelstein, R. (1996). Individual differences in self-concept among smokers attempting to quit: Validation and predictive utility of measures of the smoker self-concept and abstainer self-concept. *Annals of Behavioral Medicine, 18*(3), 151–156.

Shadel, W. G., Mermelstein, R., & Borrelli, B. (1996). Self-concept changes over time in cognitive-behavioral treatment for smoking cessation. *Addictive Behaviors, 21*(5), 659–663.

Shadel, W. G., Shiffman, S., Niaura, R., Nichter, M., & Abrams, D. B. (2000). Current models of nicotine dependence: What is known and what is needed to advance understanding of tobacco etiology among youth. *Drug and Alcohol Dependence, 59*(Suppl. 1), S9–S21.

Shapiro, R., Ossip-Klein, D., & Gerrity, E. (1985). Perceived helpfulness of messages on a community based telephone support service for ex-smokers. *International Journal of the Addictions, 20,* 1837–1847.

Shediac-Rizkallah, M. C., & Bone, L. R. (1998). Planning for the sustainability of community-based health programs: Conceptual frameworks and future directions for research, practice and policy. *Health Education Research, 13,* 87–108.

Shepard, D. S., Stason, W. B., Perry, H. M., Carmen, B. A., & Nagurney, J. T. (1995). Multivariate cost-effectiveness analysis: An application to optimizing ambulatory care for hypertension. *Inquiry, 32*(3), 320–331.

Shiffman, S. (1982). Relapse following smoking cessation: A situational analysis. *Journal of Consulting and Clinical Psychology, 50,* 71–86.

Shiffman, S. (1986). A cluster analytic classification of smoking relapse episodes. *Addictive Behaviors, 11,* 295–307.

Shiffman, S. (1988). Behavioral assessment. In D. M. Donovan & G. A. Marlatt (Eds.), *Assessment of addictive behavior* (pp. 139–188). New York: Guilford Press.

Shiffman, S. (1989). Tobacco "chippers": Individual differences in tobacco dependence. *Psychopharmacology, 97,* 539–547.

Shiffman, S. (1993). Smoking cessation treatment: Any progress? *Journal of Consulting and Clinical Psychology, 61*(5), 718–722.

Shiffman, S., Gnys, M., Richards, T. J., Paty, J. A., Hickcox, M., & Kassel, J. (1996). Temptations to smoke after quitting: A comparison of lapsers and maintainers. *Health Psychology, 15*(6), 455–461.

Shiffman, S., Hickcox, M., Paty, J. A., Gnys, M., Richards, T., & Kassel, J. D. (1997). Individual differences in the context of smoking lapse episodes. *Addictive Behaviors, 22*(6), 797–811.

Shiffman, S., & Jarvik, M. (1976). Smoking withdrawal symptoms in two weeks of abstinence. *Psychopharmacology, 50,* 35–39.

Shiffman, S., Mason, K. M., & Henningfield, J. E. (1998). Tobacco dependence treatments: Review and prospectus. *Annual Review of Public Health, 19,* 335–358.

Shiffman, S., Shadel, W., Niaura, R., Khayrallah, M., Jorenby, D., Ryan, C., & Ferguson, C. (in press). Efficacy of acute administration of Nicorette gum against cue provoked craving. *Psychopharmacology.*

Shiffman, S., Shumaker, S. A., Abrams, D. B., Cohen, S., Garvey, A., Grunberg, N. E., & Swan, G. E. (1986). Models of smoking relapse. *Health Psychology, 5*(Suppl.), 13–27.

Shopland, D. R., & Burns, D. M. (1993). Medical and public health implications of tobacco addiction. In C. T. Orleans & J. Slade (Eds.), *Nicotine addiction* (pp. 105–128). New York: Oxford University Press.

Shumaker, S., Schron, E., Ockene, J., & McBee, W. (1998). *Handbook of health behavior change.* New York: Springer.

Skinner, C. S., Campbell, M. K., Rimer, B. K., Curry, S., & Prochaska, J. O. (1999). How effective is tailored print communication? *Annals of Behavioral Medicine, 21*(4), 290–298.

Skinner, H. A., & Allen, B. A. (1982). Alcohol dependence syndrome: Measurement and validation. *Journal of Abnormal Psychology, 91,* 199–209.

Slotkin, T. (1998). The impact of fetal nicotine exposure on nervous system development and its role in sudden infant death syndrome. In N. Benowitz (Ed.), *Nicotine safety and toxicity* (pp. 89–97). New York: Oxford University Press.

Smith, T. A., House, R. F., Croghan, I. T., Gauvin, T. R., Colligan, R. C., Offord, K. C., Gomez-Dahl, L. C., & Hurt, R. D. (1996). Nicotine patch therapy in adolescent smokers. *Pediatrics, 98,* 659–667.

Solberg, L. I., Brekke, M. L., Kottke, T. E., & Steel, R. P. (1998). Continuous quality improvement in primary care: What's happening. *Medical Care, 36,* 625–635.

Solberg, L. I., Kottke, T. E., Conn, S. A., Brekke, M. L., Calomeni, C. A., & Conboy, K. S. (1997). Delivering clinical preventive services is a systems problem. *Annals of Behavioral Medicine, 19,* 271–278.

Spitzer, R. L., Williams, J. B. W., Gibbon, M., & First, M. B. (1990). *Structured clinical interview for DSM-III-R.* Washington, DC: American Psychiatric Press.

Spitzer, R. L., Williams, J. B., Kroenke, K., Linzer, M., deGruy, F. V., Hahn, S. R., Brody, D., & Johnson, J. G. (1994). Utility of a new procedure for diagnosing mental disorders in primary care: The PRIME-MD 1000 study. *Journal of the American Medical Association, 272*(22), 1749–1756.

Stokols, D. (1992). Establishing and maintaining health environments: Toward a social ecology of health promotion. *American Psychologist, 47,* 6–22.

Strecher, V., & Rimer, B. (1999). *Freedom from smoking.* New York: American Lung Association.

Sutherland, G., Stapleton, J. A., Russell, M. A., Jarvis, M. J., Hajek, P., Belcher, M., & Feyerabend, C. (1992). Randomized controlled trial of nasal nicotine spray in smoking cessation. *Lancet, 340*(8815), 324–329.

Sutton, S. (1996). Can "stages of change" provide guidance in the treatment of addictions? A critical examination of Prochaska and DiClemente's model. In G. Edwards & C. Dare (Eds.), *Psychotherapy, psychological treatments and the addictions* (pp. 189–205). Cambridge, England: Cambridge University Press.

Swan, G. E., & Carmelli, D. (1997). Behavior genetic investigations of cigarette smoking and related issues. In E. P. Noble & K. Blum (Eds.), *Handbook of psychiatric genetics* (pp. 379–398). Boca Raton, FL: CRC Press.

Syme, S. L. (2000). *Promoting health: Intervention strategies from social and behavioral research.* Washington, DC: National Academy of Sciences.

Taylor, C. B., Houston-Miller, N., Killen, J., & DeBusk, R. F. (1990). Smoking cessation after acute myocardial infarction: Effects of a nurse-managed intervention. *Annals of Internal Medicine, 113,* 118–123.

Tiffany, S., & Hackenworth, D. M. (1991). The production of smoking urges through an imagery manipulation: Psychophysiological and verbal manifestations. *Addictive Behaviors, 16,* 389–400.

Tiffany, S. T. (1990). A cognitive model of drug urges and drug-use behavior: Role of automatic and nonautomatic processes. *Psychological Review, 97,* 147–168.

Tiffany, S. T., & Drobes, D. J. (1991). The development and initial validation of a questionnaire of smoking urges. *British Journal of Addiction, 86,* 1467–1476.

Transdermal Nicotine Study Group. (1991). Transdermal nicotine for smoking cessation: Six-month results from two multicenter controlled clinical trials. *Journal of the American Medical Association, 266,* 3133–3138.

U.S. Department of Health and Human Services. (1988). *The health consequences of smoking. Nicotine addiction: A report of the Surgeon General* (DHHS Publication No. CDC88–8406). Rockville, MD: U.S. Department of Health and Human Services, Public Health Service, Office on Smoking and Health.

U.S. Department of Health and Human Services. (1990). *The health benefits of smoking cessation: A report of the Surgeon General* (DHHS Publication No. CDC 90–8416). Washington, DC: Public Health Service.

U.S. Department of Health and Human Services. (1994). *Preventing tobacco use among young people: A report of the Surgeon General.* Atlanta, GA: U.S. Department of Health and Human Services, Public Health Services, Centers for Disease Control and Prevention, National Center for Chronic Disease Prevention and Health Promotion, Office on Smoking and Health.

U.S. Department of Health and Human Services. (1998). *Tobacco use among U.S. racial/ethnic minority groups: A report of the Surgeon General.* Washington, DC: U.S. Government Printing Office.

U.S. Department of Health and Human Services. (2001). *Women and smoking: A report of the Surgeon General.* Rockville, MD: U.S. Department of Health and Human Services, Public Health Service, Office of the Surgeon General.

Unger, J. (1996). Stages of change of smoking cessation: Relationships with other health behaviors. *American Journal of Preventive Medicine, 12,* 134–138.

Valle, S. (1981). Interpersonal functioning of alcoholism counselors and treatment outcome. *Journal of Studies on Alcohol, 42,* 783–790.

Velicer, W. F., DiClemente, C. C., Prochaska, J. O., & Brandenburg, N. (1985). A decisional balance measure for assessing and predicting smoking status. *Journal of Personality and Social Psychology, 48,* 1279–1289.

Velicer, W. F., DiClemente, C. C., Rossi, J. S., & Prochaska, J. O. (1990). Relapse situations and self-efficacy: An integrative model. *Addictive Behaviors, 15,* 271–283.

Velicer, W. F., Fava, J. L., Prochaska, J. O., Abrams, D. B., Emmons, K. M., & Pierce, J. P. (1995). Distribution of smokers by stage in three representative samples. *Preventive Medicine, 24,* 401–411.

Wall, M., Severson, H., Andrews, J., & Lichtenstein, E. (1995). Pediatric office-based smoking intervention: Impact on maternal smoking and relapse. *Pediatrics, 96,* 622–628.

Warner, K. E., Slade, J., & Sweanor, D. T. (1997). The emerging market for long-term nicotine maintenance. *Journal of the American Medical Association, 278*(13), 1087–1092.

Washton, A., Stone, A., & Hendrickson, E. (1988). Cocaine abuse. In D. M. Donovan & G. A. Gordon (Eds.), *Assessment of addictive behaviors* (pp. 325–363). New York: Guilford Press.

Wechsler, H., Levine, S., Idelson, R. K., Schor, E. L., & Coakley, E. (1996). The physician's role in health promotion revisited: A survey of primary-care practitioners. *New England Journal of Medicine, 334,* 996–998.

Wechsler, H., Rigotti, N. A., Gledhill-Hoyt, J., & Lee, H. (1998). Increased levels of cigarette use among college students. *Journal of the American Medical Association, 280*(19), 1673–1678.

Weinstein, N. (1980). Unrealistic optimism about future life events. *Journal of Personality and Social Psychology, 39*, 806–820.

Weinstein, N. (1984). Why it won't happen to me: Perceptions of risk factors and illness susceptibility. *Health Psychology, 3*, 431–457.

Weinstein, N. (1987). Unrealistic optimism about illness susceptibility: Conclusions from a community-wide sample. *Journal of Behavioral Medicine, 10*, 481–500.

Weinstein, N. (1988). Precaution adoption process. *Health Psychology, 7*(44), 355–368.

Weinstein, N., Rothman, A., & Sutton, S. (1998). Stage theories of health behavior: Conceptual and methodological issues. *Health Psychology, 17*, 1–10.

Weinstein, N. D. (1993). Testing four comparative theories of health behavior. *Health Psychology, 12*(4), 324–333.

Weissman, W., Glasgow, R., Biglan, A., & Lichtenstein, E. (1987). Development and preliminary evaluation of a cessation program for adolescent smokers. *Psychology of Addictive Behaviors, 1*, 84–91.

Wetter, D., Fiore, M. C., Young, T. B., McClure, J., DeMoor, C. A., & Baker, T. B. (1999). Gender differences in response to nicotine replacement therapy: Objective and subjective indices of tobacco withdrawal. *Experimental and Clinical Psychopharmacology, 7*, 135–144.

Wetter, D., Kenford, S. L., Smith, S. S., Fiore, M. C., Jorenby, D. E., & Baker, T. B. (1999). Gender differences in smoking cessation. *Journal of Consulting and Clinical Psychology, 67*, 555–562.

Wetter, D. W., Smith, S. S., Kenford, S. L., Jorenby, D. E., Fiore, M. C., Hurt, R. D., Offord, K. P., & Baker, T. B. (1994). Smoking outcome expectancies: Factor structure, predictive validity, and discriminant validity. *Journal of Abnormal Psychology, 103*(4), 801–811.

Willey-Lessne, C., Goldstein, M. G., Niaura, R., DePue, J., Velicer, W., & Prochaska, J. (1996, March). *Smoking cessation outcomes of a physician counseling and home-based expert system intervention.* Paper presented at the annual meeting of the Society of Behavioral Medicine, Washington, DC.

Witte, K. (1993). Managerial style and health promotion programs. *Social Science and Medicine, 36*, 227–235.

Working Group for the Study of Transdermal Nicotine in Patients with Coronary Artery Disease. (1994). Nicotine replacement therapy for patients with coronary artery disease. *Archives of Internal Medicine, 154*(9), 989–995.

Zacny, J. P. (1990). Behavioral aspects of alcohol-tobacco interactions. In M. Galanter (Ed.), *Recent developments in alcoholism: Vol. 8. Combined alcohol and other drug dependence* (pp. 205–219). New York: Plenum Press.

Zarin, D. A., Pincus, H. A., & Hughes, J. R. (1997, July). Treating nicotine dependence in mental health settings. *Journal of Practical Psychiatry and Behavioral Health*, 250–254.

Zevin, S., Jacob, P., III, & Benowitz, N. L. (1998). Dose-related cardiovascular and endocrine effects of transdermal nicotine. *Clinical Pharmacology and Therapeutics, 64*, 87–95.

Zimmerman, M., & Mattia, J. I. (2001). A self-report scale to help make psychiatric diagnoses: The Psychiatric Diagnostic Screening Questionnaire. *Archives of General Psychiatry, 58*, 787–794.

Index

Note. The titles of the reproducible handouts are shown in **boldface**.